Abdominal Pain: Essential Diagnosis and Management in Acute Medicine

Authored by

Ozgur KARCIOGLU
Department of Emergency Medicine
University of Health Sciences
Taksim Education and Research Hospital
Beyoglu, Istanbul
Turkey

Selman YENİOCAK
University of Health Sciences
Department of Emergency Medicine
Haseki Education and Research Hospital
Fatih, Istanbul
Turkey

Mandana HOSSEINZADEH
Corlu Community Hospital
Department of Emergency Medicine
Tekirdag
Turkey

&

Seckin Bahar SEZGIN
Department of Emergency Medicine
University of Health Sciences Adana City Hospital
Adana
Turkey

Abdominal Pain: Essential Diagnosis and Management in Acute Medicine

Authors: Ozgur KARCIOGLU, Selman YENİOCAK, Mandana HOSSEINZADEH & Seckin Bahar SEZGIN

ISBN (Online): 978-981-5051-78-0

ISBN (Print): 978-981-5051-79-7

ISBN (Paperback): 978-981-5051-80-3

© 2022, Bentham Books imprint.

Published by Bentham Science Publishers Pte. Ltd. Singapore. All Rights Reserved.

First published in 2022.

need for a court order if at any point you breach any terms of this License Agreement. In no event will any delay or failure by Bentham Science Publishers in enforcing your compliance with this License Agreement constitute a waiver of any of its rights.

3. You acknowledge that you have read this License Agreement, and agree to be bound by its terms and conditions. To the extent that any other terms and conditions presented on any website of Bentham Science Publishers conflict with, or are inconsistent with, the terms and conditions set out in this License Agreement, you acknowledge that the terms and conditions set out in this License Agreement shall prevail.

Bentham Science Publishers Pte. Ltd.
80 Robinson Road #02-00
Singapore 068898
Singapore
Email: subscriptions@benthamscience.net

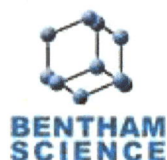

BENTHAM SCIENCE

CONTENTS

PREFACE

Almost all aspects of medicine are challenging for both healthcare providers and sufferers. Although subthemes covered by medicine can be classified as discrete systems or organs of the body, caregivers in primary and acute care prefer to conceive these with complaints, symptoms and semiological approaches. Therefore, no patient presents to the acute care area with an 'acute appendicitis' or 'acute cholangitis', instead, there comes *'a girl in her 18 with vomiting and abdominal pain for a couple of days'*, or, *'an elderly gentleman who is not looking very good recently'* in the boxes. The patient's diagnosis seems very elusive, for it can turn out to be pelvic inflammatory disease, urinary tract infection, ruptured ovarian cyst or abscess, intestinal obstruction, diverticulitis, mesenteric ischemia, etc, while the patient is screaming for emergency relief for both pain and vomiting in the acute care area.

Abdominal pain is one of the most common chief complaints in both emergency settings and primary care, which constitutes around 10% in most large studies in the world. Unlike many entities presenting to outpatient clinics and those admitted to the wards, the origin of abdominal pain is harder to diagnose provided with the complexity and closeness of the structures in the abdomen and also extra abdominal causes that can trigger the symptomatology. Nonetheless, recent decades witnessed giant leaps and advances in the recognition and treatment of patients with acute abdominal pain. Apart from advanced studies such as computed tomography, and magnetic resonance imaging, bedside point-of-care procedures like ultrasonography have eased diagnosis and facilitated the management of patients with abdominal pain. We should note that regardless of technological advances, the most important contributor to the diagnosis and management process consists of the evaluation of the patient with an elaborate history and physical examination. Using a tailored approach for evaluation, an experienced physician can not only narrow the list of differential diagnosis, but also expedite the complex pathway to definitive treatment, preventing unnecessary delays with cumbersome investigations.

The optimal management of the patients with abdominal pain warrants a multifaceted approach undertaken in harmony. COVID-19 pandemic era has brought *de novo* challenges for the delivery of 'usual' medical care into the scene for most patients. This book titled **"Abdominal Pain: Essential Diagnosis and Management in Acute Medicine"**, therefore, is intended to highlight the contemporary approaches with respect to diagnostic and therapeutic modalities for diseases of digestive tract and other entities precipitating abdominal pain. Abundant figures, tables, and radiological images have been used to render understanding easier and to illustrate key findings. We hope this project can be used as a reference and an everlasting source for caregivers facing sufferers of abdominal pain, albeit a small step in the history of medical progress lasting for thousands of years.

CONSENT FOR PUBLICATION

Not applicable.

CONFLICT OF INTEREST

The authors declare no conflict of interest, financial or otherwise.

ACKNOWLEDGEMENT

Declared none.

Ozgur KARCIOGLU
Department of Emergency Medicine
University of Health Sciences
Taksim Education and Research Hospital
Beyoglu, Istanbul
Turkey

Selman YENİOCAK
University of Health Sciences
Department of Emergency Medicine
Haseki Education and Research Hospital
Fatih, Istanbul
Turkey

Mandana HOSSEINZADEH
Corlu Community Hospital
Department of Emergency Medicine
Tekirdag
Turkey

&

Seckin Bahar SEZGIN
Department of Emergency Medicine
University of Health Sciences Adana City Hospital
Adana
Turkey

CHAPTER 1

The "Stomachache" of Medicine: Concepts and Mechanisms of Abdominal Pain

Abstract: Abdominal pain (AP) is by far among the most common complaints in healthcare institutions. Approximately every tenth patient in the acute setting is estimated to present with AP. Although cultural, geographical and sociodemographic variations exist, it is an outstanding complaint in all patient groups, independent of age and gender. Although it can be a manifestation of an intraabdominal pathology itself, a serious systemic or extraabdominal condition can be revealed following a thorough investigation of AP. Therefore, it is vital to evaluate the patient systemically, a focused but elaborate history, and extensive physical examination not confined to the abdomen in order to establish important diagnoses. Inspection, auscultation, percussion, superficial and deep palpation are important elements of the examination methods for the abdomen. Each positive or negative finding on examination should be interpreted cautiously for the individual patient. After history and evaluation narrow the list of differential diagnoses (DD), ancillary investigations including laboratory tests and radiological modalities can be ordered.

Keywords: Abdominal pain, Physical examination, Laboratory tests, Work up, Imaging, Differential diagnoses.

GENERAL CONSIDERATIONS

Abdominal pain (AP) is one of the commonest reasons for admission to emergency departments (ED) and other healthcare institutions. Considering the singular 'chief' main complaints, it is established that 8% to 10% of patients both in Turkey and in the world are admitted to the ED with AP. Since registry databases are operated inadequately in developing worlds, most data are derived from Europe and America, therefore substantial variations may occur especially in regard to entities affected by geographical properties. While the rate of hospitalization among adult patients who present to ED with AP varies between 18% and 42%, the same can be found higher, up to 65% in elderly patients.

Pearl: The main goal of the physician in the management of AP is to decide which patients can be safely discharged and which patients should be kept in the hospital.

Ozgur KARCIOGLU, Selman YENİOCAK, Mandana HOSSEINZADEH & Seckin Bahar SEZGIN

Distinction Between Acute And Chronic AP

In many sources, acute AP is noted as pain within the first 7 days. The term "chronic" mostly refers to the pain of the same character over months and years. In this case, it should be borne in mind that the patient presenting with pain for 6 or 7 days can still be diagnosed with "acute" cholecystitis or pancreatitis, although somehow difficult to be comprehended. For example, it is possible to extend this period even longer, since the pain associated with choledocholithiasis may last (and neglected) for a few days and then turn into acute cholecystitis. In brief, real-life scenarios may not fit into the encyclopedic information or what we can expect to see.

Why does My Belly Hurt?

The structure related to the digestive system in embryonic life differentiates into 3 separate parts.

- **Foregut:** It includes stomach, duodenum, liver, gall bladder, and pancreas. Upper abdominal pain is remarkable in their malfunctions or inflammations.
- **Midgut** (small intestine, proximal colon, appendix) causes periumbilical pain.
- **Hindgut** structures (distal colon and genitourinary system) cause pain in the left, midline or right lower abdomen.

Anatomophysiologic mechanisms include the splanchnic and the cerebrospinal neural pathways activated for transmission of AP. Pacinian corpuscles and free nerve endings in the visceral walls are the splanchnic afferent receptors sensitive to stretch and spasm. On the other hand, cerebrospinal receptors are sensitive to pressure, friction, cutting, burning that are discerned by the skin. In the dorsal root ganglia (DRG) the splanchnic and cerebrospinal cell bodies are in close proximity. The proximal fibers terminate around the spinal cord. The close relationship of these anatomic pathways may contribute to the fact that severe visceral pain, such as rapid distention of a viscus, may "spill over" into somatic segments (viscerosensory and visceromotor reflexes) in the absence of somatic nerve irritation (Fig. **1**).

The embryonic gut and its appendages emerge as midline organs, therefore, their splanchnic innervation is bilateral. This is why the perception of visceral pain locates in the midline. In fact, there are not any nerve fibers in the visceral peritoneum. Cerebrospinal nerves to the parietal peritoneum (T6 through T12) have the same segmental organization as the lower thoracic dermatomes.

Dichotomous Classification of Pain: Visceral or Somatic?

Visceral pain is a type of pain originating from the internal organs. This type of pain is ill-defined, not well localized, is felt in a wide area, and its changes are also felt much slower than somatic pain. With these features, it can cause pain to be felt away from the diseased or inflamed organ.

Somatic pain, on the other hand, is the stimulation of **peripheral nociceptive nerves**. Abdominal pain is essentially triggered by irritation of the parietal peritoneum. It is also provoked by infection, chemical irritation (like spilled bile, faeces or urine into peritoneal cavity), and/or trauma. When the inflammatory process expands and eventually irritates the peritoneum, the **somatic component** is activated and the pain is much better localized by the conscious patient. It is often described by patients in the form of severe 'sharp' pain. Typically, this course is observed in pathologies such as acute appendicitis (AAp) and acute cholecystitis (AC), which are very close to the peritoneum.

It has been documented in rats that there is an organ-to-organ cross-sensitization of pelvic viscera, including colon, bladder, and female reproductive organs, which may contribute to the overlap of lower abdominal pain. At the peripheral and spinal level, there are two potential pathways involved in such cross-sensitization: (1) axonal dichotomy of visceral sensory afferents (Fig. **1A**) and (2) convergence of two visceral afferents from two organs on spinal neurons (Fig. **1B**).

Pitfalls

The term "stomachache " seems to be justified as the difficulty of diagnosis in patients presenting with AP is a real challenge for physicians. Delay in diagnosis and misdiagnosis is a common problem even for the most experienced emergency physician or general surgeon. Disruptions that may be related to ancillary services such as radiology and biochemistry also increase the difficulty.

Age and Sex

Two important factors for the definitive diagnosis of AP are age and gender. Peptic ulcer, gastritis, urinary stone disease and AAp are more common causes of AP encountered in men, while nonspecific abdominal pain (NSAP), biliary tract diseases, functional bowel disorders including IBS, urinary tract infections (UTI) and pelvic inflammatory disease (PID) are outstanding in women.

As with every symptom, the cause of AP should be explained, diagnosed and resolved. Many diseases known in medicine can cause AP directly or indirectly.

The physician undertakes the difficult task to shorten the list of differential diagnoses (DD), which is very wide, *via* a logical and expedient evaluation.

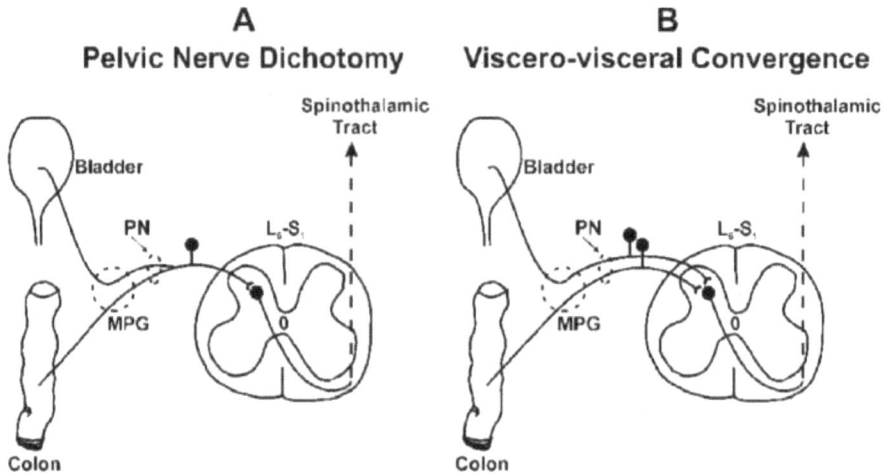

Fig. (1). Illustration of the pelvic nerve dichotomy (**A**) and viscero-visceral convergence of colon and bladder afferent fibers on to spinal dorsal horn neuron (**B**).
A: Although the primary sensory neurons are pseudounipolar cells, retrograde labeling of bladder and colon shows colabeling of dorsal root ganglion (DRG) soma in the lumbosacral spinal cord, suggesting that there are two axon collaterals innervating two pelvic organs. Sensitization of a spinal neuron by inflammation of one organ may affect the sensitivity of the noninflamed organ innervated by the axon collateral.
B: Common convergence of two primary sensory afferents from two organs a spinal dorsal neuron is another neural pathway which can exhibit cross-organ sensitization.

In an ideal world, the physician examines the patient and reduces the DD list to a single possible entity, which we call a 'diagnosis', even if it is not yet verified by pathological examination. However, real life does not operate like this. In most clinical scenarios, a definitive diagnosis can be availed quickly after an elaborate history and examination, by performing targeted biochemistry and focused radiological examinations, as prompted by the clinical findings. For example, cholelithiasis/cholecystitis can be diagnosed without doing anything other than bedside USG in a middle-aged woman with right upper quadrant pain (+/- Murphy sign) precipitated with a heavy meal.

In another vignette, a person whose stomachache after taking iron medication can be discharged without advanced investigations after administration of symptomatic treatment and a reasonable period of follow-up, should there be no guarding or another finding other than epigastric sensitivity. Another patient with constipation and AP can be discharged with relief after the enema, provided that he/she feels good (Fig. **2**).

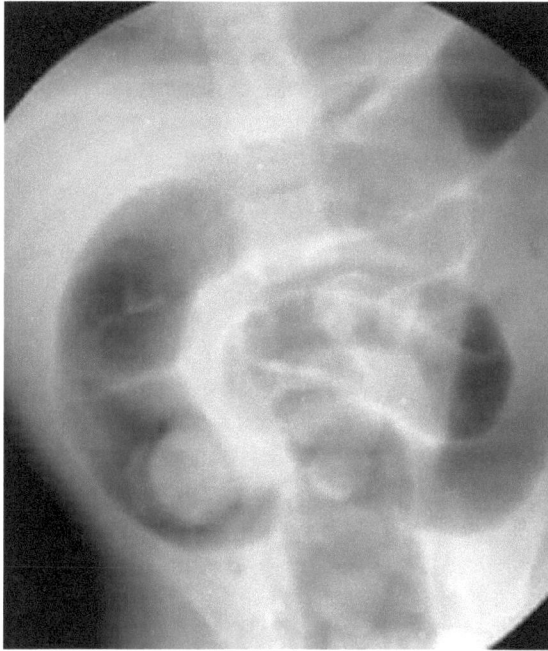

Fig. (2). In the pediatric patient with 4.5 cm invagination in the mid-abdominal segment, reduction was performed with normal saline guided by ultrasound.

Does Every Patient Presenting with AP Necessarily Receive A Specific Diagnosis?

No! Although there are many precipitating reasons inside and outside the abdomen, in an average of 34% to 52% of AP cases admitted to hospitals, a significant cause of AP cannot be elucidated, and the patients are diagnosed with NSAP. However, as age progresses, more serious diseases such as biliary system diseases, malignancy, ischemic bowel disease, and intestinal obstruction appear as causes of AP. Acute appendicitis (AAp) (28%) follows the NSAP group (the largest one); biliary tract diseases (10%), acute gynecological diseases (4%), intestinal obstruction (4%). Before considering NSAP in a patient, serious causes of abdominal pain that prompt urgent surgery must be ruled out from DD. A significant decrease in the rate of NSAP has marked the increased accessibility of laboratory and radiological modalities since the 90s. Bedside point-of-care USG (POCUS) represents a leap in expedient imaging and while creating a shortcut to the operation room (OR) in most instances within the scope of AP (*e.g.*, ruptured ectopic pregnancy, dissecting aortic aneurysms (DAA, ulcer perforation *etc.*).

The female-to-male ratio in those considered to have NSAP is around 2.4 to 3 in some studies (Lukens 1993, Koyuncu & Karcioglu, 2018). The average age is between 38 and 41. While 90% of patients with NSAP recover in the first few weeks or remain asymptomatic, up to 10% may have some disease, for example, 1/3 of them develop AAp (Gallagher, 2004). In the doctorate thesis research which had been conducted in Izmir-Turkey, it is shown sthat 46% out of 684 AP patients were discharged from the university-based ED with the diagnosis of NSAP (Koyuncu & Karcioglu, 2018). Of note, 9% of them were re-admitted within the first 3 days and there were several patients with *de novo* diagnoses of acute abdominal conditions.

Effect of Age

The rate of specific diagnoses and surgical interventions increases with the advancing age. For example, vascular causes such as aneurysm and mesenteric ischemia have a considerable share of 10% of all AP in people over 65 years of age. Only one tenth of this age group is discharged without a specific diagnosis, a.k.a., NSAP. The surgical intervention requirement in patients with AP is 33% in the population over 65 years of age, while only 16% in the others. In patients around 80 years of age, mortality due to AP is around 7%, which is 70 times higher than that of young adults.

Chronic AP with exacerbation can present acutely in the primary care or ED at any point in time.

Severity of COVID-19 and Presentation with AP

In a meta-analytic study, He *et al.* demonstrated that COVID-19 patients whose presenting complaint is dyspnea, hemoptysis, anorexia, diarrhea, or fatigue, especially AP conveyed higher odds ratios for deterioration and thus should be closely monitored (He, 2021). Presentation with AP (OR = 7.5, 95% CI: 2.4-23.4; $p < 0.001$), and anorexia (OR = 2.8, 95% CI: 1.5-5.1; $p < 0.001$) had increased likelihood for unfavorable clinical course. In another meta-analysis of the data obtained in the first phase of the pandemics, Zhu *et al.* disclosed that AP comprised 4.4% and nausea and vomiting were recorded in around one tenth of the main complaints of patients diagnosed with COVID-19 (Zhu, 2020).

ABDOMINAL PAIN AND ITS EVALUATION: HOW TO BE BOTH THOROUGH AND EXPEDIENT?

The two most important points in the approach are history and physical examination. In other words, a well-received history and a thorough physical examination are mostly sufficient to establish the preliminary diagnosis of approximately 90% of the cases. The biggest mistake that can be made is to order a broad list of biochemistry and imaging studies to approach a diagnosis without full history and examination. In this way, a patient who can be diagnosed with myocardial infarction by examining his/her ECG can even be sent to the radiology unit for abdominal tomography and his death can be caused. Or, the patient, whose chronic constipation could have been relieved by evacuating the fecaloma, may be left unnecessarily waiting for hours with fancy investigations.

The patient's history should be taken in detail, for it plays a key role in determining the cause of AP. The following characteristics of the pain, accompanying symptoms, medical diseases, and previous operation histories should be noted.

The onset of the pain: Sudden onset pain is usually due to more serious causes such as vascular problems (acute ischemia) or perforation. In inflammatory causes of pain such as cholecystitis and appendicitis, the onset is slow or insidious.

The localization and spread of pain are to be attended. For example, in 70% of patients with AAp, the pain starts from the midline and settles in the right lower quadrant over time. But these should never be considered as a *sine qua non*. As a rule, every patient exhibits a unique pathway of developing symptoms and historical features and thus different clinical pictures develop in each case. It should not be forgotten that a 'classsical' AAp presentation which is "just as we expected" is not seen in more than 25% of the verified patients.

Although gallbladder problems trigger discomfort in the right upper quadrant, some cases may present with widespread AP. Pain expressed in a well-defined localization often suggests new-onset inflammation in a specific organ, while widespread pain and development of guarding and/or rigidity covering the entire abdomen indicate that acute abdominal syndromes prompt urgent surgical intervention. For example, while localized tenderness in the epigastric area is typical in acute gastritis, rigidity develops in the entire abdomen in a perforated peptic ulcer. "Belt-like" pain that radiates to the entire abdomen and even the back associated with vomiting in the absence of guarding is mostly noted in cases with acute pancreatitis.

The Severity and Pattern of the Pain

While 90% of the patients describe the pain as very severe in peptic ulcer perforation, only 1/6 of the patients with NSAP use this definition for their discomfort. As a general rule, most patients with acute abdominal syndrome requiring operation state that they have experienced "the most severe pain of their life". Patients with acute abdominal syndrome originating from remarkable inflammation have a typical continuous (incessant) and steadily increasing pain pattern. AAp and cholecystitis are examples of this phenomenon. It should also be known that there may be a short-term relief in pain at the point of perforation which can cause confusion for the junior doctors. On the other hand, in colicky pain of hollow organs, there is pain that increases and decreases rhythmically in a "wavy" or ondular manner. Examples include bowel or biliary colic, kidney/ureteral colic, and dysmenorrhea.

The Characteristics (Qualifications) of the Pain

Pain in small bowel obstruction is mostly described as "tearing" or "ripping" in aortic dissection, and "burning" in acute erosive gastritis or duodenal ulcer. However, not every patient should be expected to explain their feelings or discomfort this way.

Pearl: The rule in evaluating a patient with acute abdomen is there is no rules fitting every patient.

Signs and symptoms accompanying AP and interpretations:

- **Loss of appetite** is often a symptom in the case of AAp, but this is absent in 10-20% of the cases. Likewise, other acute conditions can sometimes accompany near-normal appetite. Acute pancreatitis and bowel obstructions are associated with anorexia (with vomiting) almost in 100% of the cases. Those with nonocclusive mesenteric ischemia (NOMI) is mostly an elderly patient with a history of AP often aggravated by meals, which can lead to loss of appetite.
- **Nausea and vomiting** are present in three-quarters of AAp cases. For this reason, we cannot postulate precise templates in our minds and wait for the patient to comply with it. Every specific entity within the context of AP has its own rates of nausea and vomiting with the lowest rate recorded in NSAP.
- **The predominance of vomiting compared to pain** can be encountered in pancreatitis and AGE. Vomiting after prolonged colicky pain is an expected scenario in urinary stone disease and AAp. Cough, headache, fever, abdominal pain and vomiting may also be present in atypical pneumonia which may sometimes masquerade as primary abdominal and/or neurological entities. Therefore, vomiting has little diagnostic value *per se*, and should be viewed only as another star in the constellation of the presentation.
- **Dysuria and other urinary complaints** are frequently encountered in urinary system pathologies such as pyelonephritis, nephritis and cystitis. However, some patients without a urinary pathology, can complain of dysuria and the like. For instance, appendices and other inflamed organs irritate the bladder ureters and bowels, resulting in urinary and intestinal symptoms. It should also be

underlined that female patients with PID, vaginitis or other gynecological problems can feel and describe it as dysuria.

- **Shortness of breath:** AP may be the main symptom for some cardiopulmonary diseases such as pneumonia, pulmonary embolism, aortic catastrophes, pericardial tamponade, and acute coronary syndromes. AP associated with shortness of breath requires the urgent exclusion of extra-abdominal causes including life-threatening ones as exemplified above. Sepsis and septic shock can also be manifested with dyspnea and tachypnea, especially in the elderly.
- **Cold sweating:** Hemodynamic instability is an ominous finding that should never be overlooked or underestimated in a patient with AP. Cold sweating is an important warning sign in a hypotensive and/or tachycardic patient. Cold sweating may indicate septic shock, hypoglycemia, hypovolemia (*e.g.*, excessive vomiting, bowel obstruction or diarrhea), or acute blood loss resulting from an aortic dissection, GI hemorrhage or ruptured ectopic pregnancy (REP). On the other hand, hypoglycemia should also be ruled out in all cases with cold sweating and moribund clinical status.

Medical history/previous illnesses: Some of the patients presenting with AP describe similar pain episodes from the past. Around 70% of patients with acute cholecystitis and 18% of patients with AAp fall into this group. Likewise, 70% of patients with small bowel obstruction have a history of intra-abdominal surgery. Studies pointed out that 65% of patients over the age of 70 have at least one medical disease. In typical cases of Familial Mediterranean Fever (FMF), numerous previous admissions to the hospital with AP attacks (mostly including appendectomy) and sometimes a history of multiple laparotomies are noted.

Drug-related history: Use of drugs such as salicylate and substances such as alcohol are also important for peptic ulcer disease, acute erosive gastritis and/or GI bleeding. A history of severe cough accompanied by anticoagulant use (all kinds) should suggest abdominal wall hematoma. Direct oral anticoagulants (DOACs) and vitamin K antagonists have a more direct relation with such bleeding episodes. The use of barbiturates can precipitate acute intermittant porphyria which is also manifested in severe acute AP.

Lead poisoning: Exposure to any toxin and exposure to lead in the factories and/or ateliers must be questioned in a patient with AP and chronic anemia. A typical patient is a blue-collar worker who have been working in a risky milieu (car batteries, dyes, paints, lead pipes *etc*) for at least several years without due measurements and protection in a developing country. It is a common cause of chronic AP associated with hypochrome microcytic anemia in male workers and their offsprings.

It is known that causes such as spider bite and scorpion sting can also cause acute AP. Latrodectism from black widow spider (BWS) bites is known to be a life-threatening entity which precipitate severe acute AP frequently reported in the literature (Kubena, 2021). This type of AP easily mimicks acute surgical abdomen and therefore should be kept in mind while ruling out the wide list of DD, especially systemic findings such as hypertension, tachycardia, fever, oliguria/renal failure *etc.* accompany AP. Among children signs included pain in wounded area, abdominal and thoracic, muscle spasms, fine tremor (Sotelo-Cruz, 2006). Such a constellation of signs and symptoms coupled with an erythematous wound compatible with spider bite prompts advanced investigation for BWS and latrodectism (Karcioglu, 2001).

Scorpion sting or envenomations should be taken into account in the DD. Similar to spider bites, these events need to be individualized and evaluated geographically, in accord with predominant species in the region. Tityus stigmurus is prevalent in Brazil, while Androctonus and Buthidae, Mesobuthidae, Chacthida, Iurida, and Scorpionidae species cause deaths and severe injuries in Northern Africa, Middle East and Turkey (Albuquerque 2018, Gullu, 2021). Envenomations caused by almost all species present with severe acute AP. Commonly recorded symptoms apart from AP include agitation, tachycardia, vomiting, salivation, diaphoresis, dehydration, muscle rigidity and twitching, tremor, seizures, coma, hyperthermia, tachyarrythmias and hypertension (Amital, 1998).

In evaluation of the history, the presence of kidney failure that may cause AP due to uremia, diabetes mellitus (DM) causing ketoacidosis which precipitate AP due to dehydration and hyperosmolarity should be questioned. Adrenal insufficiency and porphyria can also be associated with AP. In addition, hemoglobinopathies such as sickle cell anemia that cause occlusion of microvascular structures of spleen and some other intraabdominal organ should be remembered.

Obese patients with or without a history of bariatric surgery are at high risk for internal hernia, adhesions, anastomotic leakage and should be evaluated in this respect. Consultation with the relevant surgeon should also be prioritized in such special subgroups.

A detailed gynecological and menstrual history should be taken in all female patients after puberty. Pregnancy and ectopic pregnancy must be borne in mind in all female patients of childbearing age. Inquiry as to whether the person is married or had sexual intercourse should never be used as rule-out criteria. It is also important for all women to record the last menstrual period. Vaginal discharge can be considered essential for PID. Complaints after birth or procedures such as curettage and/or abortion warrant the relevant department consultation. AP accompanying delayed menstruation should suggest an ectopic pregnancy unless proven otherwise.

Situations that aggravate or relieve pain should also be questioned (Table **1**). For example, blunt, colicky pain that is noticed in the right upper quadrant reproduced after meals almost establishes the diagnosis of biliary colic due to gallstones or sludge. It is typical for lactose intolerance to have full abdominal discomfort and dyspepsia, often after consuming foods or beverages containing milk. "Burning-like" epigastric pain aggravated by hunger is suggestive of gastritis and pain in the same region that is precipitated by meals can indicate duodenitis. Although epigastric pain relieved with antacid intake is likely to be related to gastritis or esophagitis, the exclusion of acute coronary syndromes is essential. The relief of pain after defecation is an important finding in patients with Crohn's disease. Sharp AP that occurs with deep breathing evokes upper abdominal pathologies such as subdiaphragmatic and subphrenic abscess, while pain that is exacerbated with leaning forward suggests pancreatitis and relieved pain suggests pericarditis. Following a meal, pain is mostly reported in about one hour in chronic mesenteric ischemia and a few hours in those with a duodenal ulcer.

Table 1. Etiologies of AP with increased probability of verification of presumptive diagnosis in regard to causes which aggravate or relieve the discomfort.

Aggravating Factors	Relieving Factors	Presumptive Diagnosis
Hunger (3-4 hours)	Eating, antacids, water	Duodenal ulcer
Eating	Antacids, water	Duodenitis
-	Defecation	Crohn's disease
Eating (esp. heavy meal)	Opiates	Chronic (non-occlusive) mesenteric ischemia
Dairy products, (Food/beverages containing milk)	Lactose-free diet	Lactose intolerance
Gluten-containing food	Gluten-free diet	Gluten enteropathy (Celiac disease)
Food (mainly fatty meat, chocolate, *etc*)	Hunger, eating vegetables and fruits	Biliary colic due to stones or sludge
Hunger, some foods (varies depending on the patients)	Antacid intake (including water)	Gastritis/esophagitis
Heavy meals (not a rule)	Sitting upright, leaning forward	Pancreatitis
palpating the abdomen, percusssion	Standing still, lying supine	Peritoneal irritation (peritonitis)
-	Hot water bag application, warm showers, painkillers	Renal colic or dysmenorrhea

Can I identify those patients carrying higher risk for serious disease course?

Yes. Table **2** indicates these entities.

Table 2. Conditions that pose a risk for serious pathology in a patient presenting with acute AP include:

History of previous abdominal surgery including bariatric surgery
History of inflammatory bowel disease
Recent intervention (*e.g.* colonoscopy and/or biopsy)
Known abdominal/pelvic/retroperitoneal cancer
Active chemotherapy
Having treatments which can induce immunodeficiency (including azathiopyrine, cyclosporine, methotrexate, low dose prednisone)
Signs of infection (fever, chills, *etc.*)
Women of childbearing age
Having arrived in the country as a new immigrant
Communication problem (language problems or cognitive deficiency)
Psychiatric conditions preventing communication (excitation, delirium, psychosis)
Physical examination (abdominal and systemic)

Physical exam should start with the control of airway, respiratory (breathing) and circulatory (ABC) functions within the context of "primary survey". Systemic examination should then be performed as part of the "secondary survey". Resuscitation of vital functions should be parallel to these examinations.

Vital Signs

Fever: Measurement of body temperature can give an idea about the source of AP. Since it is generally a nonspecific finding, it should be evaluated together with other findings such as abdominal tenderness or pain in any other parts of the body, such as sore throat, sputum or flank pain, indicative of alternative causes of infection. AP may accompany fever in typhoid fever and/or some other gastrointestinal infections. Likewise, fever can be noted in AAp, cholangitis, PID, diverticulitis, inflammatory bowel diseases (IBD) such as Crohn's disease. There is no one-to-one relationship between the presence of "surgical" acute abdomen and fever. On the other hand, it should be recognized that especially elderly patients cannot produce febrile response at the expected level due to weakness of the immune system.

Consciousness: AP accompanying temporary or permanent altered mental status renders it necessary to rule out a range of serious entities which could be vital, such as diabetic ketoacidosis, acute porphyria, scorpion sting, cholangitis, and anaphylaxis.

Blood Pressure: If hypotension is associated with AP, the presence of a condition requiring emergent intervention such as sepsis, hypovolemia, and/or AMI should be considered and sought for emergently. In contrast remarkable hypertension accompanying AP can mostly be associated with AAA/DAA, scorpion and spider bites.

Pulse Rate: Bradycardia accompanying AP may be a warning sign in organophosphorus poisoning and AMI (mostly inferior AMI, RCA occlusion) or total AV block. Tachycardia with orthostatic hypotension is usually a manifestation of blood or volume loss (eg, DKA, intestinal obstruction, or GI bleeding, severe AGE).

Respiratory Rate: Respiratory functions may be impaired in patients with severe acute AP. Many conditions such as acidosis, cardiopulmonary causes of AP, and mesenteric ischemia can cause tachypnea. Developing sepsis/septic shock in those with delayed treatment of acute surgical abdomen should also be kept in mind. In addition, all causes of AP triggering generalized rigidity in the abdomen can present with impaired respiratory functions (and tachypnea) as an ominous finding for grave outcomes. Pulse oximetry should be routinely used in those with tachypnea or dyspnea. Pathological levels (<93% in previously healthy patients in room air) should prompt resuscitative measures and consultation with ICU. The clinician should check blood gases and accordingly, consider supplemental oxygen, high-flow nasal oxygen and endotracheal intubation, tailored for the individual characteristics.

Systemic Examination: A detailed systemic examination should be carried out and recorded in all patients presenting with AP. For example, in spinal cord disease, there may be abdominal pain due to compression of the nerve root. In another clinical scenario, unilaterally localized AP may be the chief complaint in the patient with zona zoster, depending on the dermatoma involved and physician can only notice vesicles if he/she examines the skin carefully.

The main purpose of the abdominal examination is to locate the problem and to shorten the DD list. The diseased area is mostly the point of maximum tenderness. The second purpose of the examination is to determine the extraabdominal causes of pain such as pneumonia, tonsillitis, *etc*.

Serial Examinations are a very important strategy in the evaluation and follow-up of the patient with AP, provided with the dynamic nature of the patient's findings over time. For example, the findings of a patient with a moderate probability of AAp on presentation can become evident after ten hours of observation.

Pill Information: We can say that the presumptive diagnosis of acute abdomen is confirmed with appropriate follow-up and the definitive diagnosis is established with a pathological examination. All the other examinations done in between are helpful in bringing us closer to our prediction.

Red flags in AP: Certain ominous findings can herald deterioration of the patient and mark high-risk groups to pay particular attention in terms of admission and operative interventions. (Fig. **3**).

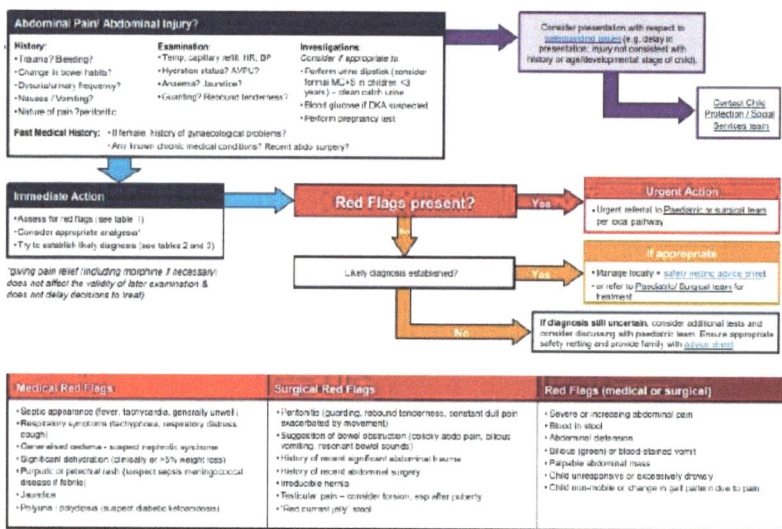

Fig. (3). Medical and surgical red flag signs should be specifically sought for and ruled out before discharge decisions are announced and recorded.

General Evaluation of Abdomen and Methods of Examination

Inspection is one of the indispensible components of examination. It is first noted how painful the patient really is. The stories and narrations of the patient, facial expressions including grimace, and general appearance are important. The obligatory position taken by the patient (writhing, standing still, lying on one side, leaning forward, moving like dancing, wrestlessness) is noted. It should be recorded whether sluggish, exhausted or lively, energetic, agitated. Detailed inspection of the abdomen (as shown in Table **3**) is known to narrow the DD and saves the patient from unnecessary work up.

Table 3. Certain features should be sought in the inspection of the abdomen.

• General appearance
• Swollen,
• Tight
• Tight
▫ Color changes in the skin,
▫ Dermatological lesions (*e.g.* vesicles of zona zoster),
▫ Petecchiae and ecchymoses +/- a history of trauma,
▫ Reduced skin turgor,
▫ Venous collaterals on the abdominal wall (suggestive of portal hypertension),
▫ Trauma scars
▫ Marks of previous surgery,
▫ Abdominal respiration pattern

Nine-quadrant System is a useful guide to use a standard language and also a systematic approach in inspection and other methods of examination (Fig. **4**).

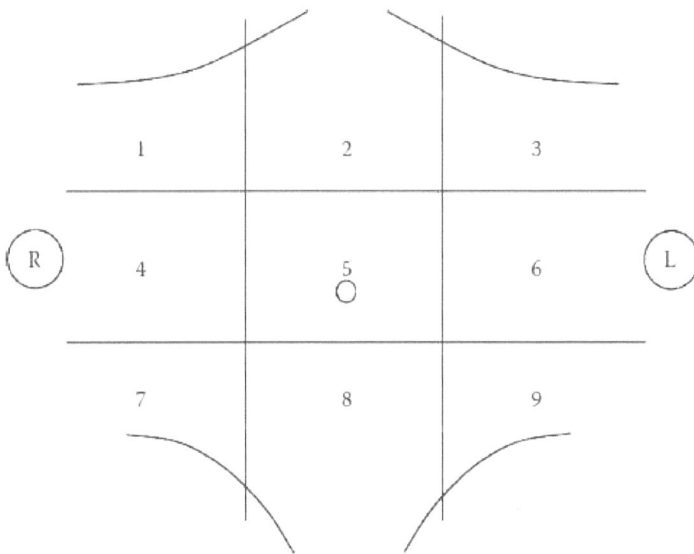

Fig. (4). Many physicians use the 9-quadrant system to localize abdominal pathologies. Referring to the embryonic system, anterior-mid-posterior intestines phenomena (foregut-midgut-hindgut) can also be conceptualized in this way, and the DD list can be narrowed substantially on a patient-specific basis.

Specific Tips: Multiple operation scars may support the presence of FMF or psychopathologic conditions. Although an appendectomy scar minimizes the possibility of AAp in the patient, it increases the probability of brid ileus and stump appendicitis. Detection of a cholecystectomy scar increases the likelihood of cholangitis in a patient with signs of the biliary tract on the right upper quadrant.

Pill Info: The most alarming finding possible on inspection is *de novo* distention with the moribund general condition. This clinical picture may be encountered in ileus, or together with hypotension-tachycardia, it may suggest abdominal aortic rupture and represent an indication for emergency intervention.

Auscultation; Increased bowel sounds are the early signs of acute gastroenteritis (AGE) or brid ileus, while the decrease or disappearance of bowel sounds is suggestive of paralytic ileus and peritoneal inflammation. Adynamic ileus may also occur resulting from some metabolic-electrolyte disorders such as hypercalcemia and hypokalemia. In weak individuals, a murmur may be heard on auscultation, which may suggest renal artery stenosis and/or some conditions related to the aorta. Lung auscultation performed in presence of AP may reveal preliminary findings of lower lobe pneumonia, pneumothorax or diaphragmatic hernia.

Percussion should precede palpation in the cascade of examination. Light percussion to be performed radially, especially starting from the distance of the painful area, is sufficient to reveal the sensitivity. Detection of **dullness** suggests collection of massive fluid or ascites in the percussion of the abdomen. This phenomenon is important in terms of cirrhosis, while obtaining **clapotage** is indicative of pyloric stenosis. As a rule, dullness in a fixed region should suggest the presence of a mass. Hepatomegaly and splenomegaly can also be detected *via* a proper percussion. **Tympanism** may suggest a dilated bowel loop.

Palpation: It is rare to have severe intra-abdominal pathology without any abdominal tenderness on palpation. The clinician should search for the presence of abdominal tenderness, guarding and/or rebound (indirect) tenderness (Fig. **5**). Specific painful points and abdominal mass(es) are sought *via* superficial and deep palpation, while pulsatile character of the mass should also be noted. Likewise, the presence of any intraabdominal organomegaly is important, for they can suggest a disease of the organ itself or a systemic process like malaria or leukemia.

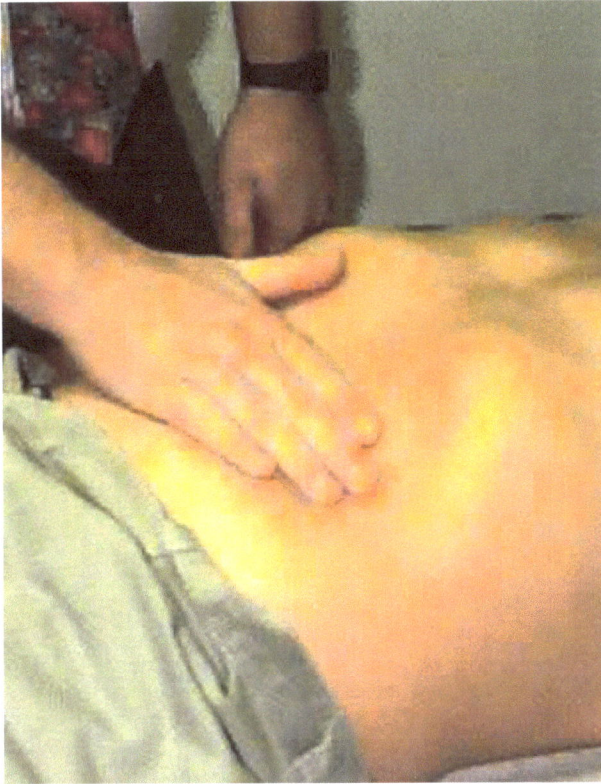

Fig. (5). Abdominal examination should begin with superficial inspection and continue with auscultation, percussion, light (superficial) and finally, deep palpation.

The tender area in the patient with AP does not always indicate the exact anatomical localization of the diseased organ. If the tenderness is limited/localized to a small area, DD is narrower and easier. However, local tenderness may not be elicited despite the presence of an inflamed organ in the abdomen. Organs located in the retroperitoneum such as kidney and pancreas will not irritate the peritoneum and thus may not be symptomatic on palpation or may give misleading findings. This is the reason one should suspect pancreatitis in a patient with persistent vomiting and near-normal abdominal examination.

Kidney stones or other urinary problems can be tested with a gentle blow to the lower ribs on the back (costovertebral angle tenderness), as shown in Fig. (**6**). However, this exam is not hundred-percent sensitive for a kidney stone.

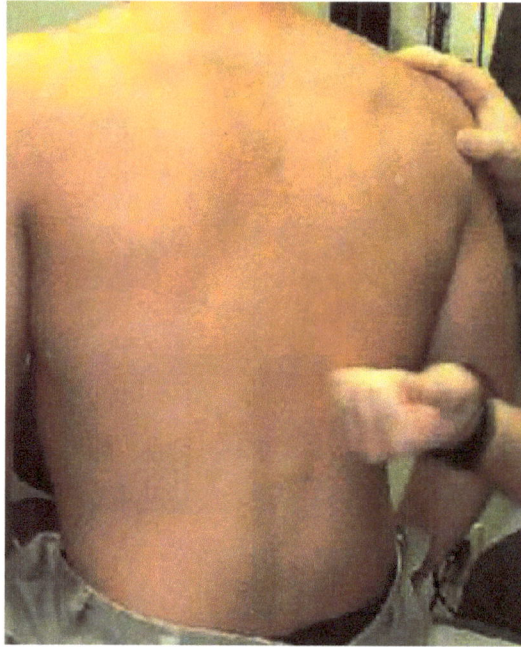

Fig. (6). Kidney stones and similar diseases that can present with abdominal pain are tested with a light blow (costovertebral angle tenderness) applied to the lower part of the ribs on the back. Severe pain produced with this maneuver suggests kidney diseases (eg, ureteral stones or pyelonephritis). Of note, similar findings can be obtained when there is a problem in the ribs.

Pain and hyperesthesia in the region conforming to a dermatomal distribution may suggest zona zoster or other neuropathies (impingement syndromes). Pathologies of the abdominal wall such as an injury or hematoma of rectus abdominis muscle can be sought for *via* Carnett's sign (Fig. **7**).

Guarding; Involuntary guarding (rigidity) is a hallmark of peritoneal inflammation that usually warrants surgical intervention. It cannot be relieved by the effort of the physician or by distracting the patient's attention *via* outer stimuli. In localized cases such as diverticular abscess or appendicitis, it is unilateral (left and right, respectively), but after peritonitis ensues, right and left cannot be discerned, it becomes widespread or generalized. Guarding is typically not evident in the case of inflammation of organs that are not directly adjacent to the peritoneum, such as the kidney or pancreas (Table **4**).

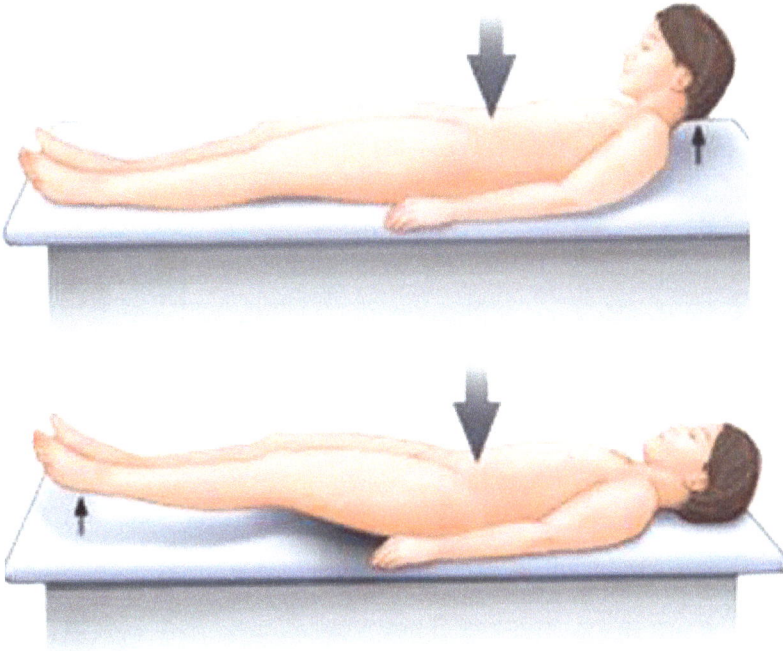

Fig. (7). Carnett's sign. When there is tenderness in palpation of the abdominal wall, we can not be sure whether its source is inside the abdomen or relate to the abdominal wall. This sign helps to distinguish whether the problem is on the abdominal wall or a pathology causing peritoneal irritation. If the pain increases when the abdominal muscles are forced to flex (head flexion or active elevation of the feet), the problem relates directly to the abdominal wall (mainly musculature).

Table 4. Features of some examination findings for differential diagnosis in patients with abdominal pain.

Examination	Unique characteristics-interpretation
Rebound tenderness	Pain aggravated once the inflamed organ hits the peritoneum: It is held stable for a while in deep palpation on the suspect side and released suddenly to allow it to float against the peritoneum. Sensitivity 37%-95%, specificity 13%-91%.
Guarding	Involuntary contraction in an area localized in the abdomen with deep palpation. Voluntary and involuntary guarding can be distinguished by distraction methods. Sensitivity 13%-90%, specificity 40%-97%.
Rigidity	Generalized involuntary contraction of the abdomen without the need for deep palpation. It indicates the presence of peritonitis in almost every case. Sensitivity 6%-66%, specificity 76%-100%.
Tenderness on percussion.	Sensitivity 57%-65%, specificity 61%-86%.

(Table 4) cont.....

Examination	Unique characteristics-interpretation
Rovsing test	Pain triggered in the right lower quadrant when the left iliac fossa is pressed firmly (mostly indicative of appendicitis). Sensitivity 7%-68%, specificity 58%-96%.
Rectal tenderness	Severe pain incited on the walls of the rectum by the digital rectal examination. It is noted in 30% of acute appendicitis, it is positive almost invariably in perirectal and/or perianal abscess. Sensitivity 22%-82%, specificity 41%-95% in detecting peritonitis
Cough test	Sudden pain triggered in the McBurney point by coughing in the supine recumbent patient. Sensitivity can be as high as 85%.
Heel tap sign	Sudden pain precipitated in McBurney by rising on the toes and suddenly falling on heels. It can also be elicited with the patient supine and the right heel (elevated by 10-20 degrees) is hit firmly with the palm of the examiner's hand (Lawrence, 2012). Sensitivity 85%-90%
Murphy's sign	Breathing is halted suddenly when the inflamed gall bladder hits the examiner's hand in deep inspiration in the right upper quadrant. Sensitivity over 90%, but only 50% specific
Obturator test	Pain triggered in the right lower quadrant by internal and external rotation of the right hip while maintained in flexion. Its accuracy is very high in diagnosing peritonitis when it is present. However, it should be borne in mind that it cannot be found positive in every patient with peritonitis (Fig. **8a**). Its sensitivity is 8%, specificity 94%.
Psoas test	Pain in the right lower quadrant is precipitated by active extension or flexion of the right leg against resistance in a patient recumbent with the left decubitus position (Fig. **8b**). It may not be found in early appendicitis. Its accuracy is very high in demonstrating peritonitis when it is present. In advanced cases of appendicitis, it is 79%-97% specific but only 13%-42% sensitive.

Note: Since these examination techniques and maneuvers can be brutal, they should all be exercised after completion of other techniques, *i.e.*, inspection, auscultation, percussion, and palpation, respectively. (Sensitivity-specificity levels are quoted from McGee, 2018).

Rebound tenderness was often seen as a sign of peritoneal inflammation. Studies showed that the sensitivity was reported as 81% and the specificity as 50% to diagnose the entity of any cause. In other words, it is an examination finding that is mostly found in surgical cases with the acute abdominal syndrome. But when found, it can only suggest acute abdomen. It should be tried to be elicited firstly by light palpation and then by deep palpation. The suffering of the patient to achieve this is seen by many authors as a crude and unnecessarily painful technique (Wyatt, 2012).

Note: Since these examination techniques and maneuvers can be brutal, they should all be exercised after completion of other techniques, *i.e.*, inspection, auscultation, percussion, and palpation, respectively.

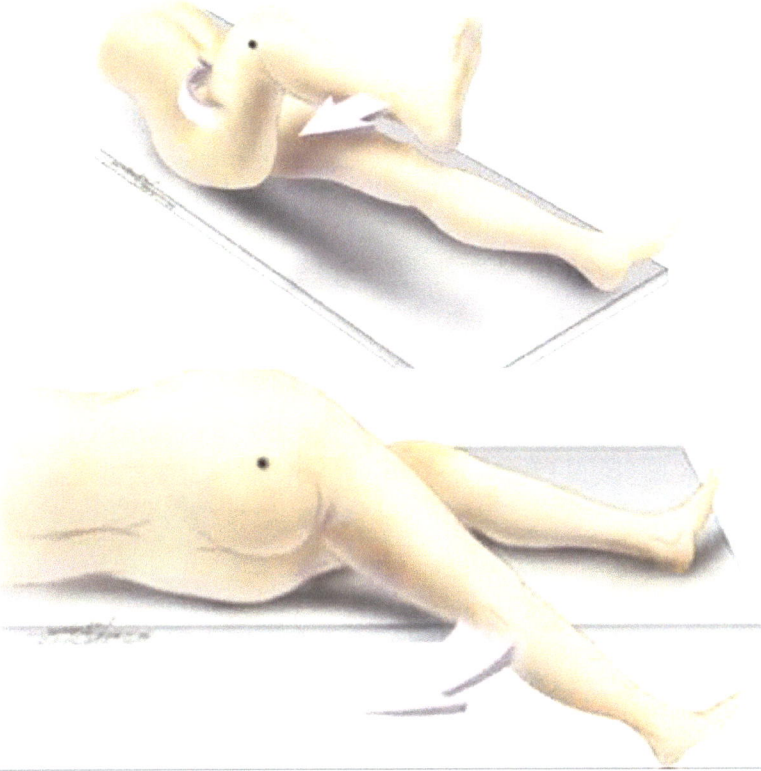

Fig. (8). A. Obturator test. Pain triggering in the right lower quadrant by internal/external rotation of the right hip in flexion. It is highly suggestive of appendicitis located in the pelvis. **B.** Psoas test. Pain in the right lower quadrant is triggered by active extension or flexion of the right hip against resistance in a patient assuming left decubitus position. When found, it suggests retrocecal appendicitis.

B. Psoas test. Pain in the right lower quadrant is triggered by active extension or flexion of the right hip against resistance in a patient assuming left decubitus position. When found, it suggests retrocecal appendicitis.

Rectal Examination: Although it is indicated in every patient presenting with AP as a rule, it is gradually neglected in line with the development of imaging modalities in contemporary medical practice. Rectal examination is inappreciable in the bedside diagnosis of GI bleeding. Sometimes a rectal mass can be identified, especially in the elderly. In others, fecal impaction is very common and can cause widespread abdominal pain. The patient will be relieved quickly by evacuation of the fecaloma(s).

Marked tenderness in the digital rectal examination is a sign of perirectal abscess or retrocecal appendicitis.

Pelvic Examination: It should be done in every woman with lower AP. PID, which is one of the most common causes of AP in the reproductive age, can be diagnosed by this examination mostly without imaging or other advanced investigations. The diagnosis is clear when adnexal/cervical tenderness is combined with purulent discharge from the cervical os. Detection of vaginal/cervical discharge does not necessarily mean that the given patient presented for PID, and the whole list of DD should still be ruled out. Generally speaking, it is performed less than necessary due to limitations such as the need for the provision of a suitable environment for the examination and having experienced physicians.

Hernias: Incarcerated/non-strangulated hernias can become easily visible, especially when the patient is standing, with maneuvers such as coughing/straining which increase the patient's intraabdominal pressure suddenly. When the hernias are incarcerated/strangulated, the patient will present with severe and sharp and incessant ischemic/inflammatory pain in the area.

The likelihood of peritonitis is estimated based on the literature data and represents an invaluable aid in the diagnostic pathways (Fig. **9**).

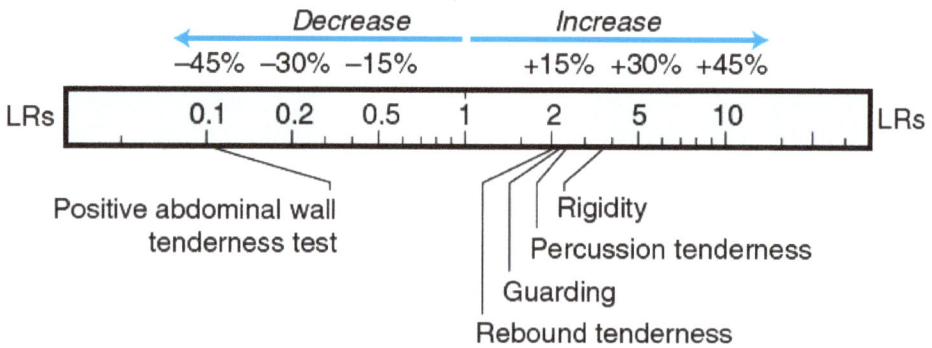

Fig. (9). Possible findings on examination and relevant likelihood ratios significantly change the probability of peritonitis.

CONCLUSION

The main goal of the assessment of the patient with AP is both to eliminate the possibility of missing an operative or life-threatening diagnosis and to expedite establishing the diagnosis before definitive treatments such as operative interventions. There are rare instances in which the physician can easily narrow the DD list to place a good first shot on the target. Therefore, we can conclude that a successful abdominal evaluation warrants a combination of a systemic and specific one.

REFERENCES

Albuquerque, P.L.M.M., Magalhaes, K.D.N., Sales, T.C., Paiva, J.H.H.G.L., Daher, E.F., Silva Junior, G.B.D. (2018). Acute kidney injury and pancreatitis due to scorpion sting: case report and literature review. *Rev. Inst. Med. Trop. São Paulo, 60*(0), e30.
[http://dx.doi.org/10.1590/s1678-9946201860030] [PMID: 29972468]

Amitai, Y. (1998). Clinical manifestations and management of scorpion envenomation. *Public Health Rev., 26*(3), 257-263.
[PMID: 10444963]

Gallagher, E.J. (2004). Acute abdominal pain.*Emergency Medicine: A Comprehensive Study Guide.* (6th ed.). New York: McGraw-Hill.

Güllü, U.U., İpek, S., Dalkıran, T., Dinçer, S., Yurttutan, S., Aynacı, E. (2021). The Role of ProBNP on Prognosis in Scorpion Stings. *Wilderness Environ. Med., 32*(2), 137-142.
[http://dx.doi.org/10.1016/j.wem.2021.01.015] [PMID: 33994108]

He, X., Cheng, X., Feng, X., Wan, H., Chen, S., Xiong, M. (2021). Clinical Symptom Differences Between Mild and Severe COVID-19 Patients in China: A Meta-Analysis. *Front. Public Health, 8*, 561264.
[http://dx.doi.org/10.3389/fpubh.2020.561264] [PMID: 33520906]

Karcioglu, O., Gumustekin, M., Tuncok, Y., Celik, A. (2001). Acute renal failure following latrodectism. *Vet. Hum. Toxicol., 43*(3), 161-163.
[PMID: 11383658]

Koyuncu, N., Karcioglu, O., Sener, S. (2018). Nonspecific abdominal pain: A follow-up survey. *Niger. J. Clin. Pract., 21*(3), 332-336.
[PMID: 29519982]

Koyuncu, N. (2001). *Acil servise karın ağrısıyla başvuran ve nonspesifik karın ağrısı tanısıyla taburcu edilen hastaların kısa dönem prognoz ve takipleri..* Uzmanlık Tezi. Dokuz Eylül Üniversitesi.

Kubena, BE, Umar, MA, Walker, JD, Harper, H (2021). Case Report: Soldier With Latrodectism After Black Widow Spider Bite During a Field Training Exercise. *Mil Med,* 22;24-201.
[http://dx.doi.org/10.1093/milmed/usab201]

Lawrence, P.F., Bell, R.M., Dayton, M.T. (2012). *Essentials of General Surgery.* Lippincott Williams & Wilkins.

Lukens, T.W., Emerman, C., Effron, D. (1993). The natural history and clinical findings in undifferentiated abdominal pain. *Ann. Emerg. Med., 22*(4), 690-696.
[http://dx.doi.org/10.1016/S0196-0644(05)81849-9] [PMID: 8457097]

Sotelo-Cruz, N., Hurtado-Valenzuela, J.G., Gómez-Rivera, N. (2006). Envenenamiento en niños por mordedura de la araña "Latrodectus Mactans" (Viuda Negra). Características clínicas y tratamiento. *Gac. Med. Mex., 142*(2), 103-108. [Poisoning caused by Latrodectus Mactans (Black Widow) spider bite among children. Clinical features and therapy]. [Spanish.].
[PMID: 16711543]

Wyatt, Oxford Handbook of Emergency Medicine.. Oxford University Press.

Zhu, J., Ji, P., Pang, J., Zhong, Z., Li, H., He, C., Zhang, J., Zhao, C. (2020). Clinical characteristics of 3062 COVID-19 patients: A meta-analysis. *J. Med. Virol., 92*(10), 1902-1914.
[http://dx.doi.org/10.1002/jmv.25884] [PMID: 32293716]

CHAPTER 2

Laboratory and Radiological Investigations and Cost-effectiveness

Abstract: Abdominal pain (AP) is a very common complaint that renders it elusive to diagnose in most instances. After history and evaluation narrow the list of differential diagnoses (DD), ancillary investigations including laboratory tests and radiological modalities are ordered. Of note, these adjuncts will only help the clinician who bears a presumptive diagnosis on the mind. Non-invasive, repeatable and cost-efficient options such as ultrasound are preferred initially, although, in most instances, more specific and definitive information warrants advanced imaging techniques including computed tomography and contrast studies. Laboratory work-up needs to be tailored to the individual based on findings on evaluation. ECG, complete blood count and blood chemistry can provide inappreciable clues for specific diagnoses while none will be sufficient *per se*. Urinalysis and specific cultures including stool studies will expedite recognition of urinary tract infection, amebiasis and other infections when indicated. B-hCG level can prevent unwanted exposure to radiation and drug effects on an unrecognized pregnant woman. Thus, all these adjunctive investigations should be included in the management plan individualized to the patient, based on the history and evaluation findings.

Keywords: Abdominal pain, Computed tomography, Contrast media, Diagnosis, Imaging, Laboratory tests, Physical examination, Radiological.

There are myriad types of investigations in the medical area and they are getting more varied over time. The clinician assumes the difficult task of tailoring these tests for each patient. A focused history and thorough examination are the key features to judge the test strategy, which will prevent unnecessary testing and expedite diagnosis and management.

ECG: It should be taken and interpreted urgently in all patients over 40 years of age, especially in patients presenting with atypical presentations of AP or additional systemic signs and symptoms. Since the sensitivity of the first ECG in detecting acute coronary syndrome does not exceed 50% to 60%, serial ECG monitoring is the rule in suspected cases. It should be noted that myocardial infarctions involving the "inferior" wall of the heart, neighbouring diaphragm,

Ozgur KARCIOGLU, Selman YENİOCAK, Mandana HOSSEINZADEH & Seckin Bahar SEZGIN

often present with AP (or thoracoabdominal pain). There may be upper abdominal or epigastric pain here, not the lower abdomen. In short, AMI and ACS are in the DD of epigastric pain.

Case example: A 30-year-old male with no previous cardiac history was admitted to the ED with epigastric pain and vomiting. There was no chest pain, shortness of breath, or shoulder or jaw pain. Chest and abdomen CT scans of the patient were taken and interpreted as unremarkable for acute abdominal conditions (Figs. **A** and **B**). Although acute inferolateral AMI is recognized in the ECG (C) taken later, it is seen that the inferior wall myocardial tissue is darker than normal myocardium in the retrospective scrutiny on CT sections. This appearance was thought to be related to the lack of contrast enhancement of the infarcted tissue.

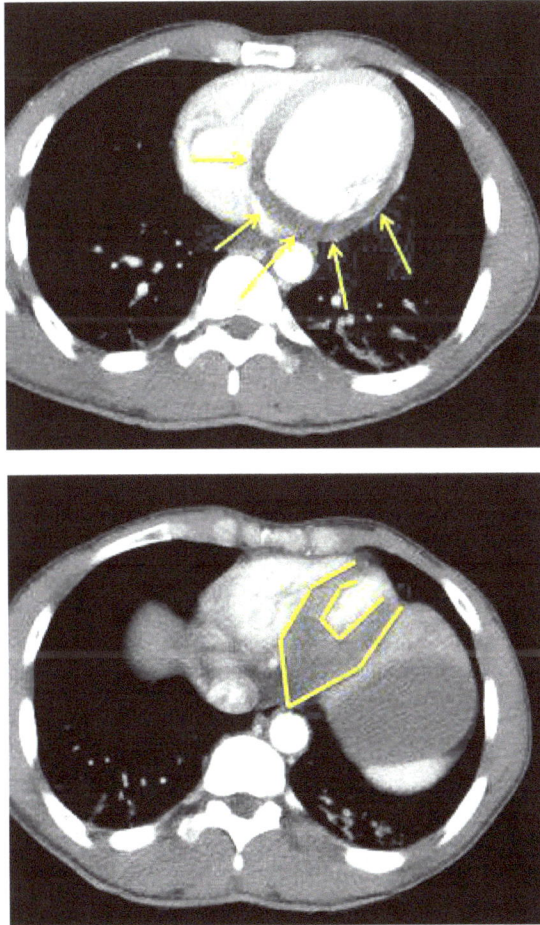

(Fig.) contd.....

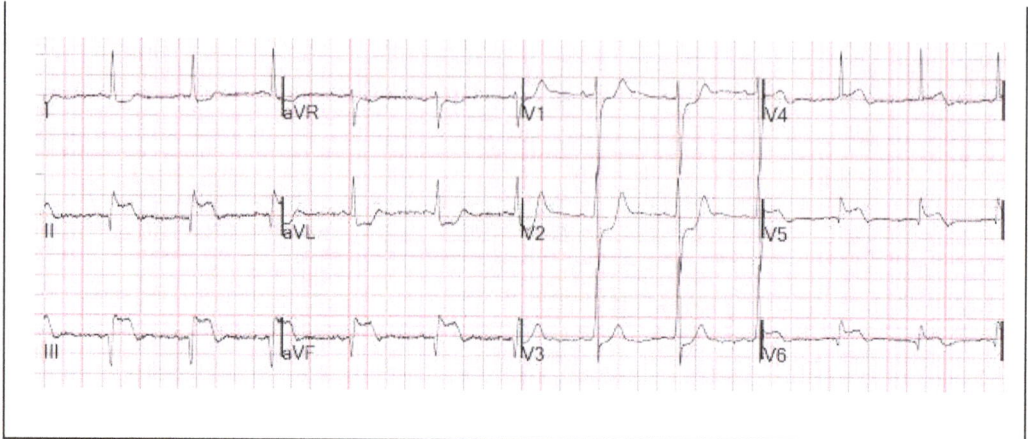

CBC: For adults, a leukocyte count of $10.000/mm^3$ and a neutrophil count above 75% are considered supranormal or pathological in most laboratories. If leukocytosis is compatible with the history and physical examination findings, it may be significant and and guide physicians in the decision making for the presumptive diagnosis. However, its sensitivity and specificity are lower than an "ideal test" in most intraabdominal conditions. For example, in 10% to 60% of AAp cases, there is no leukocytosis on presentation. If the leukocyte count is over $30,000/mm^3$, different diagnoses such as leukemia/leukomoid reaction, intraabdominal sepsis should be thought of, not the "classical" acute abdominal entities such as AAp and cholecystitis. While leukocytosis is expected in sepsis, values below $4000/mm^3$ (leukopenia) may also be encountered as an ominous sign of mortality. For these reasons, it should be tried not to rule in or out diagnoses based solely on leukocyte counts.

Amylase and Lipase: Serum amylase increases with many intra- and extra-abdominal conditions such as acute pancreatitis, peptic ulcer, ileus, ectopic pregnancy, diabetic ketoacidosis (DKA), liver diseases, small bowel ischemia/perforation, intestinal wall injury, parotid gland diseases. Serum lipase is more sensitive and specific in the diagnosis of AP and other pancreatic disorders.

Pill information: If the blood levels of amylase and lipase exceed 3 times the upper limit of normal, it indicates pancreatitis in most patients with AP or vomiting. In other situations, it can be viewed as a nonspecific test that should be verified *via* other supportive tests such as lipase and trypsinogen activation.

Liver Enzymes: AST, ALT, and bilirubin are commonly ordered tests in 'routine' biochemistry, but this is a wrong practice. Apart from acute viral hepatitis, jaundice, toxic hepatitis, cholestasis and hemolysis, there are only rare diseases in which these are useful. If these diagnoses are not considered directly, they are of little value to guide us in the maze. Since they are normal in end-stage cases with chronic hepatitis and cirrhosis, they may give a false sense of comfort to the physician. Bilirubin elevation should be confirmed by urinary urobilinogen. Since direct and indirect bilirubin is elevated in hepatic and hemolytic diseases, respectively, they should not be confused.

Ischemic Modified Albumin (IMA) may be helpful in the DD of acute AP, especially with regard to ischemic conditions due to vascular occlusions. It was noted that free radical damage in AAp and strangulated hernia would probably increase IMA values and help in diagnosis (Kadioglu, 2012). In a meta-analysis published in 2017, the sensitivity of IMA in the diagnosis of acute mesenteric ischemia was found to be 94.7% with a specificity of 86.4% (Treskes, 2017). IMA rises immediately (within minutes) after the onset of ischemia remains high for 6 to 12 hours and returns to normal levels in around 24 hours (Fig. **1**). Although it is not routinely used, it is thought to be useful in many vital clinical entities such as ACS, ischemic bowel, cerebral stroke, as its diagnostic accuracy can be high.

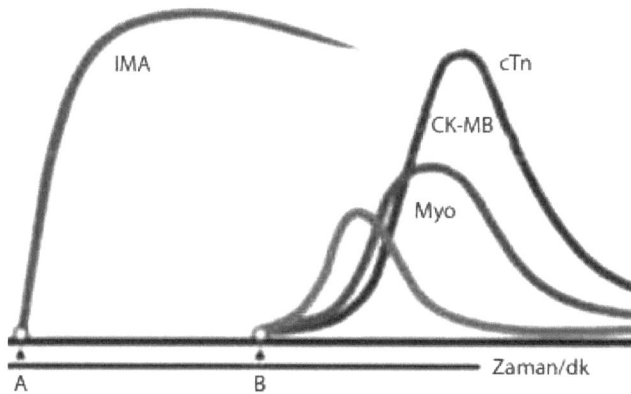

Fig. (1). Graphical demonstration of onset of organ ischemia and necrosis in accord with IMA, myoglobin, CK-MB, troponin (cTn) markers. IMA peaks much faster than others. A. Onset of ischemia. B. Onset of necrosis (30 to 60 minutes).

Urinalysis: In patients with AP, urinalysis can sometimes be misleading. In 20% to 30% of patients with AAp, there may be red blood cells, leukocytes and even bacteria in the urine. It has been stated in most publications that hematuria is detected in 30% of patients diagnosed with aortic dissection. Although **hematuria** is seen most frequently in ureter/kidney stones in men, it is not a rule (there can be patients with ureteral stones without hematuria). There is also marked **hematuria** in hemorrhagic cystitis caused by adenoviruses in women. In the case of pyelonephritis, abundant leukocytes or casts are seen in the urine, but it is not the rule. **Red blood cell or erythrocyte casts** can be seen in acute glomerulonephritis. Since almost all visible blood elements are seen in lupus nephritis, a finding called **"telescopic urine sediment"** occurs, resembling a starry sky. Although **sterile pyuria** is seen as a classical sign indicative of tuberculosis, it can also be encountered in cases with AAp and Meckel's diverticulum. Patients with urine density higher than 1.025 should be considered as dehydrated. **Ketonuria**, on the other hand, is seen as a rule in alcoholism, diabetes, malnutrition and prolonged fasting, accompanied by AP and persistent vomiting. **Glucosuria** and ketonuria accompanying AP require the exclusion of DKA.

PREGNANCY TEST (B-HCG)

Pill information: Every woman of childbearing age should be considered pregnant until proven otherwise. Pregnancy test should be performed on every female patient of childbearing age who presents with AP. Normal B-HCG level should be seen before drug administration and imaging, especially in women who will undergo tomographic scanning.

B-HCG may not be a prerequisite to be sought in investigations performed due to life threatening situations such as suspicion of aortic dissection and hemorrhagic shock. The reliability of the urine test is low, therefore, in cases where clinical pregnancy must be excluded, blood B-HCG level should be ordered. In rare cases, the test interferes with hydatidiform mole.

Laboratory markers, units, ranges, and aggravating/relieving clinical conditions frequently requested in relation to AP are given in Table **1**. Considering these, it would be appropriate to carry out a workup in accordance with the narrowed list of DD for a given patient.

Table 1. Laboratory markers, units, ranges and increasing/decreasing clinical conditions frequently ordered in the ED in patients presenting with abdominal pain.

Test	Reference range	Rises in	Declines in
Alanine aminotransferase (ALT)	5-40 U/L	Liver diseases (hepatitis, cirrhosis) Congestive hepatitis Alcoholism Pancreatitis Myocarditis Renal/pulmonary infarction Dehydration Muscle trauma or myopathies (dermatomyositis/polymyositis) Convulsion	Malnourishment Chronic alcoholic liver disease, advanced stages of cirrhosis End-stage renal disease

(Table 1) cont.....

Test	Reference range	Rises in	Declines in
Aspartate aminotransferase (AST)	10-40 U/L	Myocardial injury/cardiac surgery Cardiac contusion Muscle trauma, Liver disease (hepatitis, cirrhosis, metastasis) Burns Pancreatitis Dehydration Convulsion Myopathies	End-stage renal disease Pregnancy DKA
Alkaline phosphatase (ALP)	38-155 U/L	Bile duct obstruction Liver disease (hepatitis, cirrhosis, metastasis) Osteomalacia, rickets, bone fracture(s) Ulcerative colitis, intestinal perforation Hyperthyroidism/Hyperparathyroidism Leukemia, multiple myeloma	Hypothyroidism Hypophosphatemia Celiac disease. D hypervitaminosis
Bilirubin (Direct, conjugated) (serum)	<0.3 mg/dL	Extrahepatic bile duct obstruction Liver disease (hepatitis, cirrhosis, metastasis) Drug-related cholestasis Some hereditary liver disease (*e.g.*, Gilbert's syndrome)	-
Bilirubin (total) (serum)	<1.4 mg/dL	Hemolytic anemias Biliary obstruction Liver disease (hepatitis, cirrhosis, metastasis) Massive blood transfusions Hemolysis in the newborn, Sickle cell anemia Sepsis Congestive hepatitis Drug adverse effects Some hereditary liver diseases	-
Beta-HCG	<5 mIU/mL	Normal/ectopic pregnancy Abortion Mole hydatiform Some carcinomas	In utero fetal death, incomplete abortion
Blood urea nitrogen (BUN) (serum)	5-15 mg/dL	All diseases causing dehydration and/or hypovolemia (*e.g.*, burns, GI bleeding) Urinary tract obstructions, prostate diseases Use of diuretics Kidney failure Shock, AMI, CHF	Liver diseases Malnutrition

(Table 1) cont.....

Test	Reference range	Rises in	Declines in
Amylase	25-90 U/L	Acute Pancreatitis, pancreatic cancer Acute cholecystitis Acute appendicitis Traumatic bowel and/or parotid gland injuries DKA Peptic ulcer perforation Burns Esophagus cancer Salivary gland inflammation, parotitis Kidney failure Ruptured ectopic pregnancy Intestinal ischemia/infarction	Chronic pancreatitis Hepatic necrosis, cystic fibrosis
Lipase	13-60 U/L	Acute pancreatitis/ pancreatic cyst, pseudocyst/ Pancreatic cancer Acute cholecystitis/ cholangitis Kidney failure Spasm of Oddi sphincter	-
Ammonia (NH_3) (Plasma)	10-80 mcg/dL	Fulminant hepatitis/cirrhosis Hepatic encephalopathy Portal hypertension Reye's syndrome	-
Bicarbonate (serum)	25-32 mEq/L	Dehydration Chronic vomiting metabolic alkalosis Compensated respiratory acidosis COPD Some diuretics (esp. those including mercury)	Metabolic acidosis Compensated respiratory alkalosis Metabolic acidosis (DM or renal) Protracted diarrhea Loop diuretics Ethylene glycol intoxication
Lactate (venous)	0.6-2.2 mmol/dL	Shock (esp. septic or hemorrhagic) Acute appendicitis, mesenteric ischemia Nonketotic DM Overt exercise CO poisoning Liver disease Some metabolic diseases Tissue ischemia (tourniquet)	-

DIFFERENTIAL DIAGNOSIS; IMAGING PRINCIPLES

One of the essential questions for DD appears to be "Should I send this patient to the operating room?" In other words, "Does my patient have a surgical acute abdominal syndrome?" Other questions should include (but not limited to) those dichotomous thoughts: "Is the main problem of my patient in the abdomen, or could there be a presentation of a systemic problem as abdominal pain?" and "Is my patient stable or unstable."

The severity of the symptoms stated by the patient should not lead us to a definite conclusion about the severity or seriousness of the disease. Very severe symptoms may accompany benign disease (such as food intolerance or splenic flexure syndrome), while mild symptoms may represent severe disease (such as end-stage cancer, acute exacerbation over chronic pancreatitis). Some practical pathways can be devised to culminate entities in the scope of DD easily (Table **2**).

Table 2. The 3G+V formula in DD may help the clinician to consider all possible diagnoses.

• **Gastrointestinal:** Appendicitis, biliary colic/cholecystitis, small bowel diseases, pancreatitis, diverticulitis
• **Genitourinary:** Ureter/renal colic, postrenal obstruction/acute urinary retention, acute scrotal conditions (*e.g.*, torsion)
• **Gynecological:** PID, ectopic pregnancy (with or without rupture); ovarian cyst torsion/rupture, endometriosis
• **Vascular:** Aortic aneurysm/dissection, occlusive/nonocclusive mesenteric ischemia, ischemic colitis

Certain patterns and/or types of AP can be interrelated with certain specific diagnoses, even if not with a hundred-percent accuracy rate (Table **3**).

Table 3. Patterns of AP and attributes to specific diagnoses.

Patterns/types of Abdominal Pain	Definitions- Notes	Suggestive of Diagnoses
Crampy- colicky	Crescendo-decrescendo (there may be periods of complete relief in between)	urinary stone disease, biliary tract disease. intestinal colic, dysmenorrhea
Insidiously rising periumbilical	Constant pain without relief or cessation	Peritoneal irritation; acute appendicitis, diverticulitis, tuboovarian abscess
Severe, sudden, explosive	Sudden increase in persistent pain (rarely with sudden relief)	Hollow organ perforation (perforated acute appendicitis, gallbladder, ischemic bowel)
Progressive, severe (non-periumbilical)	progressively worsening event (never relieved, progressive)	Ischemic bowel, mesenteric ischemia, cholecystitis
Generalized after localized pain	Postinflammatory perforation,	Acute appendicitis, cholecystitis, ischemic bowel perforation

The relationship between pain and its spread is often not stable and thus changes over time. These changes give clues in diagnostic decision making. For example, urethral stones can cause pain in the scrotum in males and labia in females. The pain caused by gallstones is reflected in the right shoulder region and lower tip of the scapular area. The physician should bear these reflection points in mind and be able to direct to the region that is the source of the actual pain.

The etiological reasons that should be considered in line with the localization or extent of pain are listed in Table **4**.

Table 4. Etiologies that should be presumed according to the localization or extent of pain.

Ill-defined, diffuse abdominal pain	Right upper quadrant	Left upper quadrant	Right lower quadrant	Left lower quadrant
Peritonitis Pancreatitis Sickle cell crisis Appendicitis (initial phase) Mesenteric venous thrombosis Gastroenteritis Aortic aneurysms (dissecting or ruptured) Bowel obstruction DKA Inflammatory bowel disease Irritable bowel syndrome (IBS)	Biliary tract disease (cholelithiasis/ cholecystitis/ cholangitis) Gastritis Hepatic abscess Acute hepatitis Congestive hepatomegaly Ulcer perforation Pancreatitis Retrocecal appendicitis Acute coronary syndromes	Gastritis Ulcer perforation Pancreatitis Acute coronary syndromes Carditis (pericarditis/ myocarditis) Lower lobe pneumonias Pleuritis/ effusion	Acute appendicitis Meckel diverticulitis Caecal diverticulitis Aortic aneurysms (dissecting or ruptured) PID, ectopic pregnancy; ovarian cyst torsion/ rupture, endometriosis Mesenteric lymphadenitis Strangulated/incarcerated hernias Urinary tract infection/ pyelonephritis Ureteral stones	Epiploic appendicitis Aortic aneurysms (dissecting or ruptured) PID, ectopic pregnancy; ovarian cyst torsion/ rupture, endometriosis Mittelschmerz Mesenteric lymphadenitis Strangulated/ incarcerated hernias Urinary tract infection/ pyelonephritis Ureteral stones Psoas abscess Sigmoid diverticules

The pain-time relationship can be important. Sudden-onset AP is usually a symptom of a serious disease such as hollow viscus perforation, ruptured ectopic pregnancy, and aortic dissection. While heavy physical exertion or lung biopsy preceding AP suggest pneumothorax, a strong blow to the left lower part of the thoracic wall or abdomen will implicate splenic rupture. If the AP wakes the patient from sleep, it is more logical to consider an organic cause. Pain secondary to irritable bowel syndrome (IBS) tends to start early in the morning. Increasing severity of AP during the menstrual period, disproportionate to the previous periods, suggests endometriosis.

Which diseases can we miss most often? The clinicians are mostly focused on the most life-threatening and complicated diseases, therefore, some entities can be disguised and overlooked, especially in the chaotic environment of ED or other acute settings (Table **5**).

Table 5. Specific diagnoses, special groups and some clues can be used to help the recognition of these entities.

Diagnosis	In whom it can be missed?	Which clues are to be used to recognize it?
Acute appendicitis	- In the extremes of age (children and the very old) - pregnant women, - people with communication problems (lingual or cognitive)	It should be considered and excluded first in any case with continuous pain pattern and abdominal pain that started in the last 7 days (Alvorado score should be calculated)
Ruptured ectopic pregnancy (REP)	- New onset rupture, - - Teenage females with an unclear history,	REP should be ruled out in every woman with abdominal pain, regardless of sexual history and last menstrual period (USG + B-HCG should be ordered)
Ruptured aortic dissection/ aneurysm	- The young patient - patients whose haemodynamic findings have not yet developed - those who cannot describe their pain well due to neuropathy such as DM	It should be excluded in whom severe pain disproportionate to the findings on examination is associated with hemodynamic instability (POCUS and CT-angiography if needed)
Mesenteric ischemia/ thrombosis	- New onset ischemia, - It should be excluded in the elderly patient with moribund general condition	- Patients prone to cardiac thrombosis (previous MI or atrial arrhythmia) or in a poor general condition who has severe pain disproportionate to the findings on examination (Doppler USG and/or CT-angiography are to be ordered)
Intraabdominal abscess/ Perirectal or perianal abscess	- Elderly patient with poor general condition - Those who cannot explain their pain well due to their neuropathy such as DM - In an immunosuppressed or debilitated patient who cannot react with fever.	If there is no diagnosis that can be easily reached in an elderly, febrile, or afebrile patient, an abdominal, anal, and rectal abscess(es) should be ruled out.
Peritonitis related to tuberculosis (TB)	A patient who cannot give a satisfactory history of TB and/or cannot communicate easily	It should be tried to be ruled out in a patient with low socioeconomic level and with inconsistent findings not matching with other entities. It should be excluded in every patient with a history of TB.

(Table 5) cont.....

Diagnosis	In whom it can be missed?	Which clues are to be used to recognize it?
Pain secondary to systemic disease (DKA, porphyria, sepsis)	In patients with an unclear or inconsistent history such as newly diagnosed diabetes,	The patient's findings should be evaluated carefully and differential diagnosis should be made meticulously.
Diagnoses in neuropathic patients (DM, RF)	Almost all of them can be missed. In patients with impaired communication, therefore, inconsistent history In an immunosuppressed or debilitated patient who cannot react to fever. In patients with opiate/other substance addicts, partly due to stigmatization and prejudice	Patients with risk of neuropathic pain due to masking/stigmatization should be evaluated carefully and further investigations should be ordered.

Should we Request Imaging in the Diagnosis of AP?

First of all, diagnostic tests are not a substitute for careful physical examination and history. Laboratory examinations should only be requested according to the DD you focus on (pancreatitis: lipase + CT, ruptured ectopic pregnancy: USG, B-HCG, *etc.*). Thus, one must first conceptualize a preliminary diagnosis and order a test accordingly (*e.g.*, not to overlook ileus in a patient who is thought to have discomfort in the intestines, and therefore ordering a direct abdominal X-ray.

However, the clinician's evaluation of the complaints and findings together with the examination in the DD will negate this need, *i.e.* the possibility of ileus in a patient without persistent vomiting is almost negligible.

In principle, testing strategy should go from noninvasive and cheap testing to invasive and expensive.

Radiographs (Plain Films)

To cite the final words at the beginning, the use of abdominal graphs in acute AP typically has very low sensitivity and specificity to recognize certain acute abdominal conditions, including AAp. Direct X-rays have little clinical use in visualization of the appendiceal tissue. In brief, the added value of direct x-rays is almost negligible to employ this modality in routine practice in the work up of patients with acute AP.

Abdominal X-rays are still ordered more than necessary in most parts of the world, especially in developing countries. Robust indications may be searching for catheter location, ileus, foreign bodies, and imaging of the bullets in firearm injury. In most of the indications, even if a diagnosis is approached with X-ray, another modality for further examination (USG and/or CT) is often required. For example, you can never send a patient for whom you have evidence of ileus in X-rays to the operation room (OR) with this film alone. X-ray may be beneficial, albeit partially, in the imaging of toxic megacolon, volvulus, opaque urinary stones. X-rays may rarely image a calcified fecalith in those with suspected AAp, albeit this is a nonspecific finding. Pneumoperitoneum can also be rarely noted in complicated AAp; *e.g.* following ruptured hollow viscus. Specifically, the visualization of bowel obstruction (*i.e.*, large air-fluid levels) or subdiaphragmatic free air can help identify other serious diagnoses. In a well-designed study on 1021 patients, a small minority of the patients' diagnoses changed after X-rays and the level of confidence were mostly not affected (van Randen, 2011).

In conclusion, there is no indication for abdominal X-rays in a patient with AAp, UTI, cholecystitis, constipation, GI bleeding, *etc*.

Chest Radiography/X-Ray (CXR) can give clues for cardiopulmonary causes in the etiology of abdominal pain. The increased cardiothoracic index raises suspicion for congestion in congestive heart failure. Lower lobe pneumonias can directly cause upper quadrant pain on the affected side. A diaphragmatic hernia can directly lead to abdominal and chest pain and other problems. A view indicating the presence of subdiaphragmatic free air (SDFA) suggests hollow organ perforation in the abdomen. The flip side is, a CT of the abdomen still needs to be ordered to visualize the extent of the damage, fluid collection and to prepare for the operative interventions

Bedside/Point-of-Care Ultrasound (POCUS): It is very efficient and cost-effective in demonstrating gallstones, cholecystitis, common bile duct occlusion, perforations, free fluids (such as ruptured ectopic pregnancy), urinary stone disease, and aortic aneurysm with or without dissection (Fig. **2**). The only disadvantage may be that it requires training and is not available everywhere. Although its sensitivity is not satisfactory in some diseases, noninvasive bedside application boosted its use in the recent decades. In cases such as mechanical bowel obstruction where USG was not preferred in the past, new generation USG devices may be advantageous.

Abdominal Computed Tomography (CT): Due to its high sensitivity and superior accuracy rate, it is used as the gold standard diagnostic tool in many intraabdominal entities. With the development of multidetector CT (MDCT), its accuracy approaches 100%. It is selected especially in retroperitoneal pathologies such as pancreatitis because its accuracy is considerably higher than USG.

Inarguably, it gives more detailed information not only about the presence of inflammation, damage or rupture in an abdominal organ, but also about its extent and complications. It can be ordered as a "final" examination in a patient whose diagnosis is suspected *via* USG. Another advantage is that it can also demonstrate diseases in neighboring structures such as lower lobe pneumonia with high accuracy.

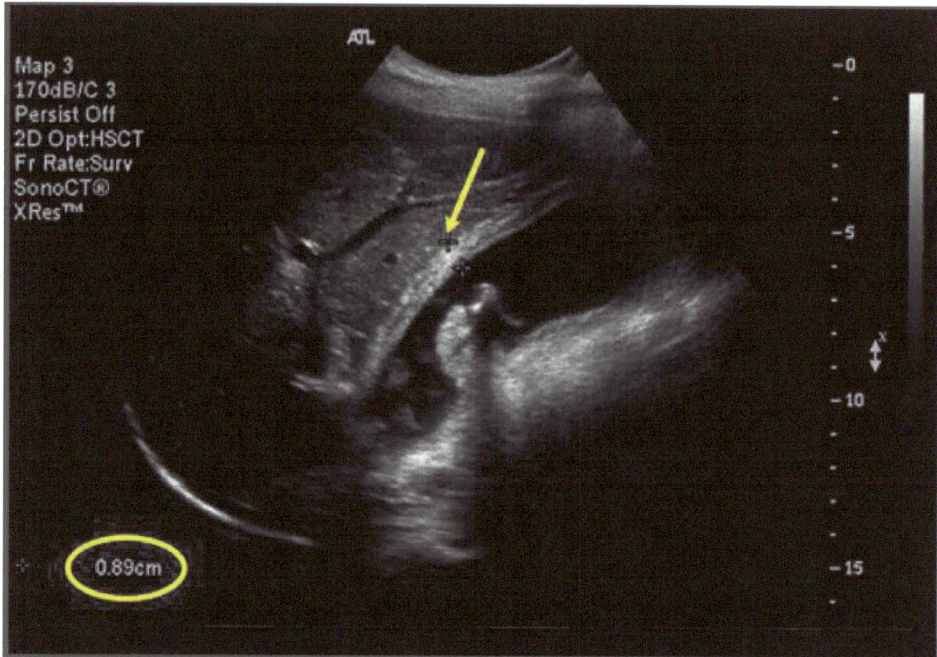

Fig. (2). USG findings of acute cholecystitis: choledochal enlargement, presence of stones, pericholecystic fluid collection, positive sonographic Murphy sign, wall thickness >4 mm (arrow), and target sign (edematous/hyperemic gall bladder wall). Among these, visualization of the stone(s) and sonographic Murphy sign are the ones that have the strongest predictivity for cholecystitis.

Any contrast? In context of CT obtained in the emergency setting, oral and rectal contrast add no diagnostic benefit in acute abdominal conditions. This is why an IV contrast-enhanced CT is the modality of choice for accurate diagnosis (Figs. **3** and **4**) (Table **6**).

Table 6. Routine CT protocols recommended in the acute abdomen to establish a specific diagnosis.

Variables/Media	Recommended Protocols
Oral contrast	750 - 1000 mL iodinated contrast media
IV contrast	100–120 mL iodinated contrast media, injection rate 2 ml/sec
Timing of imaging	70 - 90 sec (portal venous phase)

(Table 6) cont.....

Variables/Media	Recommended Protocols
Targeted area of imaging	Between superior part of the diaphragm and symphysis pubis
Section width	5 - 8 mm
Pitch	1.5
Reconstruction intervals	5 - 8 mm

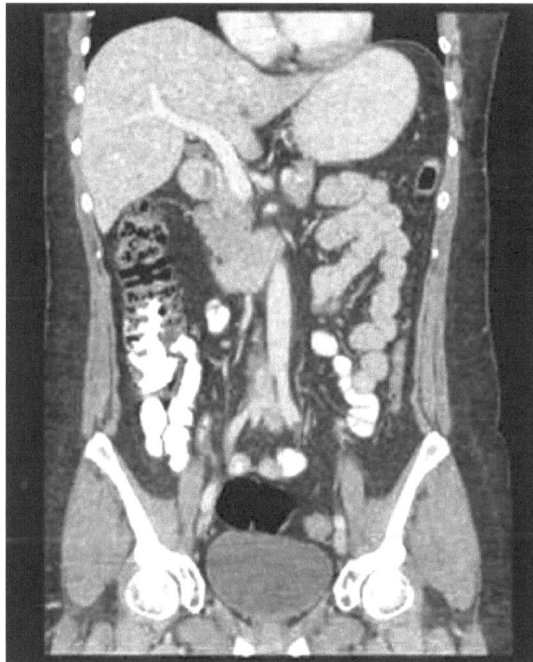

Fig. (3). The appearance of acute appendicitis in coronal section abdominal tomography (Oral + IV contrast enhanced CT).

Routine *Versus* Selective CT in Case of AP? A meta-analytic study revealed that the routine use of CT does not increase the accuracy rate of diagnoses or reduce death rates compared to the selective use of CT in adults with AP (Hajibandeh, 2020). Length of hospital stay also remained unchanged with a routine application of CT. Of note, the findings of the analysis did not comprise elderly patients.

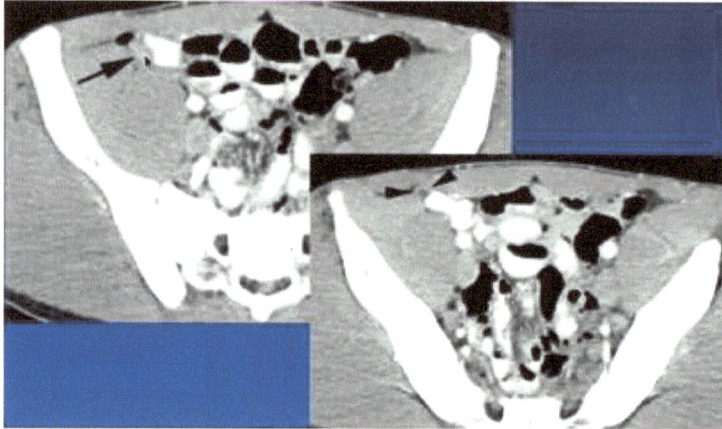

A.

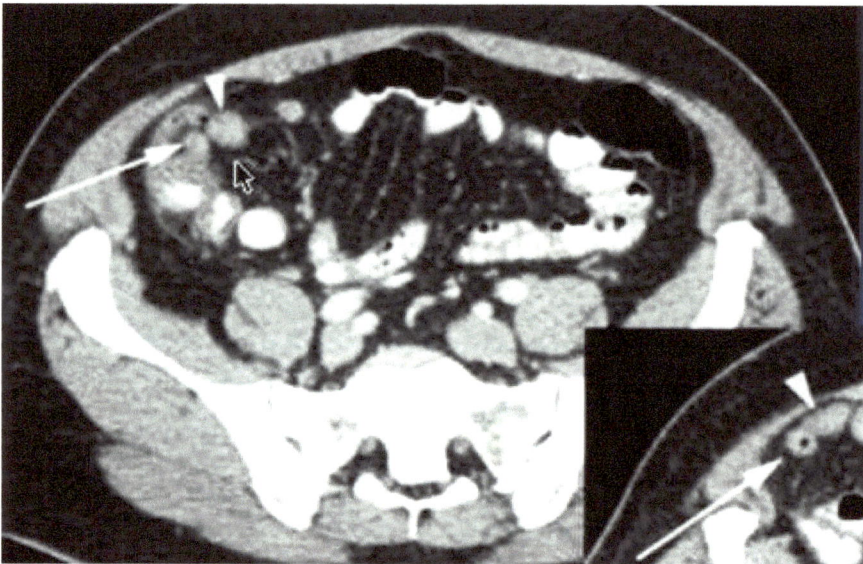

B.

Fig. (4). A. The appearance of acute appendicitis in a thin patient in his 20s on abdominal tomography (Oral + IV contrast enhanced CT). **B.** On the contrary, the heterogeneity in mesenteric fat tissues in the overweight patient in his 40s and the appearance of more remarkable appendicitis due to heterogeneity draws attention.

Is CT or MRI the Best To Diagnose AAp? Fig. (**5**) shows that both CT and MR images can accurately demonstrate appendiceal wall thickening, periappendiceal stranding, and mucosal enhancement (Repplinger, 2018). Other examples of advanced imaging exhibit invaluable information to guide the diagnosis of the patients with AP (Figs **6-8**).

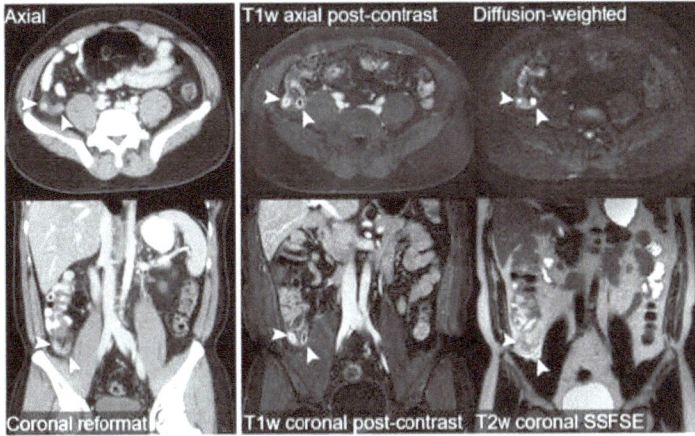

Fig. (5). Adapted from Repplinger, 2018) IV contrast-enhanced CT and IV contrast-enhanced MR images in a 41-year-old woman with abdominal pain and uncomplicated appendicitis (arrowheads). Thin axial and reformatted coronal CT images acquired after administration of iodinated contrast material are shown. Selected images from MR imaging protocol are also shown, including coronal and axial postcontrast T1-weighted (T1w) images acquired after administration of gadolinium-based contrast material, a coronal T2-weighted (T2w) single-shot fast spin-echo image, and an axial diffusion-weighted image. The T2-weighted MR image also depicts periappendiceal fluid, and the inflamed appendix is very conspicuous on the diffusion weighted MR image.

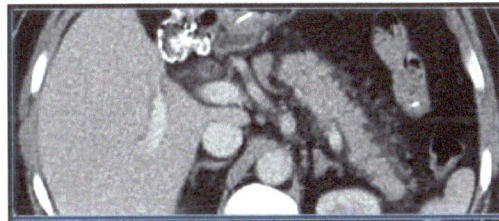

CT severity index

Pancreatic Inflammation Score

-	Normal pancreas	0
-	Increased volume in pancreas	1
-	Peripancreatic inflammation	2
-	1 peripancreatic fluid collection	3
-	>1 peripancreatic fluid collection	4

Pancreatic necrosis:	
None	0
<30%	2
30%-50%	4
> 50%	6
Total:	Maximum 10 points

Fig. (6). Interstitial pancreatitis.

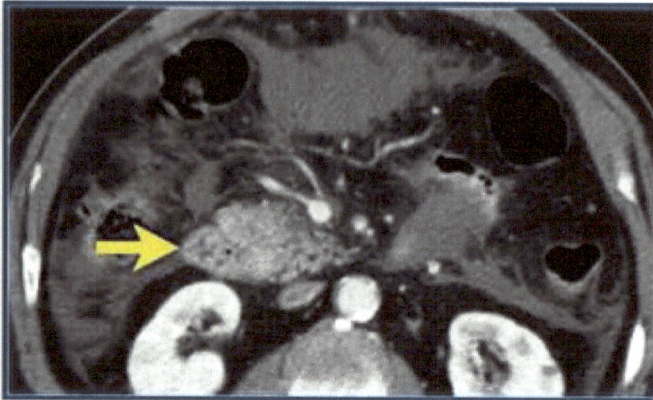

Fig. (7). Acute necrotizing pancreatitis. Non-enhancement is remarkable in the corpus and tail. Since more than 50% of the pancreas is necrotic, the index score is 10.

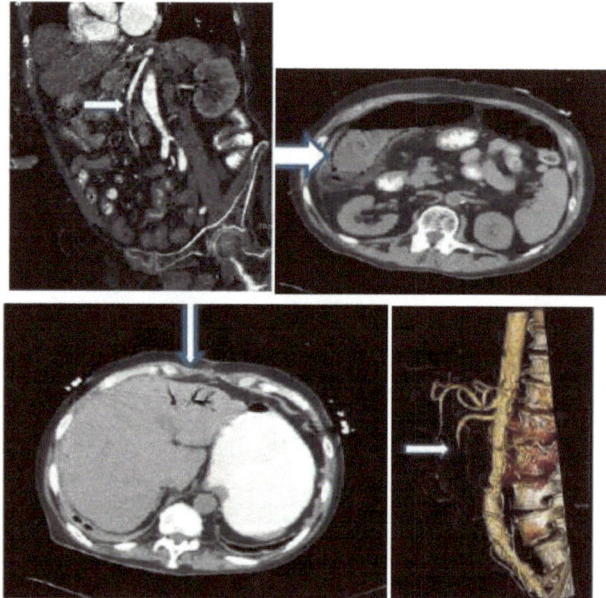

Fig. (8). Contrast-enhanced CT image obtained after acute onset AP in a patient with AF on ECG, not using any treatment agents. Embolic distal SMA occlusion is visualized in the vein track (arrow). Ischemia in the ileum and colon and air is noted in the portal venous system. Occlusion is seen more clearly in 3-D reconstruction.

Thoracoabdominal MRI: Since most cases can be diagnosed practically and accurately with USG/CT in the ED, the indications of MRI are very limited in the acute setting. It is superior to other modalities in very few diseases such as diaphragmatic injury or spinal pathologies. In chronic diseases, however, MRI can be inappreciable in some elusive diagnoses, like pancreatic cancer, and decision making and follow-up of some important procedures like MRCP.

COVID-19 and Abdominal Imaging Findings: Pandemic disease changed everything on earth as "it will be never like before". Attributed imaging features have included bowel wall thickening, fluid-filled colon, pneumatosis, pneumoperitoneum, intussusception, and ascites (Lui, 2021). Of note, many patients exhibited evidence of COVID-19 caught incidentally through abdominal CT imaging at the lung bases. Typical GI findings have included nonspecific intestinal and colonic wall thickening and liquid stool throughout the bowels.

CONCLUSION

Remarkable elements in medical history and positive findings on examination should constitute a basis for planning a management plan including the radiological, laboratory and microbiological investigations in patients with AP, together with sociodemographic factors such as age and gender.

REFERENCES

Can, Ü., Yosunkaya, Ş. (2017). İskemide Yeni Bir Marker: İskemi Modifiye Albumin. *Koşuyolu Heart J, 20*(2), 148-152.
[http://dx.doi.org/10.5578/khj.10257]

Hajibandeh, S., Loutfi, M., Hajibandeh, S., Abulkhir, A., Rehman, S., Mansour, M., Arsalani Zadeh, R. (2020). Routine *versus* selective computed tomography in non-traumatic acute abdominal pain: meta-analysis of randomised trials. *Langenbecks Arch. Surg., 405*(3), 283-291.
[http://dx.doi.org/10.1007/s00423-020-01884-1] [PMID: 32388716]

Kadıoğlu, H, Kaptanoğlu, L. (2012). *İskemik Modifiye Albüminin Acil Cerrahide Kullanımı J Kartal TR.*

Lui, K., Wilson, M.P., Low, G. (2021). Abdominal imaging findings in patients with SARS-CoV-2 infection: a scoping review. *Abdom. Radiol. (N.Y.), 46*(3), 1249-1255.
[http://dx.doi.org/10.1007/s00261-020-02739-5] [PMID: 32926211]

Karcioglu, O., Koyuncu, N. (2020). Acilde biyokimyasal tesler.

Treskes, N., Persoon, A.M., van Zanten, A.R.H. (2017). Diagnostic accuracy of novel serological biomarkers to detect acute mesenteric ischemia: a systematic review and meta-analysis. *Intern. Emerg. Med., 12*(6), 821-836.
[http://dx.doi.org/10.1007/s11739-017-1668-y] [PMID: 28478489]

User, N.N., Karcioğlu, Ö. (2002). Acil servis hastalarında kan biyokimya incelemelerinin istenmesinde Lowe klinik kriterlerinin yeri ve değeri. *Türkiye Tıp Dergisi, 9*(2), 77-83.

van Walraven, C., Naylor, C.D. (1998). Do we know what inappropriate laboratory utilization is? A systematic review of laboratory clinical audits. *JAMA, 280*(6), 550-558.
[http://dx.doi.org/10.1001/jama.280.6.550] [PMID: 9707147]

Yılmaz, F.M., Kahveci, R., Aksoy, A., Özer Kucuk, E., Akın, T., Mathew, J.L., Meads, C., Zengin, N. (2016). Impact of Laboratory Test Use Strategies in a Turkish Hospital. *PLoS One, 11*(4), e0153693.
[http://dx.doi.org/10.1371/journal.pone.0153693] [PMID: 27077653]

CHAPTER 3

Pain: Methods for the Assessment

Abstract: International Association for the Study of Pain defines pain as an unpleasant subjective sensation that includes the past experiences of the person with or without tissue damage.

Acute pain, generally lasting for hours to days, is the primary complaint at a rate of up to 70-80% at first admission. Headache, myalgia, arthralgia, back pain, local pain induced by minor trauma (such as sprains), thoracoabdominal pain, ear, facial pain, etc. are the most common types of presentations in the acute setting related to pain. Analgesia, on the other hand, is the relief of the perception of pain without causing sedation or any change in vital signs.

It is one of the few areas a physician can make a difference to implement more efficient patient care. The subjective and multidimensional nature of the pain experience make pain assessment really challenging. Patients' evaluation of pain should be the main reference for decision-making to provide analgesics or not. Implementation of dimensional recording of pain in clinical practice include the addition of pain as the "fifth" vital sign to be noted during initial assessment; the use of pain intensity ratings; and posting of a statement on pain management in all patient care area.

Our motto should be "pain cannot be treated if it cannot be assessed". The most important principle is that clinicians should somehow assess their patients' pain levels, independent of the specific method or scale to achieve this. Although all pain-rating scales are valid, reliable and appropriate for use, the VAS has somehow appeared more difficult than the others. Pain reassessment should be guided by pain severity reported by the patients themselves.

Keywords: Assessment, Evaluation, Multidimensional, Pain, Pain rating, Physical examination, Unidimensional.

Pain is the most common reason for presenting to EDs, regardless of age, gender, occupation or education level (Cordell, 2002, Wheeler 2010). Researchers cited that pain was the main complaint of more than 80% of patients admitted to the ED. In the last three decades, the Joint Commission on Accreditation of Healthcare Organizations (JCAHO), which has issued the accreditation principles of health institutions in many items, has announced that appropriate assessment and management of pain is mandatory and therefore, standard care rules have

Ozgur KARCIOGLU, Selman YENİOCAK, Mandana HOSSEINZADEH & Seckin Bahar SEZGIN

commenced to be established in ED setting all over the world.

Pain is not simply a response to physical injury, instead, it is a behavioral pattern that is affected by anxiety, depression, expectations and other psychological changes, together with current and past experiences. Thus, the International Association for the Study of Pain (IASP) has described pain as a "sensory and emotional experience originating from any part of the body, accompanied by tissue damage or potential tissue damage, or defined in the process of such damage" (Raja, 2020).

Furthermore, JCAHO stated that **pain should be measured and recorded as a 5th vital sign** in the ED evaluation of the patients in the acute setting.

THE TERMINOLOGY OF PAIN

The IASP published the terminology for pain in 1979. In routine clinical practice, many different terms are used to describe different pain syndromes and patterns. These terms and their explanations are given below:

- **Analgesia**: Absence and sensation of pain caused by painful stimulation.
- **Anesthesia Dolorosa**: Pain in an anesthetic site or area.
- **Causalgia**: Burning pain that persists after a traumatic nerve lesion.
- **Central pain**: Pain associated with a central nervous system lesion.
- **Dysesthesia**: An unpleasant (undesirable) abnormal sensation (feeling).
- **Hyperalgesia**: Increased sensitivity and responsiveness to painful stimuli.
- **Hyperesthesia**: Increased sensitivity to stimulation.
- **Hyperpathy**: Painful syndrome characterized by hyperalgesia and overreaction.
- **Hypoalgesia**: Decreased sensitivity and responsiveness to painful stimuli.
- **Hypoesthesia**: decreased sensitivity to stimulation.
- **Neuralgia**: Pain that radiates to a nerve.
- **Neuritis**: An inflammation of the nerve itself.
- **Neuropathy**: Pathological change or dysfunction in a nerve.
- **Nociceptor**: Specific receptor sensitive to painful or potentially painful stimulus.
- **Paresthesia**: Abnormal sensation (in the absence of a stimulus)
- **Stimulus**: A material effect that causes a change or damage in the tissue.
- **Pain threshold**: The intensity of the smallest stimulus that causes pain in the person.
- **Pain tolerance level**: The largest stimulus triggering pain that the person can tolerate.

Acute Pain and its Perception

Acute pain is provoked by harmful stimuli produced by abnormal muscle or organ function, deep somatic structures, organs, skin disease, or trauma. The corresponding mechanisms in the clinical practice are muscle contraction, tissue ischemia, and traumatic tissue destruction.

Individual perception of pain differs according to continents, countries, or smaller geographical units, whilst age and gender also affect perception and management.

In brief, perception of and response to pain vary from person to person. The clinician should not expect a standard pattern of pain behavior. Another important point is that perceived pain intensity does not appear to be directly related to the degree of tissue damage that occurred.

One of the most commonly used pain classifications is given in Fig. (**1**).

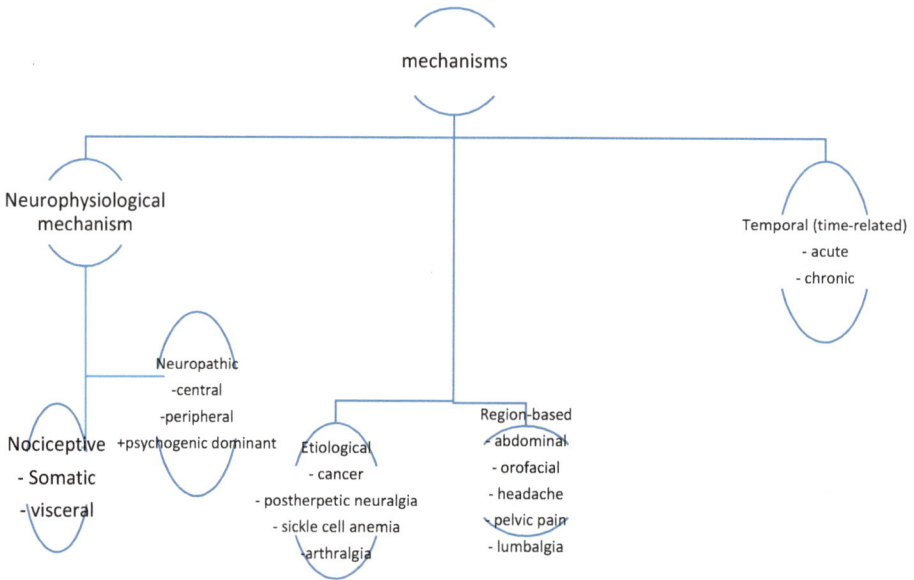

Fig. (1). Types and subtypes of pain.

Pain in the Clinical Practice

It is known that pain is one of the most common problems in daily practice, since most of the diagnostic or therapeutic procedures in medical practice are painful, in addition to the patients who present to the hospital specifically due to pain. Hence, it is thought that it should be incorporated into the evaluation patterns of all patients in the acute setting as the "fifth vital sign" apart from body temperature, blood pressure, pulse rate, and level of consciousness. With the contemporary approach formulated as 'if you do not assess the pain, you cannot manage it', the pain will be able to be recorded and treated individually in all acutely ill and injured.

Evaluation and Monitoring of Pain

The patient should be asked by the physicians and nurses whether there is pain or not. Pain is not a unidimensional parameter that can be easily measured, but a complex and multidimensional concept. It has been established that a majority of physicians do not use objective measures to assess pain level or pain relief in most instances (Ho, 1996).

Does Pain have Physiological Consequences?

Yes, it has. Physiological cues such as tachycardia and hypertension may assist in the assessment of pain in intubated or uncooperative patients (Albrecht, 2012). Abdominal and thoracic pain can result in decreases in tidal volume, vital capacity, and alveolar ventilation (Ossewaarde, 1997). Secretions and smooth muscle sphincter tone increase in the gastrointestinal tract, sometimes leading to paralytic ileus and bowel necrosis. Clinicians should be aware that increased systemic vascular resistance and changes in sympathetic tone may mask hypovolemia with "normal-appearing blood pressures". Cerebral functions of patients with increased intracranial pressure can be impaired by increased vasoconstriction in response to acute pain which is detrimental in certain conditions especially attributed to bleeding.

Does Every Patient Describe Pain in the Same Way?

No. Age, gender, ethnicity, previous experiences, accompanying psychiatric problems and socioeconomic status affect the way the patient describes pain. Therefore, pain is unique to each patient. There are no definite physiological or clinical findings that can be used to measure pain objectively. According to the National Institute of Health (NIH) in the USA, the patient's self-report is the most reliable indicator of the presence and severity of pain.

Gender effect: In studies, it has been observed that women perceive and express the severity of pain higher than men and therefore are better treated (Raftery 1995, Jones 1996). This is so remarkable that men have a major disadvantage compared to women in the management of pain. In addition, children and the elderly are also disadvantaged and receive suboptimal treatment in this regard.

Many sociodemographic variables can affect the perception and narration of pain (Table **1**).

Table 1. Patient groups who are disadvantaged in evaluation and management of pain because of difficulty in describing/perceiving pain.

• Babies and toddlers
• Men
• Elderly
• Diseases causing autonomic neuropathy such as DM, kidney failure, lupus (SLE)
• Debilitated individuals
• Those with communication and language problems, *e.g.* immigrants
• Patients who cannot get along due to intelligence and psychiatric problems

In a study we conducted in Turkey in 2006, the behavioral practices before and after the training is given to emergency medicine residents focusing on the administration of analgesia in victims of extremity trauma were compared (Akarca, 2012). The mean NRS scores of women were found to be significantly higher than men (7.4±2.3 and 6.7±2.5, respectively) (p=0.020). It was noted that the patients included in the study received significantly more analgesia in the post-training period than before the training (p<0.001), and the treatment times were significantly shortened in the post-training period (mean 19.3±8.3 minutes) compared to the pre-training period (mean 41.3±27.6 minutes). (p<0.001). Accordingly, an increase was observed in the rate of administration of analgesia within 30 minutes, furthermore, analgesia was administered to all patients within one hour in the post-training period.

In addition, a study conducted on 12,860 ED admissions in the USA revealed that self-reported pain intensity had a minimal effect on waiting times (Wheeler, 2010). In the literature review, it is seen that the inadequacy of pain assessment in the acute setting is not limited to a country or region, but is a global problem.

Pain Measurement Tools: Is 1 kg of Cotton or Iron Heavier?

In a systematic review we published in 2018, we examined 3 types of measurement tools (VAS, NRS, VRS) commonly used in acute setting in terms of ease of use and effectiveness (Karcioglu, 2018). As a result of the analysis of 19 studies that met the criteria, it was revealed that all three scales are valid and usable tools in clinical practice. On the other hand, VAS is less feasible in practice due to its difficulty in use, while NRS is more widely used because it is practical and does not require pen-paper and manual dexterity.

In the evaluation of pain in the ED, record-keeping is essential, and these ratings should be based on the patient's perceptions and self-expression on this issue. Valid and practical assessment tools should be used in this context.

How should be an ideal pain measurement tool? An "ideal tool" should encompass detection of pain as well as tracking pain and treatment effectiveness over time. In addition, it should be applicable to everyone, regardless of the individual's psychological, emotional, sociocultural characteristics. The ideal measurement tool for acute pain should definitely be practical, reliable, sensitive, valid, and conform to proportional scale specifications.

Unidimensional pain scales were developed with these concerns. Due to their ease of use, they have become popular tools used to measure pain intensity. Pain can be measured with pain assessment scales such as Numeric Rating Scale (NRS), Visual Analog Scale (VAS), and qualitative assessment scales (*i.e.*, Adjective/Verbal Rating Scale-ARS/VRS) (Fig. **2**) (Berthier 1998, Ho 1996, Liebelt 2000).

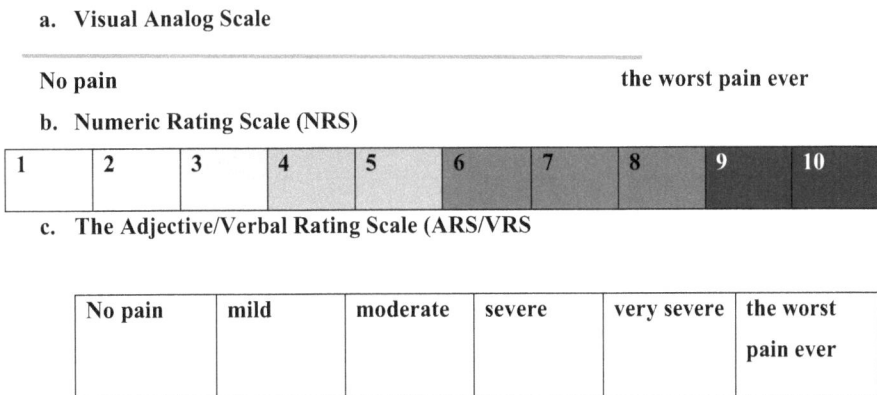

a.　**Visual Analog Scale**

No pain　　　　　　　　　　　　　　　　　**the worst pain ever**

b.　**Numeric Rating Scale (NRS)**

1	2	3	4	5	6	7	8	9	10

c.　**The Adjective/Verbal Rating Scale (ARS/VRS**

No pain	mild	moderate	severe	very severe	the worst pain ever

Fig. (2). Unidimensional pain measurement tools: **(a)** Visual Analog Scale; **(b)** Numeric Rating Scale (NRS); **(c)** The Adjective/Verbal Rating Scale (ARS/VRS).

VAS has been one of the most widely used pain assessment tools for research in acute medicine for decades due to its ease of use and simple structure. Its use in sequential pain assessment is very favorable, while allowing statistical evaluation (Ho 1996, Bodian 2001).

Adjective/Verbal Rating Scale-ARS/VRS is also a very practical scale but does not provide detailed information. The patient indicates how he/she evaluates his/her pain by choosing one of the adjectives in front of him: None, mild, moderate, severe.

The Brief Pain Inventory (BPI) is also a self-contained, valid multidimensional scale that is widely used in research. Validity studies have also been carried out in different languages. It is a scale that reveals both the severity and location of pain and its functional effects in almost all patient groups. In recent years, with the development and widespread use of technology, its use in pain assessment has come to the fore.

In a cross-sectional observational study, Kos et al. evaluated conditions and complaints such as fatigue, pain and anxiety, and quality of life by self-scoring using smartphones and tablets. They reported that this application called **"electronic visual analogue scale (eVAS)"** is valid and useful for evaluation, especially in those with chronic diseases.

Pediatric pain assessment is a practice with its own challenges. The stress and anxiety caused by the injury that brought the child to the ED render communication difficult *per se*. Sometimes the situation becomes even more difficult when the parent is not yet there, with feeling in a foreign environment, and the stress created by past experiences.

The FACES scale is commonly used in pediatric pain assessment. Children are asked to choose the most appropriate caricature expression for them with 6 different shapes scoring between 0-10.

MULTIDIMENSIONAL PAIN ASSESSMENT TOOLS

According to the concept put forward by the 'socio-economic pain model', preconditioned by experiences together with *in utero* pain reflexes determine the human being's response to pain. Multidimensional methods aim to evaluate not only the severity of pain but also other factors affecting the perception of pain. Because of the complexity of this situation, these tools are more difficult to use and interpret. It is impractical to use in the ED as it takes a long time to complete. The best-known example in this group, McGill Pain Questionnaire (MPQ). Since completion of this scale takes approximately 20 minutes from the patient, it is mostly used for research purposes or in private office practices. The most advantageous aspect of MPQ can be reliability and consistency in the assessment of various types of pain. The system has been validated in different languages.

Preparation and Operation: The MPQ is read to the patient by the physician, and the patient is asked to choose the words describing the current pain. As a result of the query, three basic variables are sought for:

1. Pain Rating Index (PRI): Each selected word is given a score, starting with the least. The collected scores are determined separately for each group (for example, the sub-class score totals of the sensory, affective, and assessment classes).

2. Pain Intensity at that Moment: It is found by summing the scores assigned to the words describing pain intensity.

3. Number of selected words: With this number, the difference between measurements in the number of selected descriptive words for pain is determined.

Further research is needed to develop correct methods in the use of pain measurement tools, to reveal the problems in practice, and to determine the psychometric properties in the acute setting.

There are many deficiencies in acute patient care with special regard to pain management. Analgesics are routinely administered in primary care and acute setting mostly without measuring the initial pain level and keeping records. Similarly, the effectiveness of analgesic treatment at discharge is not addressed in routine practice.

CONCLUSION

1. In emergency conditions, it should be patients who will decide whether there is pain, not physicians. The same is true for the severity of discomfort.

2. Pain should be measured with tested and validated pain assessment scales such as Numeric Rating Scale (NRS), and Visual Analog Scale (VAS).

3. Patients' perceptions of pain differ in accord with continents, countries, or smaller geographical units. Similarly, age and gender have an impact on the perception and management. In the evaluation of pain in the emergency, records should be kept taking the patient's perception and expression into account.

4. Healthcare professionals often fail to assess and manage patients' pain, or do not prioritize it necessarily. There is a need for more education, training and practice in patient management prioritizing acute pain assessment. The first step is to note the presence of pain and determine its severity.

REFERENCES

Akarca, F.K., Karcioglu, O., Korkmaz, T., Erbil, B., Demir, O.F. (2012). Analgesic Treatment in Patients with Acute Extremity Trauma and Effect of Training. *Türkiye Acil Tıp Dergisi,* *12*(2), 69-76.

Albrecht, E., Taffe, P., Yersin, B., Schoettker, P., Decosterd, I., Hugli, O. (2013). Undertreatment of acute pain (oligoanalgesia) and medical practice variation in prehospital analgesia of adult trauma patients: a 10 yr retrospective study. *Br. J. Anaesth.,* *110*(1), 96-106.
[http://dx.doi.org/10.1093/bja/aes355] [PMID: 23059961]

Cordell, W.H., Keene, K.K., Giles, B.K., Jones, J.B., Jones, J.H., Brizendine, E.J. (2002). The high prevalence of pain in emergency medical care. *Am. J. Emerg. Med.,* *20*(3), 165-169.
[http://dx.doi.org/10.1053/ajem.2002.32643] [PMID: 11992334]

Dworkin, R.H., Turk, D.C., Revicki, D.A., Harding, G., Coyne, K.S., Peirce-Sandner, S., Bhagwat, D., Everton, D., Burke, L.B., Cowan, P., Farrar, J.T., Hertz, S., Max, M.B., Rappaport, B.A., Melzack, R. (2009). Development and initial validation of an expanded and revised version of the Short-form McGill Pain Questionnaire (SF-MPQ-2). *Pain,* *144*(1-2), 35-42.
[http://dx.doi.org/10.1016/j.pain.2009.02.007] [PMID: 19356853]

Jones, J.S., Johnson, K., McNinch, M. (1996). Age as a risk factor for inadequate emergency department analgesia. *Am. J. Emerg. Med.,* *14*(2), 157-160.
[http://dx.doi.org/10.1016/S0735-6757(96)90123-0] [PMID: 8924137]

Karcioglu, O., Topacoglu, H., Dikme, O., Dikme, O. (2018). A systematic review of the pain scales in adults: Which to use? *Am. J. Emerg. Med.,* *36*(4), 707-714.
[http://dx.doi.org/10.1016/j.ajem.2018.01.008] [PMID: 29321111]

Melzack, R. (1975). The McGill Pain Questionnaire: major properties and scoring methods. *Pain,* *1*(3), 277-299.
[http://dx.doi.org/10.1016/0304-3959(75)90044-5] [PMID: 1235985]

Melzack, R. (1987). The short form McGill pain questionnaire. *Pain,* *30*(2), 191-197.
[http://dx.doi.org/10.1016/0304-3959(87)91074-8] [PMID: 3670870]

Raftery, K.A., Smith-Coggins, R., Chen, A.H. (1995). Gender-associated differences in emergency department pain management. *Ann. Emerg. Med.,* *26*(4), 414-421.
[http://dx.doi.org/10.1016/S0196-0644(95)70107-9] [PMID: 7574121]

Raja, S.N., Carr, D.B., Cohen, M., Finnerup, N.B., Flor, H., Gibson, S., Keefe, F.J., Mogil, J.S., Ringkamp, M., Sluka, K.A., Song, X.J., Stevens, B., Sullivan, M.D., Tutelman, P.R., Ushida, T., Vader, K. (2020). The revised International Association for the Study of Pain definition of pain: concepts, challenges, and compromises. *Pain,* *161*(9), 1976-1982.
[http://dx.doi.org/10.1097/j.pain.0000000000001939] [PMID: 32694387]

Wheeler, E., Hardie, T., Klemm, P., Akanji, I., Schonewolf, E., Scott, J., Sterling, B. (2010). Level of pain and waiting time in the emergency department. *Pain Manag. Nurs.,* *11*(2), 108-114.
[http://dx.doi.org/10.1016/j.pmn.2009.06.005] [PMID: 20510841]

Abdominal Pain, 2022, 51-105

CHAPTER 4

Specific Diagnoses and Management Principles of the Upper Digestive Canal

Abstract: Acute abdominal conditions which frequently necessitate emergency interventions and/or surgery include visceral perforations *i.e.*, gastric and duodenal ulcer, bleeding and rarely, ingested foreign bodies causing tissue damage, *e.g.*, button batteries. However, the differential diagnosis (DD) of patients presenting with acute abdominal pain is much broader than this, including many benign conditions as well. Acute gastroenteritis, acute gastritis and peptic ulcer disease are benign and mostly temporary diseases which may be relieved with simple treatments and follow-up. Gastrointestinal bleeding (with or without esophageal varices) may cause hemorrhagic shock unless expedient management is pursued. Ingested foreign bodies can constitute emergency conditions with tissue damage, especially when lodged in a specific site. The most important thing about button batteries is the prevention of their ingestion. Complications increase in direct proportion to time wasted.

Keywords: Acute abdominal pain, Esophageal varices, Gastrointestinal bleeding, Peptic ulcer, Surgical abdomen, Visceral perforation.

ACUTE GASTROENTERITIS (AGE)

Diarrhea or acute gastroenteritis (AGE) is defined as the passage of loose or watery stools typically at least three times in 24 hours. Every individual experiences this condition in one way or another throughout his life. Diarrhea represents one of the top five causes of death worldwide and is the second leading cause of death in children under the age of five (following only acute respiratory infections). Although seasonal variability is remarkable, diarrhea constitutes a substantial rate of 3-4% in the ED patient population (Yılmaz S, 2018). In a number of studies, the average age was around 35 and more than half (up to 2/3) of the cases were women in Turkey (Yilmaz S, 2018, Bozdemir MN, 2014, Tiryaki O, 2005). Its incidence is higher in rural areas than in cities.

Diarrhea is usually caused by a viral or bacterial infection that is relieved within a few days. Most children and adults with AGE are associated with contaminated

Ozgur KARCIOGLU, Selman YENİOCAK, Mandana HOSSEINZADEH & Seckin Bahar SEZGIN

food and water supplies (WHO). Paying attention to some basic principles in treatment will provide satisfactory results for patients and physicians.

Why do we have diarrhea? Apart from bacteria, viruses and fungi, emotional factors such as stress and anxiety can precipitate diarrhea. In some susceptible individuals, consumption of alcohol or caffeine, and overt ingestion of sweet or heavy foods have also been reported to be among factors for diarrhea which is mostly short-lived and self-limiting. Diarrhea occurs when babies cannot digest lactose-containing foods and beverages, especially feeding with cow's milk. Diarrhea can spread rapidly due to unhygienic pools used in the summer period. In general, toilet hygiene and infrastructural factors are prominent variables causing a surge in diarrhea incidences worldwide, especially in developing countries and regions.

Causative Agents and Spread: Campylobacter, Salmonella, Shigella and *E. coli.* are among the most common bacterial agents detected in developing countries related to diarrhea. Differences in rates vary depending on age, eating habits, socioeconomic level and geographical distribution. For example, it spreads rapidly among young children who have not fully learned hygienic toilet principles at home and in schools.

The most common etiologies of diarrhea are given in Table **1**.

Table 1. The most common causes of diarrhea.

Microbial diseases (virus, bacteria, fungus, protozoa) ingested with water and food
Consumption of milk and dairy products other than breastfeeding in infants.
Parasites
Use of agents such as laxatives and purgatives
Other drug-related untoward effects, *e.g.*, chemotherapy
Radiotherapy
Diseases that impair intestinal structure or absorptive functions, such as inflammatory bowel disease (Crohn's disease, ulcerative colitis).

Inadequate Storage of Foods: Most often, milk, cream, mayonnaise, and meat-containing foods that were left out for a long time cause diarrhea. Minced meat is much more likely than bulk meat to get infected. Quick-melting and corruptible foods such as ice cream and chocolate can also cause diarrhea if not stored properly.

Chronic Diarrhea lasting more than two weeks may be inflicted by a more serious condition and requires further investigation. Conditions such as immunodeficiency, AIDS, radiotherapy and some specific GI diseases can cause this. Chronic diarrhea can also be caused by diseases such as untreated dysentery, irritable bowel syndrome (IBS), and pancreatitis.

Large Bowel Infection (Infectious Colitis, IC)

IC can be precipitated by bacterial or viral agents, or parasites and represents a form of inflammatory diarrhea. Most cases with IC manifest with acute purulent, bloody, and mucoid types of diarrhea. Fever, tenesmus, and AP are also encountered in a majority of patients with IC.

Causative Agents for IC: Table **2** summarizes the agents isolated in patients with IC.

Table 2. Causative agents isolated from stool samples of patients with infectious colitis.

Bacteria	Viral	Parasitic Infestation	Sexually Transmitted Diseases in Rectum
Campylobacter jejuni (most common) *Shigella Salmonella, Escherichia coli, Clostridium difficile, Yersinia enterocolitica Mycobacterium tuberculosis*	*Norovirus, Rotavirus, Adenovirus, Cytomegalovirus (CMV)*	*Entamoeba histolytica*	*Chlamydia trachomatis Neisseria gonorrhoeae, Treponema pallidum* Herpes simplex,

Short Notes on Specific Agents

Campylobacter Jejuni is the leading causative agent among bacterial agents inciting diarrhea throughout the world with a prevalence of around 30 / 100000 people (Azer, 2020).

Salmonellae are another commonly isolated agent which is responsible of 1.2 million patients with non-typhoidal salmonellosis diagnosed in the US every year.

Shigellosis is also important with severe clinical course and systemic complications. Although the global incidence is still high (around 170 million patients), attributed death rates are estimated to have decreased nowadays. Huge developments in laboratory techniques in recognition and management are thought to have resulted in this achievement.

Shiga Toxin-producing *E. coli* O157: H7 represents a prominent food and waterborne agent that causes diarrhea, hemorrhagic colitis, and hemolytic-uremic syndrome (HUS) in human beings (Ameer, 2021). The expression of Shiga toxins is critical for the development of HUS. Enterohemorrhagic *E. coli* (EHEC) O157: H7 induces illnesses with Shiga toxin which precipitates a wide variety of entities, from temporary acute diarrhea to persistent hemorrhagic colitis. The systemic illness is described as HUS (induced by EHEC 0157: H7) and presents with a triad consisting of hemolytic anemia, thrombocytopenia, and acute kidney injury/renal failure (Atnafie 2017).

Clostridium difficile infection is prevalent in severe diarrhea, *e.g.*, 8.2 cases per 1000 discharge in 2010 and a mortality rate of 7% (Reveles, 2014). Of note, the incidence of *Clostridium difficile* infection among hospitalized adults in the US doubled in the first decade of the millennium. *Pseudomembranous colitis* is also encountered as a complication of toxin-producing *Clostridium difficile*. Cephalosporin and beta-lactam antibiotics are the most blamed agents associated with *pseudomembranous colitis* (Slimings, 2014).

A typical patient with colitis triggered by *Yersinia enterocolitica* is a small child presenting to the ED in the winter. Clinical findings are an excellent masquerade of AAp, encompassing severe acute AP associated with tenderness on palpation, anorexia, and vomiting. Laboratory examination typically reveals inflammatory changes, ulcerations in the cecum and terminal ileum areas, hyperplasia of Peyer patches, microabscesses, and granulomas (Azer, 2021).

Mycobacterium Tuberculosis is also among common causative pathogens isolated in diarrhea specimens, especially in developing countries. Infections involving the gut account for one-eighth of all cases with verified extra-pulmonary tuberculosis (Cherian, 2017). The prevalence of the agent in developing countries is closely related to the distribution of AIDS cases. Widespread problems of the century, namely, rising census of migrant population, deterioration in social conditions, cutbacks in public health services, and increased prevalence of immune-suppressed individuals (AIDS, those receiving immune suppressive) are effective factors for boosting incidences of tuberculosis (Karagiannis, 2008).

Entamoeba Histolytica is a protozoan parasite that is capable of invading the colonic mucosa and causing colitis. Amebiasis ranks as the second leading cause of death due to protozoan infection after malaria, Chagas disease, and leishmaniasis (Stanley, 2003). In an Iranian population-based study, the weighted prevalence of *E. histolytica/dispar*, *G. lamblia*, and *Cryptosporidium* spp. infection among Iranian general population were calculated to be 1.3% (95% CI 1.1-1.5%), 10.6% (95% CI 9.6-11.5%) and 2% (95% CI 1.5-2.5%), respectively (Mohebali, 2021).

Treatment options depend on the location of the infectious process. Amoebiasis in tissue is treated with metronidazole and tinidazole

Apart from hydration, the primary therapy for symptomatic amebiasis requires the administration of metronidazole and/or tinidazole (Zulfiqar, 2021). These two agents are dosed as follows:

- Metronidazole dosing for adults is 500 mg orally every 6 to 8 hours for 7 to 14 days.
- Tinidazole adult dosing is 2 g orally each day for 3 days.

Nitazoxanide, dehydroemetine, or chloroquine are also alternative regimens. A luminal infection is treated with diloxanide furoate or iodoquinoline.

An amoebic liver abscess can be managed by aspiration using CT guidance in combination with metronidazole (González-Alcaide, 2017). Surgery is sometimes required to treat massive gastrointestinal bleeding, toxic megacolon, perforated colon, or liver abscesses not amenable to percutaneous drainage

CMV infection is a serious health problem in immune compromised patients, while it is mostly asymptomatic in the immunocompetent. CMV colitis is among the DD of patients with diarrhea in the immune compromised. The prevalence of *Cytomegalovirus* (CMV) infection in those with IC ranges between 21% and 34% (Wada, 2003). Colonic mucosal biopsies may reveal specific findings for CMV, that is, "owl eye appearance" inclusion bodies as typical inclusion associated with CMV colitis.

Sexually transmitted diseases (STD) can also involve the rectum. These diseases are mostly diagnosed in HIV (+) patients and men who have sex with men. Causative agents comprise *Neisseria gonorrhoeae, Chlamydia trachomatis, Herpes simplex,* and *Treponema pallidum.*

Stool microscopy and culture constitute a major starting point for expedient diagnosis, while endoscopic exam provides more insight for IC. Of note, stool cultures yield accurate information in only a half of patients with bacterial IC, and endoscopic examinations usually reveal non-specific pathological changes.

Traveler's diarrhea (TD) occurs following ingestion of half cooked meat, and/or milk and vegetables with poor hygiene. Enterotoxigenic *E. coli* (ETEC) is known to be the primary cause of TD, followed by Enteroaggregative *E. coli*. ETEC expresses heat-labile (HL) and heat-stable (ST) toxins. EHEC can trigger outbreaks in developed regions, with its serotypes *EHEC* O157: H7 and non-O157: H7 (Uhlich, 2008).

Evaluation: In addition to microbiological factors, the severity of diarrhea is determined by the patient's age, physiological reserves, immune status and adequacy of treatment. As the age of the patient increases, comorbid diseases such as diabetes, cancer and COPD are more prevalent and entities with higher mortality risk are encountered more frequently.

Studies are carried out on how accurately the data obtained from the vital signs of patients in ED referrals can predict the mortality and morbidity of patients. Many scoring systems have been developed and used efficiently in patient triage and follow-up. Pazar *et al.* conducted a study and reported that the early warning score system (EWS), which consists of vital signs, enables faster intervention in complications that may develop in patients (Pazar, 2013).

History should reveal whether the complaint has emerged acutely or has been going on for a while, presentation complaints (severity, frequency and volume of diarrhea, accompanying fever, nausea, vomiting, abdominal pain, presence of blood or mucus in the stool) should be recorded. Previously known comorbid diseases of the patient (DM, HT, CAD, CRF, COPD, cirrhosis) should be questioned and recorded. Recent antibiotic use for other reasons (such as URTI, bronchitis, sinusitis, pneumonia, UTI) should be questioned. Only in this way can antibiotic-associated diarrhea be recognized.

Physical examination: As in all patient encounters, ABC sequence and resuscitation of life-threatening conditions take top priority. In severe diarrhea cases, up to 13-14 liters of fluid can be lost per day. Vital signs, and level of consciousness should be measured and recorded first. The most important point is the general condition and the degree of dehydration. Without using any laboratory data, findings such as a fever, moribund appearance, absence of tears, sunken eyeballs, decreased turgor tone of the skin, remarkably dry tongue and mucous membranes, and tendency to sleep (lethargia) suggest significant dehydration due to diarrhea or other reasons. This data is more appreciable than any laboratory result and should prompt aggressive intervention.

On physical examination, increased bowel sounds, intermittent cramping, waxing-and-waning (colicky) pain, and increased tenderness on deep palpation of some parts of the abdomen can be expected in AGE, although not a rule. On the contrary, inflammatory or ischemic processes that irritate the peritoneum (such as diverticulitis, appendicitis, cholecystitis) should be sought and definitely excluded, if the patient exhibits findings such as guarding, rebound tenderness, and rigidity. It should be borne in mind that symptoms resembling AGE can be noted in the course of acute abdominal syndrome which can mandate operative procedures. The clinician should be highly suspicious about 'something other than simple AGE' if something is not consistent with it. For example, abdominal pain associated with frequent copious vomiting without diarrhea can be seen in a mechanical bowel obstruction or pancreatitis, rather than AGE.

In the bedside/point-of-care USG (POCUS) to be performed as part of the examination, the volume status of the inferior or superior vena cava and the degree of dehydration of the patient can be monitored with more objective criteria by looking at the caval index and distensibility of the vessels. In doubtful cases, the patient's immediate response to the administration of fluids can also be evaluated *via* the VCI with the passive leg lift test or the fluid load test. This is also important for the effectiveness and titration of fluid therapy.

Antibiotic-associated diarrhea (AAD) has been most commonly associated with clindamycin, amoxicillin and ampicillin in the acute phase, and with erythromycin, ciprofloxacin and clarithromycin in the delayed phase. It leads to an increase in the length of stay in hospital and increased use of diagnostic work up. In case of suspected AAD, the culprit antibiotic should be discontinued and fluid resuscitation should be performed as needed. In addition to supportive treatment, the administration of probiotics, *e.g.*, S. Boulardii at a dose of 200 mg [4 × 109 cfu/day] was found to be significantly effective in preventing AAD (17.5% vs. 4.5%) (McFarland, 2010).

Laboratory: Since a significant percentage of patients with diarrhea are caused by agents such as rotavirus, norovirus, and adenovirus, in most cases, the severity of diarrhea is alleviated rapidly and complete recovery is expected within a few days without any laboratory abnormalities. For this reason, many patients do not need to undergo any work up. Electrolytes such as Na and K, urea, creatinine, glucose, and leukocyte values should be checked in more severe cases, those with IBD, those who had been using diuretics, diabetics, immunosuppressed, and the frail elderly. In some cases, such as amoebic dysentery, these metabolic disorders can ensue with acute and severe diarrhea even in previously healthy young people. It should not be forgotten that more serious conditions such as acute coronary syndrome or diabetic ketoacidosis may also be triggered due to the sudden stress and imbalance caused by diarrhea. Since the fluid intake is traditionally low in some countries, the incidence of renal failure secondary simple volume loss can be substantial.

Blood count: Most patients with colitis induced by EHEC 0157:H7 will have a leukocytosis (>10,000/microL).

In cases of prolonged diarrhea, a **stool sample** may be taken to rule out bacterial infections and parasitic agents. The bloody macroscopic appearance of the stool may suggest infection with more virulent agents such as E. Histolytica, enteroinvasive *E. coli*. Mucous and/or oily appearance should also be noted in these cases.

Stool Microscopy

It may be a useful diagnostic tool for the identification of protozoa, helminths and fecal leukocytes. Normally, erythrocytes and leukocytes should not be detectable in the stool. As a rule, they are not expected to be seen in diarrhea due to viruses and parasites, either. If leukocytes are present, they are visible in the examination performed on the samples from the mucous area of the stool (Kasirga, 2019). The presence of leukocytes is highly suggestive of bacterial infections. Fresh feces should be examined immediately *ex vivo* for motile organisms. If the stool will not be examined immediately, it can be kept in 10% formalin not to denaturate the organisms. At least three consecutive stool samples are required to rule in or out the parasitic infestation.

Cysts and trophozoites of Entamoeba histolytica should be searched in stool samples in the diagnosis of patients who are thought to have intestinal amebiasis, which varies in clinical picture and treatment.

Shiga toxin induced Escherichia Coli (STEC) and bloody diarrhea: In a meta-analytic Iranian study, Hooman *et al.* aimed to determine the prevalence of STEC (Hooman, 2019). In conclusion, patients with bloody diarrhea are less likely to have positive STEC than patients with non-bloody diarrhea (pooled OR = 0.33, 95% CI: 0.10-1.02). STEC was prevalent in diarrheic patients and the rate increased in recent years. In subgroup analysis, the pooled prevalence was 8% (95% CI, 4 - 13; I2 = 97.55%) in children but 4% (95% CI, 2 - 7; I2 = 97.66%) in adults. The mean interval following interaction with STEC to illness is approximately 3 days, although this can vary between 2 and 12 days (Talarico, 2016).

Shall we use a rapid antigen test? Yes and no. It can be very helpful in diagnosis in some cases. For example, the Giardia Rapid antigen test may be more useful than microscopy in the diagnosis of Cryptosporidium and Entamoeba infections. Kits using ELISA, radioimmunoassay or immunofluorescence methods have been developed for antigen tests (Uyar, 2009). Again, adenovirus stool antigen test is also used in the first step.

It is a useful review. The ELISA method is 78% sensitive and 100% specific for adenovirus infection.

Searching for Clostridium Difficile Toxin in Stool

Toxin B is clinically important. The sensitivity of the enzyme immunoassay for toxins A and B is about 75%, and the specificity is almost 100%. Since false positivity can be encountered in young children, it should be interpreted with caution (Deshpande, 2011).

Multiplex Molecular Panels

It was developed for the detection of digestive tract pathogens from stool samples by PCR methods. It is used to detect a variety of pathogens (bacteria, viruses and parasites) within an hour (Liesman, 2016).

Imaging: Although not indicated in simple diarrhea, additional examinations such as rectosigmoidoscopy, colonoscopy, and contrast-enhanced CT may be requested in cases such as Crohn's disease, ulcerative colitis, suspected cancer, and bloody diarrhea to exclude certain diagnoses with serious outcomes.

Subgroups that Require Special Attention

Diarrhea is more dangerous in extremes of age (infants and the elderly) as it causes dehydration much more easily.

Can Training Change the Test-ordering Behavior of Emergency Physicians in the Management of Adults with Acute gastroenteritis?

Yes. We have analyzed physicians' test ordering behavior in patients admitted to our metropolitan ED with AGE in Turkey. The physicians underwent a one-hour focused training on the management of patients with AGE (Yilmaz, 2021). Data abstracted from a total of 1430 ED patients were analyzed. More than half of the patients (54.1%) were women and the mean age was 35 years. In the month following the education session, there was a small but significant decrease (6%) in the rate of tests (Na, K, urea, creatinine, amylase, lipase, glucose, leukocytes) ordered for the patients. Likewise, an increase of 11% in the rate of pathological findings on the laboratory work up was observed. Another interesting finding is the rate of the patients receiving IV treatment among those with AGE tends to decrease after the training session. A majority (¾) of the patients in the sample were administered IV treatment.

What to eat in case of diarrhea? The main principle is that the patient maintains a normal diet. Hard-to-digest fatty foods, fibrous foods such as meat are not recommended. Soup, water, vegetable dishes with potatoes can be suitable for adults. Food rich in carbohydrates is recommended for infants. If the child is breastfed, the best strategy is to continue as before, or even more frequently.

Bananas are a rich source of minerals, used especially against potassium loss. Babies who are not breastfed must continue their feeding with the milk or formula they normally take, with more frequent meals.

The following formula can be prepared for children or adults in stable general condition and without persistent nausea and vomiting: 1 tablespoon of sugar, 1 teaspoon of table salt and 1 teaspoon of baking soda are added to 1 liter of boiled chilled water, and the mixture prepared is drunk by the patient as often as he or she can.

Apart from this, the foods that are edible and preferable to the patient are ideal because forced food intake is never recommended. Forcing can aggravate nausea and vomiting, especially in children. Consuming carbohydrate foods (without fat) such as potatoes, rice and bread is beneficial as it is easy to absorb from the intestine.

Treatment Principles: Regardless of the etiological agent, the priority in the approach to the patient with severe acute diarrhea is to restore the fluid-electrolyte balance and to improve the general condition. Then, the nutritional balance is restored and specific treatment is provided against the presumed or diagnosed etiological agent.

Emergency treatment is not prompted in cases without high-risk predictors such as fever, dehydration, poor general condition, and persistent vomiting. Increasing fluid intake, avoiding hard-to-digest foods rich in fat, and clinical monitoring for signs of severe AGE—*e.g.*, persistent vomiting and fever- will suffice for the management.

The most important step is to prevent dehydration by drinking plenty of fluids. Tap water, fruit juices, and isotonic (sports) drinks that restore the body's lost salt and minerals can be favourable choices. Children with diarrhea and nausea (*i.e.*, without persistent vomiting) can often drink water or oral rehydration fluids (ORS), which can be made at home or available at the pharmacy.

In case of high fever, paracetamol tablets (syrup for children) and ibuprofen/ketoprofen/dexketoprofen can be used in addition to fluid therapy. If a newborn or infant has had diarrhea, it may be helpful to temporarily use low-lactose or lactose-free milk formulas. If the mother is breastfeeding her baby with diarrhea, she should not consume milk at this stage, otherwise lactose residues may be found in her milk and disturb the child.

Prevention of HUS: A recent Cochrane analysis investigated if Shiga toxin-producing Escherichia coli (STEC) infection-induced HUS can be prevented by traditionally cited recommendations such as antibiotics, bovine milk, and Shiga toxin inhibitor (Synsorb Pk) and monoclonal antibodies (Urtoxazumab) (Imdad, 2021). The authors cited that no firm conclusions about the efficacy of these interventions can be drawn given the small number of included studies and the small sample sizes of the studies.

Treatment of Vomiting: Antiemetics can be used in patients presenting with persistent vomiting and who may suffer from dehydration. It is well known that the 5HT3 receptor antagonists including ondansetron and granisetron, can significantly reduce the frequency and volume of vomiting secondary to AGE in both children and adults. They have a safe profile and predictable efficacy. Ondansetron can be started at 4 mg IV in children and 8 mg in adults. It can be used cautiously in the presence of robust indications by considering the benefit / harm balance in pregnancy.

Metoclopramide: It is not expected to be useful in AGE as it has mainly prokinetic properties. It can be given in cases such as adynamic ileus-subileus, and in other cases such as migraine who have also decreased bowel movements. It should not be used otherwise. Many patients will develop akathisia when the usual dose (10 mg ampoules) is given as an IV infusion in less than 15 minutes.

Antibiotics should be reserved for highly suspected or documented bacterial or parasitic infection and/or if there are significant signs of infection or sepsis such as fever, leukocytosis and moribund condition. Antibacterial therapy is particularly indicated in cholera, Shigella dysentery, as well as in children under 3 months of age, immunocompromised patients or Salmonella infections with systemic involvement. In general, ampicillin is preferred against Shigella and Salmonella, metronidazole is used against Lamblia and amoeba, and erythromycin for Campylobacter jejuni. Villous atrophy and secondary infections may occur in the intestine with unnecessary and long-term antibiotic treatment.

Antimicrobial Resistance: The microorganisms that demonstrated the highest percentage of resistance were Helicobacter pylori, Clostridioides difficile, Campylobacter jejuni and Campylobacter coli, Escherichia coli, Entamoeba histolytica. Clostridioides difficile had resistance to clindamycin (8.3%-100% and cephalosporines (51%), Campylobacter jejuni and Campylobacter coli (fluoroquinolones 85%), Escherichia coli (ampicillin 76.5%), Entamoeba histolytica (metronidazole 50%), and bacterial peritonitis (third-generation cephalosporines 40%, methicillin 85%).

Agents that Reduce Intestinal Motility: Diphenoxylate + atropine (Lomotil) and Loperamide are synthetic opiate agents. Loperamide is a derivative of piperidine. It is effective as a calcium antagonist and reduces enterocyte secretions. While

Lomotil may be beneficial in some bacterial AGEs, it may also be harmful and has the potential to worsen the infectious process. Their effects in the treatment of viral AGE are not fully enlightened. CNS side effects can ensue. Small children under 2 years of age can develop paralytic ileus, necrotizing enterocolitis with decreased intestinal motility associated with use of loperamide.

Antiperistaltic agents may increase the risk of systemic complications, therefore, clinicians should avoid their utilization in the setting of AGE (Thomas, 2013).

Secretion-reducing agent: Bismuth has been reported to reduce the duration of diarrhea, stool volume, fluid requirement, and rate of hospitalization. Its mechanism of action is not fully understood. It is known that it prevents microorganisms from adhering to the mucosa and inactivates enterotoxins. It is recommended to use 100-150 mg/kg/day for 5 days.

Agents changing the intestinal flora:

Probiotics: *Lactobacillus acidophilus* **and** *Saccharomyces boulardii***:** After the adhesion of heat-killed Lactobacillus acidophilus to the intestinal cell membranes, the adhesion and invasion of the pathogens responsible for enteritis into the same cells is prevented. It is thought that these dead lactobacilli increase the normal acid flora in the intestine, and therefore create an immunological barrier by increasing the level of IgA, which is the local immune factor. It was found that the frequency and volume of stool normalized in 85-94% of children from the second day of treatment, and the symptoms disappeared in most cases from the first day. It was observed that stool cultures that were positive before treatment turned negative at around 48 hours.

Similarly, it has been shown that S. boulardii, known as nonpathogenic yeast, inhibits the secretion of cholera toxin and enterotoxigenic E. coli, and neutralizes cholera toxin through a yeast protein. It is also known to reduce the frequency of antibiotic-associated diarrhea (AAD). In a large study conducted in Ankara, around 19% of children using antibiotics reported AAD, while diarrhea was reported to be statistically significantly less (5.7%) in children using S. Boulardii as a probiotic (Erdeve, 2002).

Many clinical and experimental studies have shown that S. boulardii has an important role in both the prevention and treatment of not only diarrhea but also various inflammatory GI diseases (Kelesidis, 2012, Gareau *et al.* 2010; Szajewska *et al.* 2006). It appears that the agent acts as a preventive factor by mediating effects similar with the protective effects of normal healthy intestinal flora. No serious adverse effects have been reported in clinical studies to date. However, caution should be exercised in immunocompromised patients (Whelan, 2010).

It was determined that a daily dose of 500 mg was associated with reduction of the frequency of diarrhea, the amount of stool, and the intestinal passage, while the stool consistency increased with the treatment.

Management of Specific Agents

The use of antiviral agents is not recommended in viral AGEs. Fluid and electrolyte losses should be corrected in accord with the severity of the patient's findings and symptomatic treatment should be prioritized. Antiemetics can be used if necessary.

***EHEC* 0157: H7–induced AGE** is mostly managed with supportive care and rehydration. Most EHEC-inflicted diarrhea usually recover without specific treatment in around 10 days. Antibiotics are not indicated. Patients with manifest HUS may be managed with hemodialysis to restore volume and electrolyte imbalances and to treat acute renal failure. Some literature findings indicate that eculizumab (monoclonal antibody) can be useful against *EHEC* 0157: H7-induced HUS (Ameer, 2021).

Clostridium difficile: Diarrhea due to C. difficile is significantly relieved with appropriate and careful treatment, use of probiotics and appropriate antibiotic. Hygiene measures, proper isolation of sick individuals, thorough washing of hands are important protective factors. Drugs that reduce peristalsis are not recommended. The frequency of AAD has decreased with the use of Saccharomyces boulardii. It is known to inhibit colonization and toxin production of the bacteria, and its benefit has also been shown in pseudomembranous colitis. In treatment, vancomycin 20-60 mg/kg/day or metronidazole 15 mg/kg/day can be used for 10 days. In general, the response to treatment is expected to be remarkable in a short time. Otherwise, another disease entity or a complication such as toxic megacolon, ileus, and perforation should be considered.

Campylobacter jejuni: Although most of them are self-limiting and heal spontaneously, macrolide antibiotics (erythromycin 20-40 mg/kg/day for 7-10 days) or ciprofloxacin can be used. Diarrhea ceases within a week in 2/3 of untreated cases and within two weeks in 90% of cases. There are also more persistent cases.

In addition to symptomatic treatment, antitoxin should be administered in the GI infection of Clostridium botulinum.

Prevention: Since most AGE agents are transmitted *via* fecal-oral route, proper toilet hygiene and hand-washing practices are expected to prevent the transmission of diarrhea from person to person. Hands should always be washed after using the toilet, after playing with pets, after gardening, and before handling food. For the same reasons, sick individuals should rest at home till remarkable relief is noted. It has also been revealed that in specific risk groups (eg, in people who use antibiotics and are immune-defective, or in children), the administration of effective probiotics such as S. Boulardii in appropriate doses can prevent diarrhea or provide faster improvement.

Vaccination: Rotavirus vaccine is recommended for children. The first dose should be given to the infants between 6 weeks and 4 months. The vaccine is repeated at intervals of 4 to 8 weeks. It is administered orally in the form of drops.

Gastric Hyperacidity and Peptic Ulcer Disease

Peptic ulcer (PU) is the loss of gastric and duodenal mucosal tissues within certain limits, traversing beyond the muscularis mucosa layer, due to the harmful effects of hydrochloric acid and pepsin. Potential etiological factors are listed in Table **3**.

Table 3. Factors shown to play critical roles in the etiology of PU.

• *H. pylori* infection,
• Use of salicylates (aspirin) and NSAID
• Acute traumatic conditions, including:
• Burns
• Operations,
• Major trauma (stress ulcers),
• Zollinger-Ellison's syndrome,
• Mastocytosis,
• Antral G-cell hyperplasia,
• Genetic predisposition.
• 0 blood group

Aggressive and Defensive Factors in Mucosa

• Acid and pepsin are the aggressive factors in the stomach.
• Mucus, bicarbonate secretion, integrity, regeneration and blood supply of gastric epithelial cells are defensive factors.

A balance is achieved between these two sets of factors. If the balance is disturbed in favor of aggressive factors, gastritis and consequently PU ensue.

Bleeding occurs in approximately ¼ of PU patients. The mortality rate increases from 10% to 25% with increasing age and the emergence of comorbidities.

Bleeding is the most common and important complication of PU. Ulcers bleed by eroding the vessel wall. Bleeding of ulcers on the curvatura minor or posteroinferior wall of the duodenal bulb is more common than other sites. This is due to the rich vascular support in the region.

- The bleeding risk of duodenal ulcers is twice that of gastric ulcers.
- The frequency of PU is higher in men. 70% of those who were admitted to the ED with upper GIB are male.
- GIB is commonly identified in men in their 40s and later. The incidence of bleeding is higher in patients with duodenal ulcer and O blood group. Some scientists pointed out that people with blood group A have higher tendency to develop gastric malignancies.

In studies conducted in Turkey, it was determined that mean age of the patients with upper GIB was around 55 to 60 years, and 68% of them were male. The most common presenting complaints were melena (60%), hematemesis 16%, and both 19% (Karadag, 2008). Hematochezia was noted in only 2.2%. The length of stay is between 1 and 5 days in 3/4 of the cases. 5.2% of the cases died in the short term.

Role of Proton Pump Inhibitors (PPIs) in the Treatment of Stomach/ Duodenal Ulcer Disease, Acid Reflux and Others

Proton pump inhibitors (PPIs) have been studied for a long time in the management of gastric hyperacidity, acute and chronic gastritis, gastric ulcer disease, gastroesophageal reflux disease (GERD) *etc.* Today, we know that the PPI group is much more effective in treating heartburn than H2 receptor blockers such as ranitidine (Jamshed, 2020).

Dex-rabeprazole (D-R, rabeprazole, ilaprozole and vonoprazan (potassium-competitive acid blocker) have a significantly longer lasting acid inhibitory effect (Takeuchi, 2020, Fan, 2019).

Why do we use them? Mechanism of action: A highly specialized transport system - the proton pump - triggers acid production (*i.e.* hydrochloric acid, HCl) in the stomach. This essentially replaces potassium ions (K+), releasing hydrogen protons (H+), thereby precipitating acid secretion. A PPI agent covalently binds to this pump, irreversibly inhibiting it and stopping HCl release. The secretory process can only restart with *de novo* PP synthesis, but not earlier than 24 hours (Strand, 2017). In short, PPI agents suppress gastric acid production, independent of the source of the stimulus, and are therefore widely used around the world.

Here are Some Tips for using PPIs in Everyday Medical Practice

- Pre-emptive administration of PPI before starting antibiotics is not an effective practice, therefore it is not recommended.
- Prescribing the highest possible dose of PPI by doubling the dosage may improve clinical outcome and has been recommended in rescue therapy strategies for extreme cases with high risk of bleeding or severe symptomatology of erosive gastritis or ulcers.
- New generation agents (rabeprazole, D-R and esomeprazole) can be more effective than the first-generation agents (omeprazole, lansoprazole). One possible explanation for this is their metabolism, which has proven to be less dependent on cytochrome P450 (CYP) 2C19 genetic variants which are considerably prevalent.
- Liver metabolism of PPIs is an important parameter because PPIs are pro-drug/prodrug and therefore metabolized rapidly (Ierardi, 2019). Enzymes mostly involved in PPI metabolism include CYP3A4 and CYP2C19, with genetic differences in enzymatic activity.

Effect of CYP2C19 on PPI Treatments: The success of PPI treatment is greatly influenced by CYP2C19 with respect to efficiency of eradication (Kirsch, 2006). Most of the antibiotics used in the eradication of HP are acid sensitive. PPIs increase the activity of some antibiotics by reducing acid secretion, but also have natural anti-HP activity (Spengler, 2004).

PPIs are metabolized by the cytochrome P450 system, particularly S-mephenytoin 4 φ-hydroxylase (CYP2C19) (Furuta, 2005). Compared with the remaining poor metabolizers (PM) treated with standard triple or dual therapies, significantly lower HP eradication rates were found in homozygous extensive metabolisers (HomEM) (Padol, 2006). On the other hand, current guidelines recommend antimicrobial susceptibility testing after a second treatment failure (Malfertheiner, 2007, Maastricht III Consensus Report). In conclusion, choosing a PPI less affected by CYP2C19 (next generation) than others in second-line therapy may have favorable outcomes.

In quadruple therapy, rabeprazole-containing regimens are more effective than esomeprazole-based regimens (Kuo CH, 2010). The CYP2C19 polymorphism has played an important role in quadruple therapy. It seems reasonable to replace the old generation PPI with rabeprazole in second-line quadruple therapy.

The Third Maastricht Consensus Conference recommended that the eradication rate should be greater than 80% for an intention-to-treat analysis for an effective treatment of HP infection (Malfertheiner, 2007).

Factors in eradication failure: The most important cause of eradication failure is considered to be antibiotic resistance. Other reported causes include treatment non-compliance, drug-related side effects, bacterial load, smoking and underlying comorbidities, and genetic variations in PPI metabolism (Sezgin, 2019). Studies in developing countries have shown that antibiotic resistance is very common, especially against clarithromycin and metronidazole (Sezgin, 2008, Cagdas, 2012).

PPI in the treatment of gastritis, ulcers and GERD: GERD is a common disease caused by reflux of stomach contents into the esophagus. PPIs are recommended for first-line agents in treating GERD. Prospective randomized controlled studies have shown that rabeprazole facilitates the healing process following endoscopic submucosal dissection (ESD) (Komori, 2019).

Triple therapy against *H. pylori* (HP) infection: Eradication of *H. pylori* infection is one of the critical points in the treatment of peptic ulcer and the prevention of gastric cancer (Atherton, 2013). A regimen of 2x1 20 mg rabeprazole, 1,000 mg amoxicillin, and 500 mg clarithromycin for 14 days is recommended as a first-line effective regimen in eliminating HP infection (Herardi, 2020).

Antimicrobial resistance: The microorganisms that demonstrated the highest percentage of resistance were HP (metronidazole 50%-80%, clarithromycin 20%-40%, and levofloxacin 30%-35%) (Contreras-Omaña, 2021).

Shall we do quadruple therapy? Xie *et al.* conducted a multicenter, randomized, parallel controlled clinical trial in China to investigate the efficacy and safety of 10-day quadruple therapy containing amoxicillin, tetracycline or clarithromycin and different doses of rabeprazole and bismuth for the first-line treatment of HP infection (Xie, 2018). They reported that quadruple therapy with low-dose (10 mg daily) rabeprazole, amoxicillin, and tetracycline plus bismuth is a favorable choice for first-line treatment of HP infection in a population with high antibiotic resistance. In another study, amoxicillin-modified bismuth-containing quadruple therapy (PAM-B therapy) was as effective as concomitant therapy for the eradication of HP with similar safety profiles (Choe, 2018). The authors concluded that PAM-B therapy could represent a promising alternative to standard triple therapy for first-line eradication.

Treatment of non-ulcer dyspepsia (NUD): Amoxicillin and clarithromycin were combined with esomeprazole (EAC) or rabeprazole (RAC) for the eradication of HP in NUD patients in Hong Kong (Lee, 2010). Triple therapy with EAC or RAC is effective in NUD patients with *H. pylori* infection. Successful eradication was associated with clarithromycin resistance, but not with the CYP2C19 genotype.

Which PPI is more effective against HP? Rabeprazole is thought to be more active against HP than most PPIs (Tsutsui, 2000, Tsuchiya, 1995). One reason is the higher pKa for conversion of rabeprazole to sulfonamide, resulting in faster inhibition of proton pumps (Sachs, 2007). Rabeprazole and its thio-ether metabolite inhibit the motility and urease activity of HP (Tsutsui, 2000, Tsuchiya, 1995).

How often should PPIs be administered? BID or QD? PPIs given BID are superior to QD in the two-month period in the treatment of GERD. In a meta-analysis and systematic review, Zhang *et al.* reported that BID administration of PPIs improved the endoscopic recovery rate at week 8 more effectively than QD (Zhang, 2017). However, there was no significant difference in symptom relief, 24-hour pH monitoring, sustained symptomatic relief, and endoscopic response in BID administration four weeks.

Dexrabeprazole (D-R) (https://go.drugbank.com/drugs/DB13762): Pai *et al.* were the first authors to highlight the efficacy of D-R in patients with acid reflux disease (Pai, 2007). The recommended daily dose for the treatment of adults with GERD, gastric and duodenal ulcers ranges from 5 to 10 mg (the efficacy of which is twice that of the same dose of rabeprazole). It has been reported that 10 mg of D-R daily is more effective against GERD than 20 mg of rabeprazole daily (Kanakia, 2008).

The effect from 10 mg of D-R daily is equivalent to 20 mg of D-R daily against GERD in adults. Furthermore, a dose of 10 mg of D-R is sufficient to inhibit most of the proton pump receptors without needing to double the dose as recommended with rabeprazole. None of the patients reported any adverse drug reactions and no differences in baseline laboratory variables were seen after treatment, suggesting that D-R at different doses was well tolerated. In 2014, Bhandare *et al.* studied D-R and rabeprazole in terms of efficacy and safety and reported a shorter time (8.4 ± 1.57 days) onset of symptom improvement ($P < 0.0001$) with D-R compared to rabeprazole at 12.2 ± 2.3 days (Bhandare, 2014). There was no significant difference between the groups in the improvement of symptom scores. In GERD, D-R provides significantly better results than rabeprazole in terms of onset of symptom improvement and has a similar safety and efficacy profile even when used at half the usual dose.

Table **4** demonstrates improvement in VAS scores of symptoms.

Side Effects: The safety profile of PPIs in short-term administration is favorable (Table **5**). However, the situation is changing with the increase in long-term uses that are becoming common for patients with different indications.

Table 4. Improvement of symptoms as demonstrated *via* Visual Analogue Scale (VAS) scores (values mean ± SD) (adapted from Kanakia, 2008).

	Day 0			Day 14			Day 28		
	D10-OD (A,*n*= 74)	**D10-BD (B,*n*= 34)**	**D20-OD (C,*n*= 28)**	**D10-OD (A,*n*= 74)**	**D10-BD (B,*n*= 34)**	**D20-OD (C,*n*= 28)**	**D10-OD (A,*n*= 74)**	**D10-BD (B,*n*= 34)**	**D20-OD (C,*n*= 28)**
Heartburn	48.5 ± 22.2	59.7 ± 12.4	58.2 ± 13.6	25.1 ± 16.2[b]	38.2 ± 13.1[b]	32.1 ± 15.5[b]	7.6 ± 15.2[b]	13.8 ± 10.7[b]	12.9 ± 14.4[b]
Between group	0.007[1]	0.007	0.033	0.0001[1]	0.0001	0.052	0.034[1]	0.034	0.114
P values	0.033[2]	0.652[3]	0.652	0.052[2]	0.078[3]	0.078	0.114[2]	0.779[3]	0.779
Regurgitation	45.9 ± 20.4	57.6 ± 12.6	56.4 ±14. 5	21.9 ± 16.2[b]	35.9 ± 12.1[b]	30.7 ± 16.8[b]	6.2 ± 14.2[b]	11.8 ± 10.3[b]	10 ± 13.6[b]
Between group	0.003[1]	0.003	0.014	< 0.0001[1]	< 0.0001	0.017	< 0.0001[1]	< 0.0001	0.225
P values	0.014[2]	0.729[3]	0.729	0.017[2]	0.162[3]	0.162	0.225[2]	0.556[3]	0.556

[b]*P* < 0.001 *vs* baseline values (Tukey-Krammer Multiple comparison test). Between-group difference (*T*-test): [1]A *vs* B; [2]A *vs* C; [3]B *vs* C.

Table 5. Adverse effects (AE) reported in PPI-treated patients (adapted from Kinoshita 2018).

Most common AEs (short-term use)	Most common AEs not associated with acid inhibition (long-term use)	AEs associated with acid inhibition (long-term use)
Headache Nausea Diarrhea, abdominal pain, Constipation Dizziness, fatigue Rash and itches	Allergic reactions Collagenous colitis Acute interstitial nephritis, chronic renal disease Drug interactions (clopidogrel) Ischemic cerebrovascular diseases, coronary artery disease, Dementia / senility	Gastric cancer Gastric fundic mucosal hypertrophy and polyps Pneumonia Gastrointestinal infection Iron and/or magnesium deficiencies Vitamin deficiencies (*e.g.*, B12) Fractures

Drug interactions: The U.S. Food and Drug Administration (FDA) issued three safety announcements between January 2009 and October 2010 to warn against the combined use of clopidogrel and PPIs due to a potential drug-drug interaction that could impair the antiplatelet activity of clopidogrel. There is evidence to support that the addition of a PPI may have a weakening effect on the antiplatelet properties of clopidogrel and may be relevant in certain clinical situations (Przespolewski, 2018). A recent Korean study showed a similar antiplatelet effect compared to famotidine with the use of rabeprazole, even in patients sensitive to clopidogrel (Ahn, 2020). This may support the similar effect of rabeprazole and famotidine on the antiplatelet effect of DAPT (clopidogrel plus aspirin). Some studies in East Asian cohorts show that the potential of PPIs to reduce the efficacy of clopidogrel can be minimized *via* use of new PPs with weaker affinity for the CYP2C19 isoenzyme, namely pantoprazole, dexlansoprazole and rabeprazole (Zou, 2017).

GASTROINTESTINAL BLEEDINGS (GIB)

It is estimated that one in 1000 adults worldwide suffers from GIB each year.

Classification: In recent years, general term of GIB was divided into three anatomophysiological areas:

1. **The upper GIB** define those areas accessible to upper endoscopy, namely the area proximal to Ampulla Vateri;
2. **The middle GIB** is small bowel bleeding (SBB), or events occurring between the Ampulla Vateri and the terminal ileum; and
3. **The lower GIB** is used for hemorrhages originating from the colon.

Hematemesis and melena are found in 2/3 of those with upper GIB, while only melena is found in the remainder. A minority of the patients with lower GIB can present with hematemesis in case of profuse hemorrhage.

The clinical picture in patients with GIB can be very elusive. While completely asymptomatic or mildly fatigued patients can be seen, there are also those who present directly with hypovolemic shock.

The incidence of upper GIB is increasing gradually in the elderly. In studies, it has been reported that 30% of patients with upper GIB are over 65 years of age. Prominent causes of upper GIB have been listed in Table **6**. Likewise, etiologies of obvious and occult bleeding were given in Table **7**.

Table 6. Etiologies of upper GIB.

• Peptic ulcer (in 3/5 of the cases)
• Varices: Cirrhosis / Portal hypertension / Bleeding from esophagogastric varices (in 1/5 cases)
• Acute hemorrhagic erosive gastritis
• Malignancies
• Mallory-Weiss lesion
• Angiodysplasia
• Dieulafoy lesion
• Abdominal aortic aneurysm/ aortoenteric fistula

Table 7. Etiologies of obvious and occult bleeding.

Obvious Bleeding	Occult Bleeding
Angiodysplasia	

(Table 7) cont.....

Obvious Bleeding	Occult Bleeding
Crohn's disease	
Amoebic dysentery	Lymphoma
Hemangioma	Adenocarcinoma
Tumors: Leiomyosarcoma, leiomyoma	NSAID and other drugs
Diverticulum (jejunal)	Infections
Zollinger-Ellison syndrome	Vasculitis
Aortoenteric fistula	Carcinoid
Meckel's diverticulum	-

Factors predisposing to GIB were summarized in Table **8**, and poor prognostic factors in cases of acute upper GIB were provided in Table **9**.

Table 8. Factors predisposing to GI bleeding.

- Ulcerogenic drugs: Aspirin, NSAIDs, corticotropin, cortisone, butazolidine *etc.*
- Excess gastric acid
- Presence of *H. pylori*
- Emotional stress
- Excessive physical exertion and fatigue
- Some infections (especially upper respiratory tract)
- Smoking, alcohol, "cola" drinks
- Diseases causing coagulopathy, anticoagulant drugs, Factor Xa inhibitors (NOACs)
- Arterial hypertension
- Cirrhosis/ portal hypertension

Table 9. Poor prognostic factors in cases of acute upper GIB.

- Advanced age
- Presence of comorbidity
- Varicose bleeding
- Bright red hematemesis or hematochezia
- Shock or hypotension at primary survey
- Large number of blood transfusions (more than 6 units in 24 hours)
- Presence of active bleeding in endoscopy
- Bleeding from ulcers larger than 2 cm
- The onset of bleeding in the hospitalized patient
- Need for urgent surgical intervention

Evaluation Tips

Who has hematemesis? In hemorrhages proximal to the ligament of Treitz, the symptom may be vomiting blood (hematemesis). It is called bleeding that comes out with vomiting, comes into contact with gastric acid and looks like "coffee grounds", but has not been fully digested (not transformed into melena). It can be a small volume or a large amount.

In SBB, melena or chestnut-colored stools are expected. In the lower GIB, there can be hematochezia.

Notes for Melena: Melena is the excretion of digested blood with faeces. Bleeding usually proximal to the ligament of Treitz causes melena. In order for the stool to acquire the melena characteristics, there must be at least 60 ml of bleeding. For example, 1 liter of blood given to the upper GIB causes melena to continue for 3-5 days. After a bleeding, there are slow changes in the character of the stool over time. Fecal blood positivity can last for seven to ten days.

Iron, bismuth, activated charcoal treatment *etc.* may masquerade melena.

Hematochezia defines the physical properties of the blood in the GIS which is unchanged by defecation. Typically, it is found to be bright/red blood, although the volume and frequency vary from patient to patient. Approximately 2% to 10% of those with upper GIB manifest with hematochezia.

Hematochezia is seen in lower GIB, especially in colorectal hemorrhages.

In patients with SBB, hemorrhage flow rate is high and hematochezia can be seen in the distal focus. It can also be seen rarely in rapid and severe upper GIB. More than 1000 ml of bleeding is required to produce hematochezia in the upper GIB.

Tips in physical examination: Evaluation of general condition is of utmost importance in the stage of inspection.

The pale-looking patient with cold sweats is in hemorrhagic shock until definitely ruled out. The tachycardic patient is in Class II hemorrhagic shock until proven otherwise. Hypoglycemia, dissecting aortic aneurysm, aortoenteric fistula or acute coronary syndromes should be taken into consideration emergently.

In an elderly, cachectic patient, malignancy can be considered in the foreground. Cachexia may also be a sign of alcoholism. Operation scars are noted on the abdominal skin.

Abdominal distention accompanied by hypotension, is primarily suggestive of aortic aneurysm, while it can be a manifestation of aortoenteric fistula if it is accompanied by GIB, which prompts emergency surgery.

A functional murmur on cardiac auscultation may indicate anemia. Increased bowel sounds are an expected finding in the upper GIB.

Orthostatic hypotension (OH) should be sought. The presence of OH often suggests a loss of more than 15% to 20% of the total blood volume (almost 5 L in a 70 kg adult), although not the rule. It should be recognized that a given amount or rate of loss does not lead to the same findings in every patient.

In a young person with good hemodynamic reserve, without organ failure, tachycardia may be the only finding for a long time despite ongoing bleeding. Hypotension is a late finding and should not be considered as the only indicator of bleeding. Hypotension occurs in most patients with loss of more than 2/5 of the total volume. OH may occur with less blood loss in diabetics, people with poor cardiac reserve, and the frail elderly.

How is orthostatic hypotension recognized? After standing up for at least 5 minutes of supine rest, detection of one of the following after standing for 2-5 minutes (doing nothing else):

- A decrease of at least 20 mmHg in systolic BP
- A decrease of at least 10 mmHg in diastolic BP

The presence of cirrhosis should be investigated as it can cause both coagulopathy, esophageal varices and gastric hemorrhages. Significant ascites should be sought in the abdominal examination, though minimal ascites may go undetected in a standard examination. In abdominal radial percussion, dullness with its aperture facing upward supports fluid accumulation (ascites) but is not specific.

> While neck vein engorgement, pretibial and scrotal edema are accompanied in cardiac ascites, abdominal distension is prominent in cirrhotic ascites.

The skin is searched for spider nevus, head of medusa, palmar erythema, as well as hypothenar or other muscle atrophy, and flapping tremor.

Examination to rule in or out flapping tremor / asterixis: While the arm is in full extension, the wrist is brought to active dorsiflexion, immediately followed by the flapping motion. The finding indicates that the diencephalic motor center is involved. Apart from the early stage of hepatic encephalopathy, it is seen in CO_2 poisoning, uremia, basal ganglia infarction.

Altered level of consciousness may indicate hepatic encephalopathy (HE) or may be a sign of hemorrhagic shock. Ammonia blood levels will be helpful in distinguishing these from each other.

Revised guidelines of HE provided recommendations for the diagnosis and management including minimal hepatic encephalopathy (MHE) and overt hepatic encephalopathy, emphasizing the importance on searching for MHE in patients with liver diseases (Xu, 2019).

MHE is commonly identified in cirrhotic patients, especially those with Child-Pugh grade C cirrhosis and TIPS, which may increase the likelihood of grave outcomes. Therefore, this group of patients prompt focused screening for HE. On the other hand, MHE is a mild and sometimes undetectable cognitive dysfunction with normal findings on neurological examination but abnormal neuropsychological (NP) test results.

HE is a continuous clinical process. Based on the presence of severe liver disease, HE grades 1 through 4 can be diagnosed based on clinical manifestations (Table **10**). Neurophysiological (NP) and radiological evaluations are usually not indicated.

Table 10. Hepatic encephalopathy (HE) grading criteria were revised. When findings belonging to different stages are detected, the patient should be considered in the advanced stage.

Classification as to revised criteria	Neuropsychiatric and central nervous system (CNS) signs and symptoms
No HE	• Normal CNS signs and neuropsychological (NP) test results
Minimal HE	• Potential HE, normal CNS exam and personality / behavioral patterns • Abnormalities in NP test results
HE grade 1	• Unimportant or mild signs on exam, such as mild cognitive impairment, attention deficit, sleep disorders (including insomnia), euphoria, or depression • Asterixis and abnormal NP tests can be obtained
HE Grade 2	• Marked personality or behavioral abnormalities, lethargy or apathy, mild abnormalities of orientation, decreased cognitive ability, dyskinesia, dysarthria or slurred speech • Asterixis is positive • NP testing may not be indicated
HE Grade 3	• Marked dysfunction (time and spatial orientation), abnormal behavior, semi-coma to coma, but responsive • Asterixis usually cannot be elicited. There is ankle clonus, increased muscle tone, and hyperreflexia. • NP testing is unnecessary
HE Grade 4	• Coma (absence of responses to verbal and painful stimuli) • Increased muscle tone or positive signs of the CNS. NP testing is not necessary

Differential diagnosis of encephalopathy or altered mental status is very broad and comprises metabolic, intracranial, toxicological etiologies (Table 11) (Montagnese, 2019). Precipitating factors of overt HE were listed in Table 12.

Table 11. List of disorders that could mimic or associate with HE, and should be considered for purposes of differential diagnosis.

• Alcohol/opioids withdrawal syndromes • Electrolyte-related encephalopathy (*i.e.* hyponatremia, hyper/hypocalcemia *etc.*) • Endocrine etiologies (*i.e.* hypothyroidism and hypocorticism) • Hypercapnic encephalopathy • Hyperosmotic encephalopathy • Hypo/hyperglycaemic encephalopathy • Intoxication with alcohol or other recreational drugs • Intoxication with benzodiazepines or other psychoactive drugs (*i.e.* anticonvulsants, sedative antidepressants, opioids) • Intracranial structural injury (*i.e.* subarachnoid haemorrage, stroke, neoplastic lesions) • Meningoencephalitis • Nonconvulsive status epilepticus • Septic encephalopathy • Simulation • Uraemic encephalopathy • Vitamin deficiencies or complex malnutrition-related syndromes • Wernicke's encephalopathy

Table 12. Precipitating factors of overt HE, by decreasing frequency (Adapted from Montagnese 2018.

Episodic HE	Recurrent HE
Infections	Electrolyte disorder
GI bleeding	Infections
Diuretic overdose	Unidentified
Electrolyte disorder	Constipation
Constipation	Diuretic overdose
Unidentified	GI bleeding

Ascites is detected as a sign of chronic portal hypertension, although not specific (Fig. **1**). Beyond physical examination, radiological adjuncts will provide invaluable information on the extent of tissue damage and secondary injuries relatedto cirrhosis (Fig. **2**).

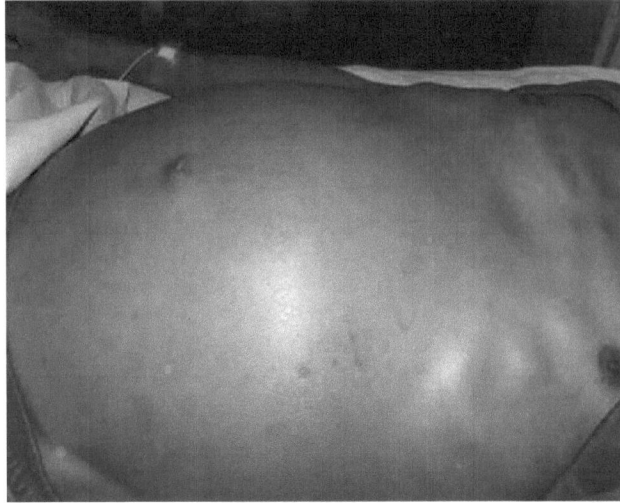

Fig. (1). The presence of ascites is a sign of chronic portal hypertension (cirrhosis and advanced right heart failure). Effaced umbilicus differentiates it from obesity, and the area of dullness must be circumscribed in percussion. Palmar erythema and flapping tremor may mark the cirrhotic patient.

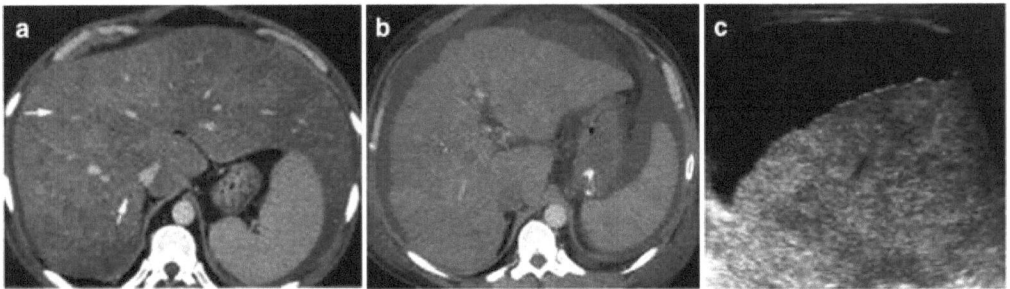

Fig. (2). CT and USG images compatible with cirrhosis. **(a, b)** Enlarged liver on axial CT, diffuse low-density fine granularity of regenerated nodules (arrows). Ill-defined diffuse fatty changes in patchy areas. **(b, c)** Axial CT and USG show surface nodularity in the cirrhotic liver and free fluid (ascites) in the abdomen in different patients. On USG, tissue images with diffuse coarse and heterogeneous echo are seen.

Esophageal Variceal Bleeding (EVB) Associated with Portal Hypertension (PHT) or Cirrhosis

Variceal bleeding is one of the most important complications of PHT and its mortality is quite high. PHT is a disease that usually occurs as a result of fibroticization, scarring and damage of liver cells and tissues due to cirrhosis.

As the disease progresses, blood flow becomes more difficult, and the resultant increase in resistance causes blood to seek for alternative routes to reach the right heart, new blood vessels evolve to overcome the blockage. The variceal dilations of the esophageal veins are the result of this process.

EVB is accused for every third death in cirrhotic patients. In fact, every patient diagnosed with cirrhosis should have an upper GI endoscopy to evaluate bleeding risk. Propranolol (beta1 beta2 antagonist) can be prescribed to patients with varicose veins for the prevention of GIB (primary prophylaxis). Varicose veins are often visualized with endoscopy only after they begin to bleed or ooze. The amount of bleeding can vary from a minor leak to life-threatening bleeding that is difficult to control.

About 90% of patients with cirrhosis develop gastroesophageal varices within 10 years. EVB accounts for up to 10% of hospital admissions with GIB. Vasculature and hemodynamics of esophagogastric varices were illustrated in Fig. (4).

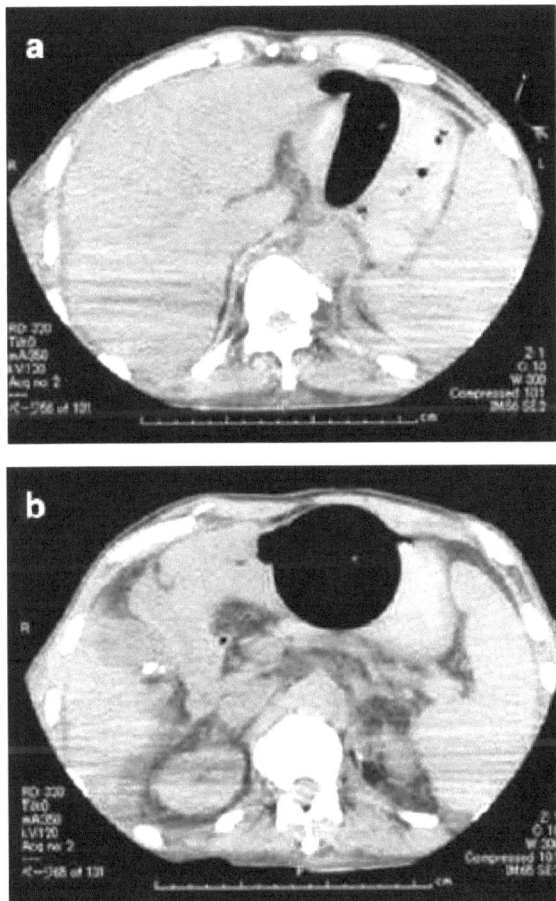

Fig. (3). CT image of misuse of Sengstaken-Blakemoore tube in the treatment of EVB. **a.** Since the esophageal balloon was not pulled sufficiently, it settled in the stomach. **b.** The gastric balloon is quite far from the esophagogastric junction.

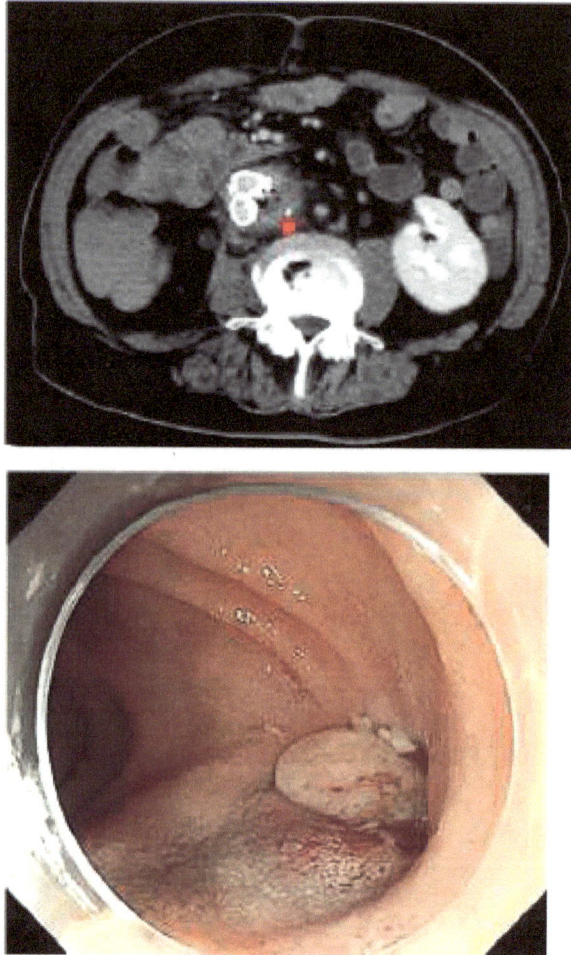

Fig. (4). A. Contrast computed tomography image of the patient with suspected GIB due to aortoenteric fistula. Arrowhead: air image in the aorta. **B.** Upper endoscopy in the 3rd portion of the duodenum. A pulsatile, granulation-like protuberance is seen.

When a cirrhotic patient is brought to the ED with an upper GIB, EVB is the first one in the DD list to rule out. Drugs that alleviate portal vein pressure (somatostatin, glipressin/terlipressin, nitroglycerin) should be initiated concurrently with ABC stabilization. Endoscopy should follow this approach, which will give a chance both to locate the bleeding and decide for endoscopic sclerotherapy (ES) or ligation. Bleeding can be controlled with these in most patients. In case of failure, shunts (TIPS or Surgical) come into play. If shunts cannot be brought into practice and drugs do not provide the desired effect, local compression should be provided with a Sengstaken-Blakemore tube (SBT).

SBT has been in clinical use since the 1950s and has saved thousands of lives. However, endoscopic sclerotherapy (ES) is more effective than application of SBT in the treatment of bleeding EVB. Using ES, complete control of bleeding is provided 90% *versus* 55% with SBT.

Mortality rates within 30 days are also in favor of ES, with 27% *versus* 10%. Of course, the implementation of SBT is valuable and will be applied in cases where ES cannot be organized in emergency situations. However, the emergency physician should expedite the necessary consultations and other preparations to facilitate the ES procedure and administration of appropriate treatment.

SBT should represent a temporary measure in the treatment of uncontrollable EVB (Fig. **3**). Apart from this, ES treatment should be expedited and organized. Gastroenterology and general surgery consultations should be obtained for these patients in all scenarios.

Teres *et al.* compared vasopressin/nitroglycerin with SBT in the treatment of EVB in an RCT (Teres, 1990). SBT was found to be 87% effective for providing hemostasis, and the drug treatment was found to be 66% effective.

One of the most important complications of SBT is aspiration and resulting pneumonia.

Contraindications for SBT consist of esophageal anatomical abnormalities, esophageal stenosis, and previous ES.

Sengstaken-Blakemoore tube placement in the emergency treatment of EVB: After the gastric balloon is inflated with air, it is gently pulled to sit on the cardia region to allow cessation of the bleed.

Occult or chronic hemorrhage: It is considered in a patient without melena or hematochezia but with (+) fecal occult blood test (FOBT). It is mostly associated with iron deficiency anemia, although not a rule (Kim *et al.* 2014).

In cases of sudden hemorrhage, the hematocrit value may not change at the beginning and may mislead the physician. A decrease in hematocrit occurs with the passage of fluid from the extravascular space to the intravascular space, in around 4-6 hours. Therefore, serial follow-up is important in a patient with suspected hemorrhage. Typically, normochromic-normocytic anemia is found in GIB cases. If hypochromic microcytic anemia is found, previously diagnosed cancer, thalassemia, renal failure, chronic lead poisoning, malnutrition, or a GI or gynecological lesion causing chronic blood loss should be considered and investigated.

Causes and Bleeding Types of Small Bowel Bleeding (SBB)

Up to three-fourths of SBBs are caused by vascular lesions, especially in the elderly. Diagnoses such as angiodysplasia (most common), telangiectasia, arteriovenous malformation, Dieulafoy lesion. vascular ectasia and angiodysplasia are mostly detected in geriatric cases. Vascular lesions that cause SBB cause 2/3 overt and 1/3 occult bleeding.

Aortoenteric fistula (AEF) is a life-threatening complication of aortic aneurysms manifested as profuse GIB. Early diagnosis of AEF can be extremely difficult (Fig. **4**). Small case series mostly reported mean ages around 65-70 years (Ichita, 2021). The entity is known to have caused high death rate.

Work up: Complete blood count, blood group, cross-match, blood sugar, urea, creatinine, electrolytes, amylase, ALT, AST are ordered. In selected patients, total protein, albumin can provide information in terms of chronic liver failure and cirrhosis.

For the upper GIB, it is important that the BUN/creatinine ratio be higher than 30 (odds ratio: 7.5).

Coagulation tests (prothrombin time, partial thromboplastin time, INR) provide inappreciable information about the severity of the condition both in liver failure, possible use of vitamin K antagonists, and use of IV heparin or similar agents.

In severe cases or those with accompanying lung disease in history or respiratory signs and/or symptoms on examination, arterial blood gases (ABG) and lactate levels can be checked for suspected intracellular hypoxia.

False (+) values are common in FOBT with Guaiac method. Foods such as red meat, broccoli, radish, horseradish, cauliflower, apples, oranges, mushrooms, and drugs such as colchicine and oxidizing drugs (such as iodine-boric acid) can result in false (+) readings. Pseudo-peroxidase activity is thought to cause this phenomenon. False positivity can also be detected in the presence of bleeding hemorrhoids and hematuria.

It gives (+) results in stool samples containing hemoglobin at concentrations of 0.06 mgHb/g by the immunochemical method, and 1.3 mgHb/g by the Guaiac method. Therefore, the immunochemical method is more accurate but expensive (Altekin E, *et al*, 2003).

An **ECG** should be obtained in all patients with GI symptoms over the age of 40. This tool will not only give clues as to previous coronary artery disease, and also acute coronary syndromes accompanying GIB. ECG can also be critical in the follow-up of cardiac rhythm and other functions in the disease course.

Goals in treatment is summarized in Table **13**.

Table 13. Approach steps to the patient presenting with a significant/overt upper GIB.

• Rapid resuscitation of the patient and stabilization of the general condition.
• Detection of the source of bleeding.
• Treatment of acute bleeding attack.
• Prevention of early and late recurrent bleeding.

Management: The vascular accesses of patients with suspected GIB should be opened as much as possible from both sides, preferably from large veins such as antecubital vein, with large diameter catheters such as 12, 14 or 16 G.

Patients with unstable general condition, who continue to have significant bleeding, who have hypovolemia or who are hypotensive should be taken to the intensive care unit.

Although fluid resuscitation is important, it should be known that aggressive fluid administration may do more harm than good. Preferably, the fluid deficit, if any, is replaced by crystalloid fluids, *i.e.*, normal saline (NS) or Hartmann's solution, and lactated Ringer's solution. It is also wrong not to give fluids in elderly patients with the fear of heart failure or possible pulmonary congestion. Under these circumstances, fluid can be given in 250 mL boluses and repeated, till any compromise occurs.

Fluid Resuscitation by evaluating the fluid response from the inferior or superior vena cava with bedside USG/POCUS stands out as the most practical and safe way today.

In addition to circulatory support, oxygenation must be corrected emergently in the resuscitation of the patient. As a rule, supplemental oxygen is given by nasal cannulae or masks. Endotracheal intubation should not be delayed for those who are in poor general condition, hypotensive, and have altered level of consciousness.

Nasogastric (NG) probe can be inserted only after intubation in patients with impaired consciousness.

Blood transfusion (BTx) should be administered to hypotensive and/or shocky patients, those with hematocrit levels below 20% to 25%, or those with Htc >25% with severe comorbidities (such as coronary artery disease, *e.g.*, unstable angina). Htc value can be increased by giving erythrocyte suspension (ES) to elderly, cirrhotic patients with coronary artery disease. Excessive transfusion should be avoided. In those with stopped bleeding, ES can be preferred to increase Htc and stabilize it, and BTx can be preferred in those with active bleeding.

Insertion of NG tube and drainage of gastric contents may be helpful in monitoring continued bleeding and evacuation of clots and bloods.

The sensitivity of NG tube+lavage in detecting the presence of upper GIB is only ~50%, so we cannot rule out bleeding just by normal appearance of the lavage fluid.

Studies have failed to show any benefit in routinely inserting NG tube in suspected GIB (Huang 2011, Pallin 2011).

Bloody lavage has very high specificity for upper GIB. It can also predict that the patient will worsen. It also indicates the need for upper endoscopy.

Although it is rarely applied in many countries, 20 G and thicker NG tubes are more suitable to evacuate blood and clots. Administration of ice water or adrenaline with NG has not been shown to have any therapeutic benefit and should not be done.

Advanced procedures: The first diagnostic and therapeutic procedure to be carried out in the patient with an upper GIB is esophagogastroduodenoscopy (EGD).

Endoscopy performed in emergency conditions and in the early period significantly reduced the length of hospital stay and safely directed 46% of nonvariceal upper GIB cases to outpatient treatment (Lee, 1999).

Endoscopic examination will be suboptimal in patients with ongoing bleeding, bloody gastric lavage, and severe bleeding with hematochezia. In these cases, resuscitation is the priority.

Endoscopy is performed as soon as possible in patients with hemodynamic stability, and after stabilization is achieved in patients with shock or ongoing hemorrhage (Fig. **5**).

Upper GI endoscopy should be performed under sedation in the patient who has not undergone endotracheal intubation. The most recommended combination for this is fentanyl and ketamine. Midazolam may also be added safely. There are also schools that recommend ketamine as a single agent, and as such it is quite safe.

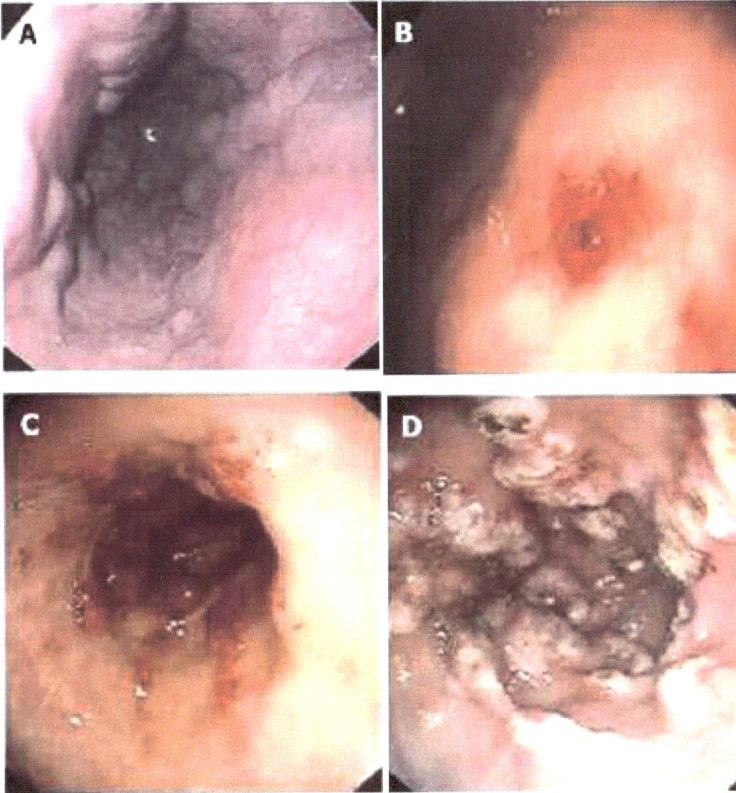

Fig. (5). Findings in cases with suspected GIB in upper GI endoscopy. Esophageal varices (**A**), Dieulafoy lesion in the stomach (**B**), gastric antral vascular ectasia (watermelon stomach) before and after argon plasma coagulation therapy (**C, D**).

In order to determine the bleeding vessel by angiography, the bleeding rate should be 0.5 mL/min and above. Intra-arterial vasopressin infusion halts ulcer bleeding in 50% of cases. The agent may cause complications such as AMI/ACS, or arrhythmias especially in the elderly.

Which Scoring System to use to Predict Rebleeding?

Rockall, Blatchford, and AIMS65 scores are not useful for predicting 6-week rebleeding or mortality in patients with acute EVB (Aluizio 2021). Child and MELD scores can identify patients at higher risk for 6-week mortality but not for 6-week rebleeding.

Budimir *et al*. compared the scores and reported that the AIMS65, GBS and pre-endoscopic Rockall score (PRS) scores are comparable but not useful for predicting outcome in patients with EVB because of poor discriminative ability.

The Glasgow Blatchford score is superior in predicting the need for transfusion compared to AIMS65 score and PRS.

Yang *et al.* analyzed findings of 955 patients with GIB due to peptic ulcer using the Glasgow-Blatchford score and shock index, as well as the Forrest classification based on their gastroscopy results (Yang, 2020). A moderate correlation was observed between the Glasgow-Blatchford score and shock index in this group, and the correlation between the Forrest classification and Glasgow-Blatchford score or shock index was relatively low.

The Rockall risk scoring system can identify 15% of all cases with acute upper GIB at the time of presentation and 26% of cases after endoscopy who are at low risk of rebleeding and negligible risk of death and who might therefore be considered for early discharge or outpatient treatment with consequent resource savings (Rockall, 1996) (Table **14**).

Table 14. Rockall scoring system combines severity indicators of the disease with endoscopic diagnosis.

Variable	Score			
	0	**1**	**2**	**3**
Age	<60 Years	60-79 Years	>=80 Years	-
Shock	'No shock', systolic BP > = 100, Pulse <100	'Tachycardia', systolic BP >= 100, Pulse >=100	'Hypotension', systolic BP < 100	-
Comorbidity	No major comorbidity	-	Cardiac failure, ischaemic heart disease, any major comorbidity	Renal failure, liver failure, disseminated malignancy
Diagnosis on endoscopy	Mallory-Weiss tear or no lesion identified	All other diagnoses (*e.g.*, peptic ulcer, erosive gastritis, esophagitis)	Malignancy of upper GI tract	-
Major stigmata of recent haemorrhage, (SRH)	None or dark spot only	-	Blood in upper GI tract, adherent clot, visible or spurting vessel	-

Maximum additive score prior to diagnosis=7. Maximum additive score following diagnosis= 11.

Blatchford scoring system was launched in 2000 to identify patients at low or high risk of needing treatment to manage their bleeding (Blatchford, 2000). Admission risk markers and associated score component values in accord with Glasgow-Blatchford scoring system is given in Table **15**.

Table 15. Glasgow-Blatchford scoring system which is used to predict the severity of the disease and therefore its prognosis.

Admission Risk Marker	Score Component Value
Blood urea (mmol/L)	
• >6·5 <8·0	2
• >8·0 <10·0	3
• >10·0 <25·0	4
• >25	6
Haemoglobin (g/L) for men	
• >120 <130	1
• >100 <120	3
• <100	6
Haemoglobin (g/L) for women	
• >100 <120	1
• <100	6
Systolic blood pressure (mm Hg)	
• 100–109	1
• 90–99	2
• <90	3
Other markers	
• Pulse >100 bpm	1
• Presentation with melaena	1
• Presentation with syncope	2
• Hepatic disease	2
• Cardiac failure	2

The use of endoscopic Doppler probe (DOP-US) identifies arterial blood flow at the ulcer base to provide a guide to treatment. In a meta-analytic study, Bhurwal *et al*. pointed out that the use of DOP-US probe decreases rebleeding, mortality, and surgical intervention as compared to Forrest Classification (Bhurwal 2021). The risk of rebleeding is significantly higher if the signal persists despite endoscopic therapy (48.5%). It can be postulated that DOP-US is a beneficial tool in the management of bleeding ulcers and adds valuable information to visual evaluation (Fig. **6**).

DSA: Angiography and embolization should be considered in treatment-resistant patients. It is considered to be advantageous over surgery. Since 85% of the upper GIB originates from the left gastric artery, extra-vascular contrast extravasation is sought in this region. This finding specifically indicates active bleeding (Figs. **7** and **8**).

I-a. Spurting artery   **I-b. Oozing vessel**   **II-a.**
Visible vessel

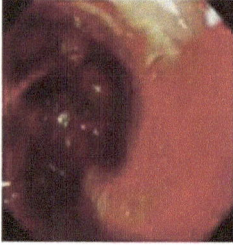

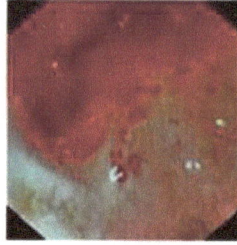

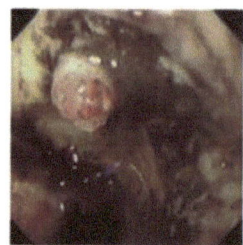

II-b. Adherent clot
II-c. Black spot (hematin-covered lesion)

III. Clean ulcer base (lesion without bleeding)

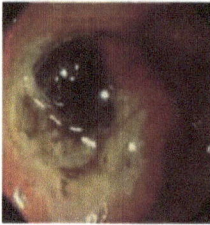

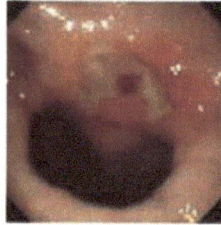

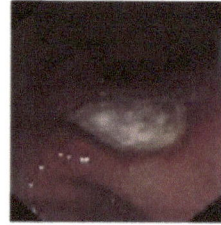

Fig. (6). Classification of bleeding severity by endoscopic findings: Forrest classification.

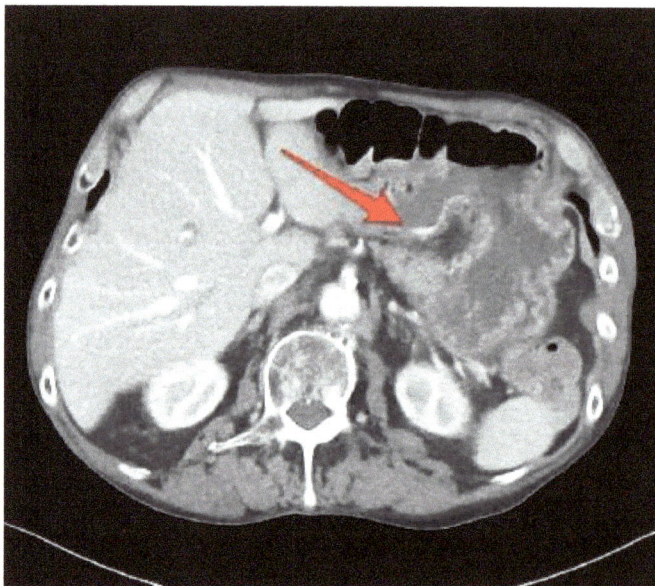

Fig. (7). Extra-vascular contrast extravasation. When it is linear, it is also called a pseudo-vein sign (arrow).

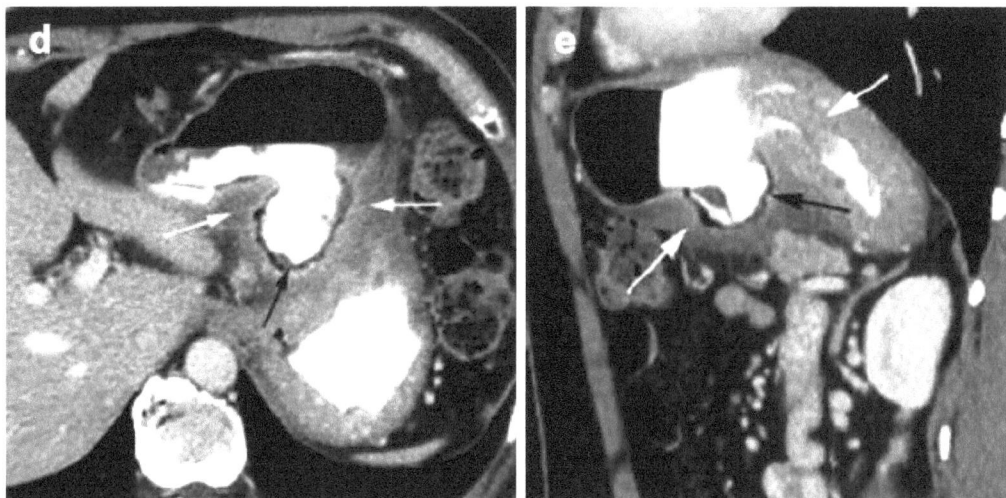

Fig. (8). The giant ulcer crater (black arrow) with positive enteric contrast-filling on axial CT **(d)** and sagittal reformatted **(e)** images are noted posteriorly as it projects onto the gastric wall (white arrows).

Empirical embolization to the gastroduodenal artery is recommended if active extravasation is not found in the presence of a bleeding duodenal ulcer and the patient tends to worsen. Otherwise, the patient may die.

Drugs Used in the Emergency Treatment of EVB

- splanchnic vasoconstrictors (vasopressin and analogues, somatostatin and analogues, nonselective beta-blockers [NSBB]),
- splanchnic vasodilators (nitrates and angiotensin receptor blockers),
- gastric acid-suppressing drugs- PPI,
- prophylactic antibiotics.

Proton Pump Inhibitors (PPI): If upper GIB is considered or suspected, IV PPI should be administered. There is no significant difference between continuous infusion and intermittent IV bolus therapy. (*e.g.* 40 mg pantoprazole IV every 12 hours).

Octreotide (50 mcg bolus followed by 50 mcg/h infusion) should be given if the physician considers varicose bleeding in the patient. There is no safety problem with this treatment. There is also weak evidence that it may also be effective in non-variceal bleeding.

Antibiotics should be given when GIB is identified in a cirrhotic patient. (Ceftriaxone 1 g/day).

Update in the 2019 Guides

According to the Guideline Recommendations in the International Consensus Report published in 2019: (Barkun 2019).

1. Patients with a Glasgow-Blatchford score of 1 and below carry very low risk for rebleeding. They do not warrant admission.

2. The hemoglobin threshold for BTx is 8 g/dL in patients without cardiovascular disease. It should be kept higher in patients with known cardiovascular diseases in history or compromise on evaluation.

3. Cases with upper GIB should undergo endoscopic examination within 24 hours.

4. High-dose IV PPI is indicated for 3 days after successful endoscopy in cases with bleeding ulcers in the presence of high-risk findings. Oral PPI is continued (mostly BID) for 14 days.

5. PPI should be given in patients with previous GIB who will receive antiplatelet therapy for cardiovascular prophylaxis.

Massive Transfusion Protocol (MTP): MTP is considered in case of severe instability (requirement of vasopressor infusion). Blood products are given at a ratio of 1:1:1 (PRBC: FFP: platelet). In addition, tranexamic acid, cryoprecipitate, IV calcium, and a warming blanket may also be considered with regard to the patient's needs.

Resuscitative endovascular balloon occlusion of aorta (REBOA) for hemorrhage control is also employed in nontrauma patients. In a case series, most common indications were GI and peripartum bleeding (Hatchimonji, 2020). A majority (24 of 30, 80%) cases with balloon inflation resulted in improved hemodynamics. More than one-third (37%) died before discharge. The technique is used in a range of patients with acute hemorrhages which require emergency surgery with low rates of complications. Mortality is high in these moribund patients; however, appropriate patient selection and early use may improve survival in these life-threatening cases.

Gastric/Duodenal Ulcer Perforation (GDUP)

The lifetime prevalence of peptic ulcer is declining and is thought to be around 10%. Three-fifths of patients are above 60 years of age. While the majority of peptic ulcers are initially asymptomatic, clinical manifestations range from mild dyspepsia to serious complications including GIB, GDUP, and gastric outlet obstruction (Stern 2021). Helicobacter pylori infection and the use of NSAIDs are known risk factors for bleeding ulcers and GDUP (Lau, 2011).

Gastric ulcers are classified into four types based on location (Stern, 2021).

- **Type 1**: in the antrum, near the lesser curvature
- **Type 2**: combined gastric and duodenal ulcer
- **Type 3**: Prepyloric ulcer
- **Type 4**: ulcer in the proximal stomach or cardia

More than half of gastric ulcers are identified in the lesser curvature, while duodenal ulcers are most commonly located in the first part of the duodenum.

Gastric ulcers have malignant potential compared to duodenal ulcers that do not have cancerous risk. A gastric ulcer greater than 3 cm is called a giant gastric ulcer which has a 6%-23% chance to turn into malignancy (Lv, 2012).

Though bleeding is a more common complication than perforation (6:1), the mortality rate is 5-fold higher with a GDUP compared with a bleeding peptic ulcer (Søreide, 2015).

History: GDUP causes sudden severe unrelenting pain, mostly in patients with a prior history of gastritis (not a sine qua non) and is an "operative" acute abdomen syndrome. Sometimes, patients may mislead you by thinking that they are experiencing just a new gastritis attack or indigestion again.

When the perforation occurs, the previously localized epigastric pain spreads to the entire abdomen. Pain that radiates to the shoulder may also be seen.

Examination: When peritonitis develops, the patient bewares of walking or moving at all. Abdominal rigidity, tenderness in the entire abdomen in response to micropercussion is typical. Opiate analgesia will facilitate patient cooperation and thus examination. Absence of bowel sounds (paralytic ileus), shock, generalized peritonitis and fever develop over time (hours to days). No painkiller is contraindicated in any patient with pain, provided with a thorough examination and elaborate documentation of the findings. Of note, NSAIDs can be avoided as their 'anti-inflammatory' features may disguise the pain from the physician.

Work up: Subdiaphragmatic free air (SDFA) can be seen in 75% of patients with perforation on upright chest X-ray, although it will be difficult to tell some patients to stand up for the X-ray. This X-ray can also be obtained in the left lateral decubitus position.

CT should be the radiological modality of choice in cases where suspicion persists with examination (Fig. **9**). ECG should be taken in every patient to rule out acute coronary syndrome.

Chilaiditi sign is radiolucency in the subdiaphragmatic space as a result of bowel interposition between a diaphragm and the liver. If GI symptoms accompany the condition, it is known as Chilaiditi's syndrome which is noted in 0.25% of all abdominal imaging studies (Sofii, 2021). It is often misdiagnosed with bowel perforation because the presence of pseudopneumoperitoneum in the plain X-Rays (Fig. **10**).

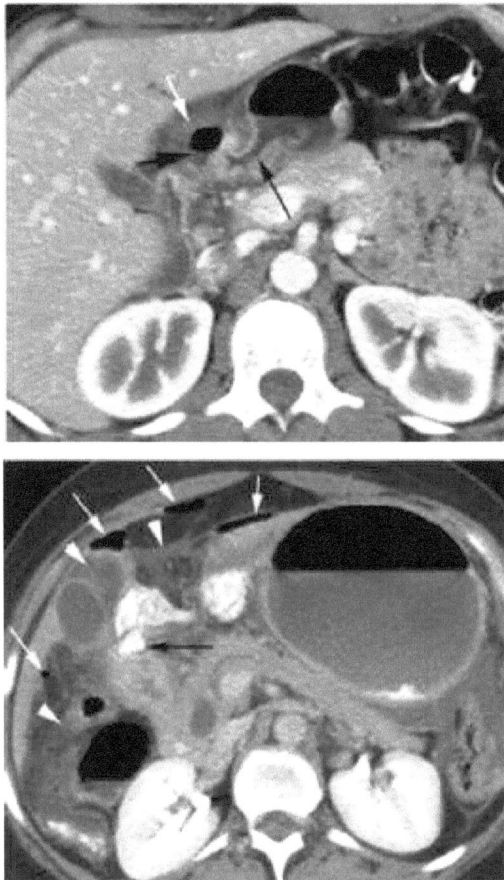

Fig. (9). A. Duodenal ulcer. Axial CT section shows fluid and gas in the ulcer crater in the bulb (thick black arrow), ensued with edema in the surrounding soft tissue (white arrow). Reactive wall thickening and narrowing of the lumen are seen in the gastric antrum (thin black arrow). **B.** Duodenal ulcer perforation. Axial CT section shows edema around the duodenum, gallbladder, colon (arrowheads) with a giant contrast-filled duodenal ulcer (black arrow) and pneumoperitoneum (white arrow) in the posterior wall of the first part of the duodenum.

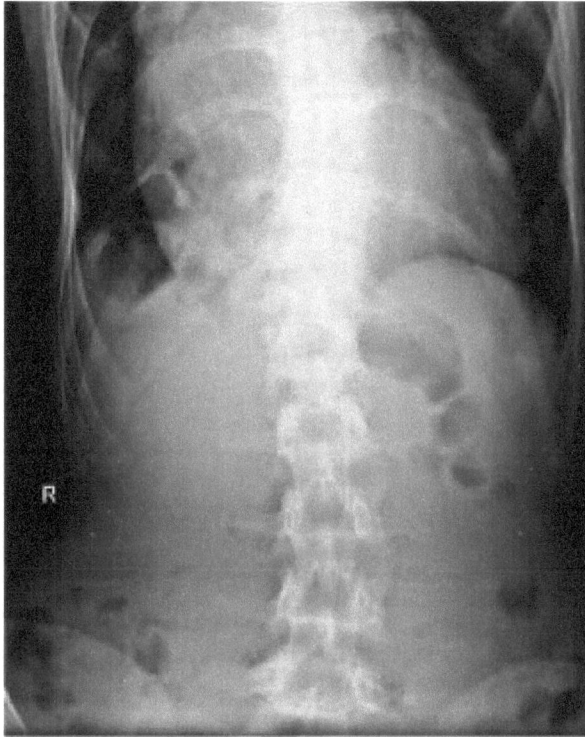

Fig. (10). Plain abdominal radiograph suggesting the presence of subdiaphragmatic air.

Treatment

GDUP is an ominous entity with a significant death rate of almost 30%. Emergent surgery and expedient management of sepsis are the mainstays of therapy (Søreide, 2015). A surgical consultation should be sought immediately in all patients with peritonitis before a specific diagnosis is established.

Around half of all mortalities of those with GDUP is attributed to sepsis and related issues. Therefore, antibiotics should be administered to all patients suspected to have GDUP (Table **16**).

Table 16. The treatment principles are similar in other GI visceral perforations (diverticulitis, bowel wall affected by cancer, trauma).

• Discontinue oral intake (nil per os, NPO) and consult with surgery.
• Broad-spectrum antibiotics with coverage of gram-negative rods and anaerobes are preferred in GDUP (Krobot 2004). Empirical treatment with a combination of a third-generation cephalosporin and a powerful anti-anaerobe (*e.g.*, metronidazole) can be chosen.
• Since most of the patients are dehydrated, IV crystalloid fluids should be started initially and then titrated to effect.
• PPI are administered via IV route to stop bleeding and facilitate tissue repair, but efficacy in GDUP is not clear yet (Satoh, 2016). PPI treatment aims to produce a neutral pH environment that helps maintain platelet aggregation and promote rapid sealing of perforation..
• Administer IV opioid (morphine/fentanyl) and antiemetics (*e.g.* ondansetron 8 mg IV) for symptomatic relief until surgery. Metoclopramide has no place in this situation, as paralytic ileus is already identifiable.

Short-term complications include hypovolemia, shock, sepsis, gastrocolic fistula formation (Stern, 2021).

Surgery will typically consist of a peritoneal lavage of 5 to 10 liters of saline followed by an interrupted sutured closure of the perforated ulcer followed by an omental patch (Roseo-Graham patch). A drain is placed in the dependent areas and the abdomen is closed. The surgical drain is removed on postoperative days 3 to 5.

Ingested Foreign Bodies (FB) as a Cause of AP

Fish bones and toothpicks were the most common FB, although local and cultural factors such as scarf needles can rank higher in some countries. Other types of. needles, blister packs, and wooden flakes and skewers are other recorded FBs. In addition, psychiatric patients ingested a wide variety of FBs (batteries, coins, and buttons) (Perkins, 1999).

More than half of the patients present with AP, followed by fever due to abscess formation, although some patients presented with GI bleeding including melena, nausea and vomiting, diarrhea and pain in the lumbar area or right iliac fossa. The diagnosis is mostly established *via* clinical suspicion and evidenced by CT, USG and/or X-ray. The relief after treatment verifies the accuracy of the diagnosis. Endoscopic intervention is suggested as the first choice (Wang, 2020). Endoscopy reportedly achieves a satisfactory (higher than a 95%) success rate in removing FBs (Li 2013). Surgical intervention is the first-line indication in only around 1% of all patients with FB in the GIS, mostly for those with unsuccessful endoscopic intervention (Webb, 1995).

Case

A fishbone stuck in the duodenal bulb, resulted in chronic AP for nearly 3 months. A 68-year-old woman was brought to the hospital with repeated right upper abdominal pain lasting for 3 months and aggravation for 9 h (Figs. **11 - 14**).

Batteries as ingested Foreign Bodies: the Hidden Threat

Injuries due to button battery ingestion (BBI) are most common in boys under 4 years of age and adults with mental retardation and other mental problems. The death and serious disability rate are 1% following the event. More than 3,500 incidents of BBI are reported to U.S. poison control centers each year (AAP Task Force, 2019). Most incidents go undetected and the whole figure is underreported.

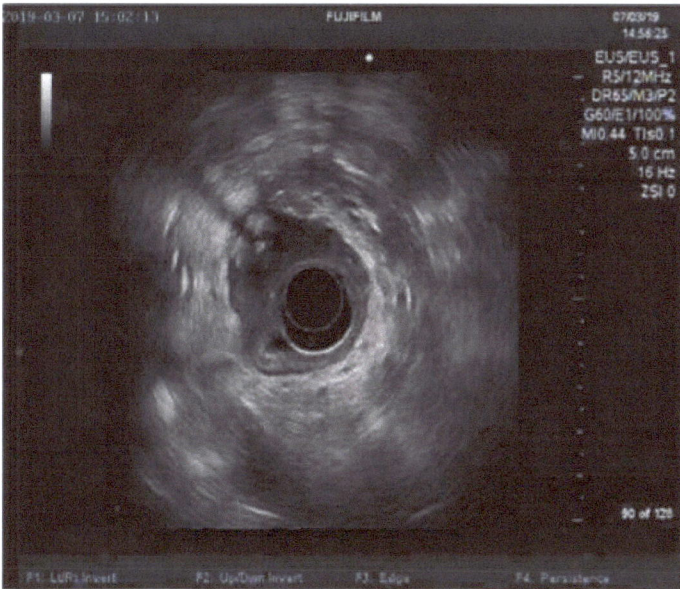

Fig. (11). Endoscopic (gastroscopic) USG demonstrates hyperechoic space with a cross-section of approximately 0.1 × 0.1 cm in the deep submucosal layer of the local stomach, accompanied by an acoustic shadow in the rear.

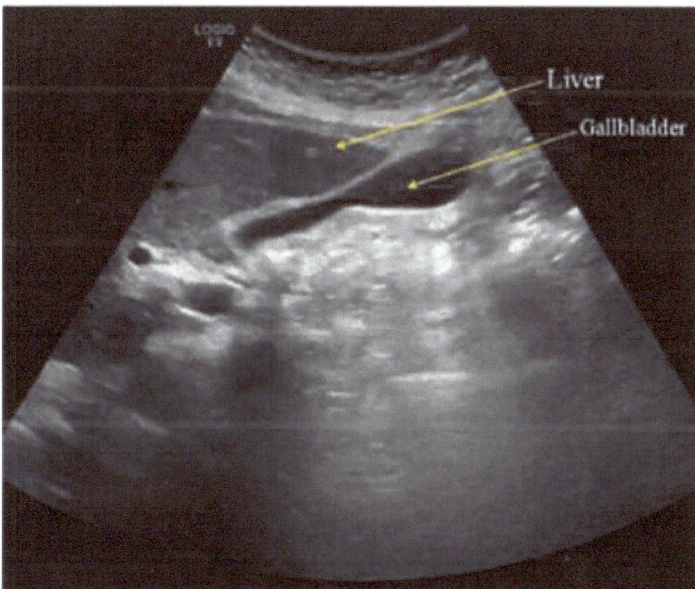

Fig. (12). USG examination is within normal limits, without any obvious abnormality in the liver, gallbladder, pancreas, spleen, and kidney.

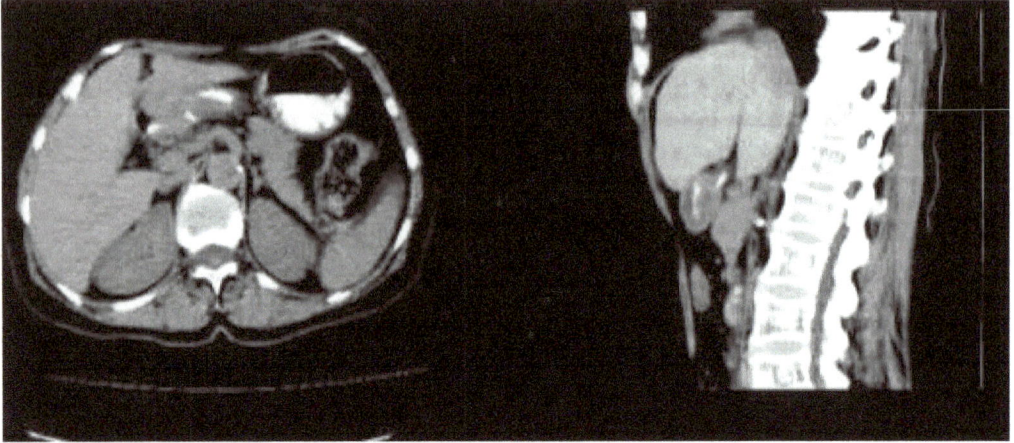

Fig. (13). CT scan revealed a streaky high-density shadow on the posterior wall of the gastric antrum extending outside the wall, with a length of about 3 cm.

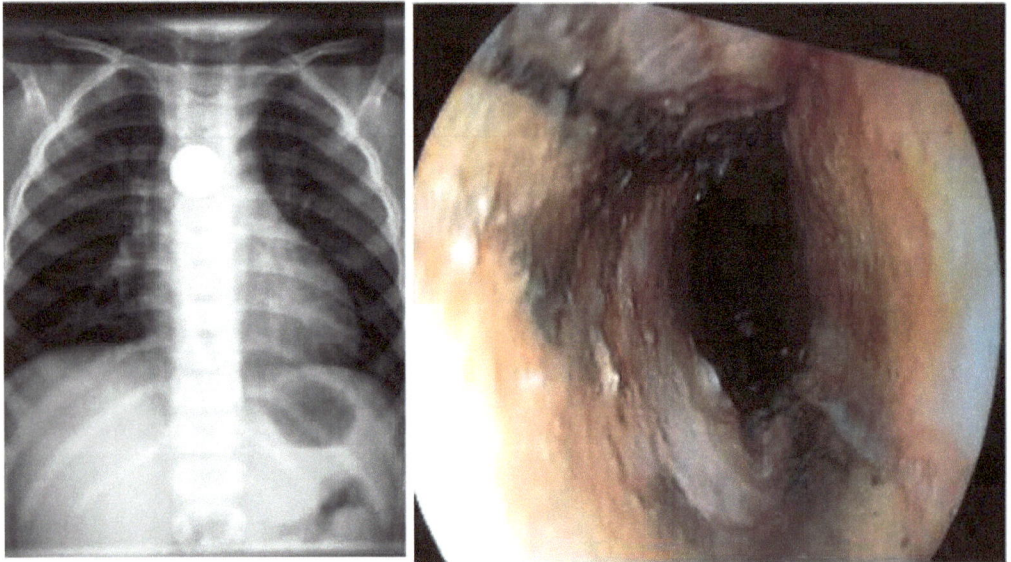

Fig. (14) A and B. Grade 3 a mucosal injury in the esophagus after being lodged in the tissue.

Most swallowed batteries can easily pass through the digestive tract and be excreted with feces. If the battery is stuck in the esophagus or another part of GIS and remains for a long time, serious complications may ensue. It has been reported that ¾ of the inserted batteries are inserted in the upper esophagus. Most of the rest remained in the middle section.

Size matters: Most batteries are smaller than 20 mm, but larger batteries have a higher rate of complications (Krom, 2018). It has also been reported that most of the batteries lodged in the tissue and removed by intervention are 2 cm and larger batteries. Litovitz *et al.* published a detailed analysis on the epidemiology of BBI: Adults most often ingested batteries that were sitting out, loose, or discarded (80.8%); obtained directly from a product (4.2%); obtained from battery packaging (3.0%); or swallowed within a hearing aid (12.1%) (Litovitz, 2010). Batteries that were intended for hearing aids were implicated in around one third of the cases (36%). Batteries were mistaken for medicines in 15% of the recorded BBI, mostly by the elderly.

As a result of BBI, the toxic content in the battery is released, and tissue damage and systemic absorption occur. Lithium batteries are the most common type of chemical content in BBI which is also the most dangerous (Ettyreddy, 2015). Pressure necrosis, formation of hydroxides by electrolysis at the negative pole of the battery, caustic damage by leakage and heavy metal toxicity are among the mechanisms put forward in the pathophysiology. As a result, necrosis, perforation and fistulas occur. Electrolysis is the most important.

The 3N abbreviation **'Negative - Narrow - Necrotic'**, sums it up.

It has been reported that the isothermal hydrolytic reaction occurring after BBI precipitates alkaline caustic damage (Jatana, 2017). They showed that CR2032, alkaline LR44 and silver oxide batteries caused severe burn damage in pig cadavers within 2 hours, and this injury progressed up to 6 hours. Tanaka *et al.* previously reported that there was visible damage to the mucosa in 15 minutes demonstrated in the living dog model (Tanaka, 1999).

Clinical Findings

It was noted that dysphagia (30%), fever and cough (26%) were the most common symptoms related to BBI. The table summarizes the symptoms and signs encountered after BBI.

Batteries remaining in the esophagus after BBI should be removed as soon as possible. The significant potential of severe damage starts within 15 minutes. Spinal erosion and tracheo-esophageal fistulae (TOF) may occur even after the successful removal of batteries. The possible sequelae are attributed to the orientation of the negative pole of the battery over time.

It has been reported that the duration of postoperative hospital stay increases significantly when button batteries remain in the esophagus for more than 15 hours (Ettyreddy, 2015). Stricture, perforation and TOF are among the factors that cause lengthened hospital stays and severe clinical courses in these patients. The development of TOF can be seen even when the battery is removed within 1 hour.

The risk of damage to the stomach is significant after ten hours.

Table **17** shows the factors that are thought to be associated with the development of complications and toxicity in patients presenting with BBI.

Table 17. Factors thought to be associated with complication development and toxicity in BBI.

Variable	Note-explanation
Time to removal	Tissue damage can begin after 15 minutes, and the risk of complications increases significantly after 24 hours. In the gastric mucosa, the damage is seen after 10 hours.
Being stuck in a narrow channel	Batteries lodged in the esophagus cause more necrosis.
Battery size (diameter)	>20 mm carries a higher risk (almost all problems occur in this group)
Chemical contents of the battery	Lithium batteries are complicated more frequently.
Battery age	New batteries cause 3.2 times more complications than old ones.
Action taken during the time until removal	Whether or not to irrigate with weak acids
Site of lodgement	Whether it is in a location suitable for the development of aortoenteric or tracheo-esophageal fistula

Evaluation, Diagnosis and Management: Physical examination is rarely helpful in locating the battery and directing the intervention. Plain radiographs are frequently employed in emergency admissions because of expedient use in diagnosis with low-radiation. Objects in the esophagus are usually seen as circular opacity on anteroposterior radiographs, while those stuck in the trachea are more vertically located (Fig. **14**).

Esophagogram is one of the best non-invasive procedures to visualize perforation and stricture development. In cases with a high risk of perforation, water-soluble contrast material should be preferred.

There is an intense debate in two main areas after BBI. One is the management of batteries that have gone beyond the esophagus in the asymptomatic patient, and the other is the management after the removal of the batteries. MRI provides important information in determining when to start enteral feeding following endoscopic removal. MRI should be used to clearly demonstrate damage to the aorta and other adjacent structures with submucosal injury. If the damaged tissue is more than 3 mm from the aorta, enteral feeding can be safely resumed. It has also been suggested that the damage to the tissue by the battery will be alleviated when irrigated with weak acidic compounds.

Endoscopic removal is recommended in selected cases in the management of batteries that cross the esophagus. A majority of deaths attributed to BBI are associated with persistent bleeding resulting from the development of aortoenteric fistula.

For cases with respiratory symptoms, tracheal erosion and other evidence of damage should be sought. ENT and surgical consultations will be appropriate in the emergency setting. Never discharge a patient with a history of BBI without a satisfactory evaluation.

Follow-up

In cases that are thought to be injured by BBI, esophagogram is performed again in the 4th week which should be specifically checked for stricture. Endoscopic dilation is recommended if there is a stricture.

Education of children and parents is critical for prevention (Eliason, 2017). Warnings on the packaging, legal measures, changing the designs of batteries and tools, making it difficult to remove the battery from the houseware tools, and awareness campaigns should take priority for an effective prevention (Litovitz, 2010).

CONCLUSION

In any case, the most important thing about BBI is protection from it. When it is lodged in the tissue, it is an emergency and should be dealt with immediately. Complications increase in direct proportion to time wasted. Prevention is of utmost importance. Permanent solutions for prevention will be found and robust protection can be provided should the industry, health professionals and educators cooperate.

REFERENCES

AAP Button Battery Task Force. *The hazards of button batteries.*https://www.aap.org/en-us/advocacy-a-d-policy/aap-health-initiatives/Pages/Button-Battery.aspx

Adamopoulos, A.B., Baibas, N.M., Efstathiou, S.P., Tsioulos, D.I., Mitromaras, A.G., Tsami, A.A., Mountokalakis, T.D. (2003). Differentiation between patients with acute upper gastrointestinal bleeding who need early urgent upper gastrointestinal endoscopy and those who do not. A prospective study. *Eur. J. Gastroenterol. Hepatol., 15*(4), 381-387.
[http://dx.doi.org/10.1097/00042737-200304000-00008] [PMID: 12655258]

Ahn, J.H., Park, Y., Bae, J.S., Jang, J.Y., Kim, K.H., Kang, M.G., Koh, J.S., Park, J.R., Hwang, S.J., Kwak, C.H., Hwang, J.Y., Jeong, Y.H. (2020). Influence of rabeprazole and famotidine on pharmacodynamic profile

of dual antiplatelet therapy in clopidogrel-sensitive patients: The randomized, prospective, PROTECT trial. *Platelets, 31*(3), 329-336.
[http://dx.doi.org/10.1080/09537104.2019.1609667] [PMID: 31037994]

Altekin, E., Solak, A., Tuncel, P. (2003). Gaitada Gizli Kan Testlerinde Guaiak ve İmmunokimyasal Yöntemlerin Karşılaştırılması. *Turk Klin. Biyokim. Derg., 3*(143-147)

Aluizio, C.L.S., Montes, C.G., Reis, G.F.S.R., Nagasako, C.K. (2021). Risk stratification in acute variceal bleeding: Far from an ideal score. *Clinics (São Paulo), 76*, e2921.
[http://dx.doi.org/10.6061/clinics/2021/e2921] [PMID: 34190855]

Ameer, M.A., Wasey, A., Salen, P. (2021).

Atherton, J.C., Blaser, M.J. (2013). Helicobacter pylori infections.*Harrison's gastroenterology and hepatology.* (2nd ed., pp. 262-268). New York: McGraw Hill Education.

Atnafie, B., Paulos, D., Abera, M., Tefera, G., Hailu, D., Kasaye, S., Amenu, K. (2017). Occurrence of Escherichia coli O157:H7 in cattle feces and contamination of carcass and various contact surfaces in abattoir and butcher shops of Hawassa, Ethiopia. *BMC Microbiol., 17*(1), 24.
[http://dx.doi.org/10.1186/s12866-017-0938-1] [PMID: 28122502]

Azer, S.A., Tuma, F. (2020). Infectious Colitis. In book: StatPearls; pp. 15.

Barkun, A.N., Almadi, M., Kuipers, E.J., Laine, L., Sung, J., Tse, F., Leontiadis, G.I., Abraham, N.S., Calvet, X., Chan, F.K.L., Douketis, J., Enns, R., Gralnek, I.M., Jairath, V., Jensen, D., Lau, J., Lip, G.Y.H., Loffroy, R., Maluf-Filho, F., Meltzer, A.C., Reddy, N., Saltzman, J.R., Marshall, J.K., Bardou, M. (2019). Management of Nonvariceal Upper Gastrointestinal Bleeding: Guideline Recommendations From the International Consensus Group. *Ann. Intern. Med., 171*(11), 805-822.
[http://dx.doi.org/10.7326/M19-1795] [PMID: 31634917]

Bhandare, B, Satyanarayana, V, Pavithra, K. (2014). *A Comparative Study of the Efficacy and Safety of Dexrabeprazole 10 mg versus* Rabeprazole 20 mg in the Treatment of GERD in A Tertiary Care Hospital.

Bhurwal, A., Patel, A., Mutneja, H., Goel, A., Palomera-Tejeda, E., Brahmbhatt, B. (2021). The role of endoscopic doppler probe in the management of bleeding peptic ulcers: a systematic review and meta-analysis. *Expert Rev. Gastroenterol. Hepatol., 15*(7), 835-843.
[http://dx.doi.org/10.1080/17474124.2021.1850261] [PMID: 33206568]

Blatchford, O., Murray, W.R., Blatchford, M. (2000). A risk score to predict need for treatment for upper-gastrointestinal haemorrhage. *Lancet, 356*(9238), 1318-1321.
[http://dx.doi.org/10.1016/S0140-6736(00)02816-6] [PMID: 11073021]

Bozdemir, M. N, Kuk, S, Yıldız, M, Ateşçelik, M, Baştürk, M, Kılıçaslan, İ. *Acil Servise Başvuran İshalli Hastaların Değerlendirilmesi.*

Budimir, I., Gradišer, M., Nikolić, M., Baršić, N., Ljubičić, N., Kralj, D., Budimir, I., Jr (2016). Glasgow Blatchford, pre-endoscopic Rockall and AIMS65 scores show no difference in predicting rebleeding rate and mortality in variceal bleeding. *Scand. J. Gastroenterol., 51*(11), 1375-1379.
[http://dx.doi.org/10.1080/00365521.2016.1200138] [PMID: 27356670]

Cağdaş, U., Otağ, F., Tezcan, S., Sezgin, O., Aslan, G., Emekdaş, G. (2012). [Detection of Helicobacter pylori and antimicrobial resistance in gastric biopsy specimens]. *Mikrobiyol. Bul., 46*(3), 398-409.
[PMID: 22951652]

Cherian, J.J., Lobo, I., Sukhlecha, A., Chawan, U., Kshirsagar, N.A., Nair, B.L., Sawardekar, L. (2017). Treatment outcome of extrapulmonary tuberculosis under Revised National Tuberculosis Control Programme. *Indian J. Tuberc., 64*(2), 104-108.
[http://dx.doi.org/10.1016/j.ijtb.2016.11.028] [PMID: 28410692]

Choe, J.W., Jung, S.W., Kim, S.Y., Hyun, J.J., Jung, Y.K., Koo, J.S., Yim, H.J., Lee, S.W. (2018). Comparative study of Helicobacter pylori eradication rates of concomitant therapy vs modified quadruple therapy comprising proton-pump inhibitor, bismuth, amoxicillin, and metronidazole in Korea. *Helicobacter, 23*(2), e12466.

[http://dx.doi.org/10.1111/hel.12466] [PMID: 29369454]

Contreras-Omaña, R., Escorcia-Saucedo, A.E., Velarde-Ruiz Velasco, J.A. (2021). Prevalence and impact of antimicrobial resistance in gastrointestinal infections: A review. *Rev. Gastroenterol. Mex., 86*(3), 265-275. [http://dx.doi.org/10.1016/j.rgmxen.2021.06.004] [PMID: 34158260]

Contreras-Omaña, R., Escorcia-Saucedo, A.E., Velarde-Ruiz Velasco, J.A. (2021). Prevalence and impact of antimicrobial resistance in gastrointestinal infections: A review. *Rev. Gastroenterol. Mex., 86*(3), 265-275. [http://dx.doi.org/10.1016/j.rgmxen.2021.06.004] [PMID: 34158260]

Deshpande, A., Pasupuleti, V., Patel, P., Ajani, G., Hall, G., Hu, B., Jain, A., Rolston, D.D. (2011). Repeat stool testing to diagnose Clostridium difficile infection using enzyme immunoassay does not increase diagnostic yield. *Clin. Gastroenterol. Hepatol., 9*(8), 665-669.e1. [http://dx.doi.org/10.1016/j.cgh.2011.04.030] [PMID: 21635969]

https://go.drugbank.com/drugs/DB13762

Eliason, M.J., Ricca, R.L., Gallagher, T.Q. (2017). Button battery ingestion in children. *Curr. Opin. Otolaryngol. Head Neck Surg., 25*(6), 520-526. [http://dx.doi.org/10.1097/MOO.0000000000000410] [PMID: 28858893]

Erdeve, Ö., Tıraş, Ü., Çamurdan, M.O., Tanyer, G., Dallar, Y. (2002). Çocuk Yaş Grubunda Antibiyotiğe Bağlı İshallerde Saccharomyces Boulardii'nin Profilaktik Etkisi. *Turkiye Klinikleri J Pediatr., 11*(3), 121-125.

Ettyreddy, A.R., Georg, M.W., Chi, D.H., Gaines, B.A., Simons, J.P. (2015). Button battery injuries in the pediatric aerodigestive tract. *Ear Nose Throat J., 94*(12), 486-493. [http://dx.doi.org/10.1177/014556131509401207] [PMID: 26670755]

(2018). http://www.adrreports.eu/

Fan, L., Xianghong, Q., Ling, W., Ying, H., Jielai, X., Haitang, H. (2019). Ilaprazole Compared With Rabeprazole in the Treatment of Duodenal Ulcer: A Randomized, Double-blind, Active-controlled, Multicenter Study. *J. Clin. Gastroenterol., 53*(9), 641-647. [http://dx.doi.org/10.1097/MCG.0000000000001186] [PMID: 30789856]

Furuta, T., Shirai, N., Sugimoto, M., Nakamura, A., Hishida, A., Ishizaki, T. (2005). Influence of CYP2C19 pharmacogenetic polymorphism on proton pump inhibitor-based therapies. *Drug Metab. Pharmacokinet., 20*(3), 153-167. [http://dx.doi.org/10.2133/dmpk.20.153] [PMID: 15988117]

Gareau, M.G., Sherman, P.M., Walker, W.A. (2010). Probiotics and the gut microbiota in intestinal health and disease. *Nat. Rev. Gastroenterol. Hepatol., 7*(9), 503-514. [http://dx.doi.org/10.1038/nrgastro.2010.117] [PMID: 20664519]

González-Alcaide, G., Peris, J., Ramos, J.M. (2017). Areas of research and clinical approaches to the study of liver abscess. *World J. Gastroenterol., 23*(2), 357-365. [http://dx.doi.org/10.3748/wjg.v23.i2.357] [PMID: 28127209]

Hatchimonji, J.S., Chipman, A.M., McGreevy, D.T., Hörer, T.M., Burruss, S., Han, S., Spalding, M.C., Fox, C.J., Moore, E.E., Diaz, J.J., Cannon, J.W. (2020). Resuscitative Endovascular Balloon Occlusion of Aaorta Use in Nontrauma Emergency General Surgery: A Multi-institutional Experience. *J. Surg. Res., 256*, 149-155. [http://dx.doi.org/10.1016/j.jss.2020.06.034] [PMID: 32707397]

Herardi, R., Syam, A.F., Simadibrata, M., Setiati, S., Darnindro, N., Abdullah, M., Makmun, D. (2020). Comparison of 10-Day Course of Triple Therapy *versus* 14-Day Course for Eradication of Helicobacter pylori Infection in an Indonesian Population: Double-Blinded Randomized Clinical Trial. *Asian Pac. J. Cancer Prev., 21*(1), 19-24. [http://dx.doi.org/10.31557/APJCP.2020.21.1.19] [PMID: 31983158]

Hooman, N., Khodadost, M., Ahmadi, A., Nakhaie, S., Nagh Shizadian, R. (2019). The Prevalence of Shiga Toxin-producing Escherichia Coli in Patients with Gastroenteritis in Iran, Systematic Review and Meta-

analysis. *Iran. J. Kidney Dis., 13*(3), 139-150.
[PMID: 31209187]

Huang, E.S., Karsan, S., Kanwal, F., Singh, I., Makhani, M., Spiegel, B.M. (2011). Impact of nasogastric lavage on outcomes in acute GI bleeding. *Gastrointest. Endosc., 74*(5), 971-980.
[http://dx.doi.org/10.1016/j.gie.2011.04.045] [PMID: 21737077]

Ichita, C., Sasaki, A., Sumida, C., Kimura, K., Nishino, T., Tasaki, J., Masuda, S., Koizumi, K., Kawachi, J., Kako, M. (2021). Clinical and endoscopic features of aorto-duodenal fistula resulting in its definitive diagnosis: an observational study. *BMC Gastroenterol., 21*(1), 45.
[http://dx.doi.org/10.1186/s12876-021-01616-9] [PMID: 33526013]

Ierardi, E., Losurdo, G., Fortezza, R.F., Principi, M., Barone, M., Leo, A.D. (2019). Optimizing proton pump inhibitors in *Helicobacter pylori* treatment: Old and new tricks to improve effectiveness. *World J. Gastroenterol., 25*(34), 5097-5104.
[http://dx.doi.org/10.3748/wjg.v25.i34.5097] [PMID: 31558859]

Imdad, A., Mackoff, S.P., Urciuoli, D.M., Syed, T., Tanner-Smith, E.E., Huang, D., Gomez-Duarte, O.G. (2021). Interventions for preventing diarrhoea-associated haemolytic uraemic syndrome. *Cochrane Database Syst. Rev., 7*(7), CD012997.
[http://dx.doi.org/10.1002/14651858.CD012997.pub2] [PMID: 34219224]

(2017). https://www.mdedge.com/infectiousdisease/ clinical-edge/summary/clinical-guidelines/id-a-guidelines-infectious-diarrhea

Jamshed, S., Bhagavathula, A.S., Zeeshan Qadar, S.M., Alauddin, U., Shamim, S., Hasan, S. (2020). Cost-effective Analysis of Proton Pump Inhibitors in Long-term Management of Gastroesophageal Reflux Disease: A Narrative Review. *Hosp. Pharm., 55*(5), 292-305.
[http://dx.doi.org/10.1177/0018578719893378] [PMID: 32999499]

Jatana, K.R., Rhoades, K., Milkovich, S., Jacobs, I.N. (2017). Basic mechanism of button battery ingestion injuries and novel mitigation strategies after diagnosis and removal. *Laryngoscope, 127*(6), 1276-1282.
[http://dx.doi.org/10.1002/lary.26362] [PMID: 27859311]

Karadağ, F. Üst Gastrointestinal Sistem Kanamalı Hastaların Genel Değerlen¬dirilmesi (Uzmanlık Tezi), İstanbul-2008.

Karagiannis, S., Papaioannou, D., Goulas, S., Psilopoulos, D., Mavrogiannis, C. (2008). Intestinal tuberculosis in a patient on infliximab treatment. *Gastrointest. Endosc., 67*(7), 1178-1179.
[http://dx.doi.org/10.1016/j.gie.2007.12.048] [PMID: 18329027]

Kasırga, E. (2019). Çocuklarda sindirim sistemi hastalıklarının tanı ve izleminde dışkı incelemelerinin yeri. *Turk. Pediatri Ars., 54*(3), 141-148.
[PMID: 31619925]

Kaufmann, H. (2019). *Mechanisms, causes, and evaluation of orthostatic hypotension.*https://www.uptodate.com/contents/mechanisms-causes-and-evaluatio--of-orthostatic-hypotension#H71186235

Kelesidis, T., Pothoulakis, C. (2012). Efficacy and safety of the probiotic Saccharomyces boulardii for the prevention and therapy of gastrointestinal disorders. *Therap. Adv. Gastroenterol., 5*(2), 111-125.
[http://dx.doi.org/10.1177/1756283X11428502] [PMID: 22423260]

Kim, B.S.M., Li, B.T., Engel, A., Samra, J.S., Clarke, S., Norton, I.D., Li, A.E. (2014). Diagnosis of gastrointestinal bleeding: A practical guide for clinicians. *World J. Gastrointest. Pathophysiol., 5*(4), 467-478.
[http://dx.doi.org/10.4291/wjgp.v5.i4.467] [PMID: 25400991]

Kinoshita, Y., Ishimura, N., Ishihara, S. (2018). Advantages and Disadvantages of Long-term Proton Pump Inhibitor Use. *J. Neurogastroenterol. Motil., 24*(2), 182-196.
[http://dx.doi.org/10.5056/jnm18001] [PMID: 29605975]

Kirsch, C., Morgner, A., Miehlke, S. (2006). Relevance of cytochrome P450 polymorphisms in the treatment

of Helicobacter pylori infection and gastroesophageal reflux disease. *Curr. Pharmacogenom.,* *4*(1), 47-56.
[http://dx.doi.org/10.2174/157016006776055365]

Komori, H., Ueyama, H., Nagahara, A., Akazawa, Y., Takeda, T., Matsumoto, K., Matsumoto, K., Asaoka, D., Hojo, M., Yao, T., Watanabe, S. (2019). A prospective randomized trial of a potassium competitive acid blocker vs proton pump inhibitors on the effect of ulcer healing after endoscopic submucosal dissection of gastric neoplasia. *J. Int. Med. Res.,* *47*(4), 1441-1452.
[http://dx.doi.org/10.1177/0300060519828514] [PMID: 30816056]

Krobot, K., Yin, D., Zhang, Q., Sen, S., Altendorf-Hofmann, A., Scheele, J., Sendt, W. (2004). Effect of inappropriate initial empiric antibiotic therapy on outcome of patients with community-acquired intra-abdominal infections requiring surgery. *Eur. J. Clin. Microbiol. Infect. Dis.,* *23*(9), 682-687.
[http://dx.doi.org/10.1007/s10096-004-1199-0] [PMID: 15322931]

Krom, H., Visser, M., Hulst, J.M., Wolters, V.M., Van den Neucker, A.M., de Meij, T., van der Doef, H.P.J., Norbruis, O.F., Benninga, M.A., Smit, M.J.M., Kindermann, A. (2018). Serious complications after button battery ingestion in children. *Eur. J. Pediatr.,* *177*(7), 1063-1070.
[http://dx.doi.org/10.1007/s00431-018-3154-6] [PMID: 29717359]

Kuo, C.H., Wang, S.S., Hsu, W.H., Kuo, F.C., Weng, B.C., Li, C.J., Hsu, P.I., Chen, A., Hung, W.C., Yang, Y.C., Wang, W.M., Wu, D.C. (2010). Rabeprazole can overcome the impact of CYP2C19 polymorphism on quadruple therapy. *Helicobacter,* *15*(4), 265-272.
[http://dx.doi.org/10.1111/j.1523-5378.2010.00761.x] [PMID: 20633187]

Lau, J.Y., Sung, J., Hill, C., Henderson, C., Howden, C.W., Metz, D.C. (2011). Systematic review of the epidemiology of complicated peptic ulcer disease: incidence, recurrence, risk factors and mortality. *Digestion,* *84*(2), 102-113.
[http://dx.doi.org/10.1159/000323958] [PMID: 21494041]

Lau, J.Y., Sung, J.J., Lee, K.K., Yung, M.Y., Wong, S.K., Wu, J.C., Chan, F.K., Ng, E.K., You, J.H., Lee, C.W., Chan, A.C., Chung, S.C. (2000). Effect of intravenous omeprazole on recurrent bleeding after endoscopic treatment of bleeding peptic ulcers. *N. Engl. J. Med.,* *343*(5), 310-316.
[http://dx.doi.org/10.1056/NEJM200008033430501] [PMID: 10922420]

Lee, J.G., Turnipseed, S., Romano, P.S., Vigil, H., Azari, R., Melnikoff, N., Hsu, R., Kirk, D., Sokolove, P., Leung, J.W. (1999). Endoscopy-based triage significantly reduces hospitalization rates and costs of treating upper GI bleeding: a randomized controlled trial. *Gastrointest. Endosc.,* *50*(6), 755-761.
[http://dx.doi.org/10.1016/S0016-5107(99)70154-9] [PMID: 10570332]

Lee, V.W., Chau, T.S., Chan, A.K., Lee, K.K., Waye, M.M., Ling, T.K., Chan, F.K. (2010). Pharmacogenetics of esomeprazole or rabeprazole-based triple therapy in Helicobacter pylori eradication in Hong Kong non-ulcer dyspepsia Chinese subjects. *J. Clin. Pharm. Ther.,* *35*(3), 343-350.
[http://dx.doi.org/10.1111/j.1365-2710.2009.01088.x] [PMID: 20831535]

Li, Q.P., Ge, X.X., Ji, G.Z., Fan, Z.N., Zhang, F.M., Wang, Y., Miao, L. (2013). Endoscopic retrieval of 28 foreign bodies in a 100-year-old female after attempted suicide. *World J. Gastroenterol.,* *19*(25), 4091-4093.
[http://dx.doi.org/10.3748/wjg.v19.i25.4091] [PMID: 23840158]

Liesman, R.M., Binnicker, M.J. (2016). The role of multiplex molecular panels for the diagnosis of gastrointestinal infections in immunocompromised patients. *Curr. Opin. Infect. Dis.,* *29*(4), 359-365.
[http://dx.doi.org/10.1097/QCO.0000000000000276] [PMID: 27191200]

Litovitz, T., Whitaker, N., Clark, L. (2010). Preventing battery ingestions: an analysis of 8648 cases. *Pediatrics,* *125*(6), 1178-1183.
[http://dx.doi.org/10.1542/peds.2009-3038] [PMID: 20498172]

Lv, S.X., Gan, J.H., Ma, X.G., Wang, C.C., Chen, H.M., Luo, E.P., Huang, X.P., Wu, S.H., Qin, A.L., Ke-Chen, , Wang, X.H., Wei-Sun, , Li-Chen, , Ying-Xie, , Hu, F.X., Dan-Niu, , Walia, S., Zhu, J. (2012). Biopsy from the base and edge of gastric ulcer healing or complete healing may lead to detection of gastric cancer earlier: an 8 years endoscopic follow-up study. *Hepatogastroenterology,* *59*(115), 947-950.
[PMID: 22469743]

Malfertheiner, P., Megraud, F., O'Morain, C. (2007). Current concepts in the management of Helicobacter pylori infection Report. *Gut, 56*, 772-781.
[http://dx.doi.org/10.1136/gut.2006.101634] [PMID: 17170018]

Memik, F. (2004). *Peptik ülser komplikasyonları.* Klinik Gastroenteroloji. Nobel Tıp Kitabevleri.

Mohebali, M., Keshavarz, H., Abbaszadeh Afshar, M.J., Hanafi-Bojd, A.A., Hassanpour, G. (2021). Spatial Distribution of Common Pathogenic Human Intestinal Protozoa in Iran: A Systematic Review. *Iran. J. Public Health, 50*(1), 69-82.
[http://dx.doi.org/10.18502/ijph.v50i1.5073] [PMID: 34178765]

Montagnese, S., Russo, F.P., Amodio, P., Burra, P., Gasbarrini, A., Loguercio, C., Marchesini, G., Merli, M., Ponziani, F.R., Riggio, O., Scarpignato, C. (2019). Hepatic encephalopathy 2018: A clinical practice guideline by the Italian Association for the Study of the Liver (AISF). *Dig. Liver Dis., 51*(2), 190-205.
[http://dx.doi.org/10.1016/j.dld.2018.11.035] [PMID: 30606696]

Novotny, M., Klimova, B., Valis, M. (2019). PPI Long Term Use: Risk of Neurological Adverse Events? *Front. Neurol., 9*, 1142.
[http://dx.doi.org/10.3389/fneur.2018.01142] [PMID: 30671013]

Padol, S., Yuan, Y., Thabane, M., Padol, I.T., Hunt, R.H. (2006). The effect of CYP2C19 polymorphisms on *H. pylori* eradication rate in dual and triple first-line PPI therapies: a meta-analysis. *Am. J. Gastroenterol., 101*(7), 1467-1475.
[http://dx.doi.org/10.1111/j.1572-0241.2006.00717.x] [PMID: 16863547]

Pai, V., Pai, N. (2007). Randomized, double-blind, comparative study of dexrabeprazole 10 mg *versus* rabeprazole 20 mg in the treatment of gastroesophageal reflux disease. *World J. Gastroenterol., 13*(30), 4100-4102.
[http://dx.doi.org/10.3748/wjg.v13.i30.4100] [PMID: 17696229]

Pallin, D.J., Saltzman, J.R. (2011). Is nasogastric tube lavage in patients with acute upper GI bleeding indicated or antiquated? *Gastrointest. Endosc., 74*(5), 981-984.
[http://dx.doi.org/10.1016/j.gie.2011.07.007] [PMID: 22032314]

Pazar, B., Yava, A. (2013). Post-Surgical Operation Care by Application of an Early Warning Scoring System and Nursing Guidance; Gülhane Askeri Tıp Akademisi Hemşirelik Yüksekokulu Cerrahi Hastalıkları Hemşireliği Bilim Dalı, Ankara, Türkiye. *Turk. J. Anaesthesiol. Reanim., 41*(6), 216-222.
[http://dx.doi.org/10.5152/TJAR.2013.37] [PMID: 27366375]

Perkins, M., Lovell, J., Gruenewald, S. (1999). Life-threatening pica: liver abscess from perforating foreign body. *Australas. Radiol., 43*(3), 349-352.
[http://dx.doi.org/10.1046/j.1440-1673.1999.433670.x] [PMID: 10901933]

Podolsky, D.K., İsselbacher, K. (2004). Gastrointestinal sistem hastalıkları. Eds. Braunwald E, Fauci AS, Kasper DL, *et al.* Harrison iç hastalıkları prensipleri. Nobel Tıp Kitabevleri. 15. baskı 2004: 1649-65.

Przespolewski, E.R., Westphal, E.S., Rainka, M., Smith, N.M., Bates, V., Gengo, F.M. (2018). Evaluating the Effect of Six Proton Pump Inhibitors on the Antiplatelet Effects of Clopidogrel. *J. Stroke Cerebrovasc. Dis., 27*(6), 1582-1589.
[http://dx.doi.org/10.1016/j.jstrokecerebrovasdis.2018.01.011] [PMID: 29449127]

Raju, G.S., Gerson, L., Das, A., Lewis, B. (2007). American Gastroenterological Association (AGA) Institute medical position statement on obscure gastrointestinal bleeding. *Gastroenterology, 133*(5), 1694-1696.
[http://dx.doi.org/10.1053/j.gastro.2007.06.008] [PMID: 17983811]

Reveles, K.R., Lee, G.C., Boyd, N.K., Frei, C.R. (2014). The rise in Clostridium difficile infection incidence among hospitalized adults in the United States: 2001-2010. *Am. J. Infect. Control, 42*(10), 1028-1032.
[http://dx.doi.org/10.1016/j.ajic.2014.06.011] [PMID: 25278388]

Rockall, T.A., Logan, R.F., Devlin, H.B., Northfield, T.C. (1996). Risk assessment after acute upper gastrointestinal haemorrhage. *Gut, 38*(3), 316-321.

[http://dx.doi.org/10.1136/gut.38.3.316] [PMID: 8675081]

Sachs, G., Shin, J.M., Vagin, O., Lambrecht, N., Yakubov, I., Munson, K. (2007). The gastric H,K ATPase as a drug target: past, present, and future. *J. Clin. Gastroenterol., 41* (Suppl. 2), S226-S242.
[http://dx.doi.org/10.1097/MCG.0b013e31803233b7] [PMID: 17575528]

Satoh, K., Yoshino, J., Akamatsu, T., Itoh, T., Kato, M., Kamada, T., Takagi, A., Chiba, T., Nomura, S., Mizokami, Y., Murakami, K., Sakamoto, C., Hiraishi, H., Ichinose, M., Uemura, N., Goto, H., Joh, T., Miwa, H., Sugano, K., Shimosegawa, T. (2016). Evidence-based clinical practice guidelines for peptic ulcer disease 2015. *J. Gastroenterol., 51*(3), 177-194.
[http://dx.doi.org/10.1007/s00535-016-1166-4] [PMID: 26879862]

Sezgin, O., Aslan, G., Altıntaş, E., Tezcan, S., Serin, M.S., Emekdaş, G. (2008). Detection of point mutations on 23S rRNA of Helicobacter pylori and resistance to clarithromycin with PCR-RFLP in gastric biopsy specimens in Mersin, Turkey. *Turk. J. Gastroenterol., 19*(3), 163-167.
[PMID: 19115151]

Sezgin, O., Aydın, M.K., Özdemir, A.A., Kanık, A.E. (2019). Standard triple therapy in Helicobacter pylori eradication in Turkey: Systematic evaluation and meta-analysis of 10-year studies. *Turk. J. Gastroenterol., 30*(5), 420-435.
[http://dx.doi.org/10.5152/tjg.2019.18693] [PMID: 31060997]

Slimings, C., Riley, T.V. (2014). Antibiotics and hospital-acquired Clostridium difficile infection: update of systematic review and meta-analysis. *J. Antimicrob. Chemother., 69*(4), 881-891.
[http://dx.doi.org/10.1093/jac/dkt477] [PMID: 24324224]

Sofii, I., Parminto, Z.A., Anwar, S.L. (2021). Differentiating Chilaiditi's Syndrome with hollow viscus perforation: A case report. *Int. J. Surg. Case Rep., 78*, 314-316.
[http://dx.doi.org/10.1016/j.ijscr.2020.12.029] [PMID: 33387865]

Søreide, K., Thorsen, K., Harrison, E.M., Bingener, J., Møller, M.H., Ohene-Yeboah, M., Søreide, J.A. (2015). Perforated peptic ulcer. *Lancet, 386*(10000), 1288-1298.
[http://dx.doi.org/10.1016/S0140-6736(15)00276-7] [PMID: 26460663]

Spengler, G., Molnar, A., Klausz, G., Mandi, Y., Kawase, M., Motohashi, N., Molnar, J. (2004). Inhibitory action of a new proton pump inhibitor, trifluoromethyl ketone derivative, against the motility of clarithromycin-susceptible and-resistant Helicobacter pylori. *Int. J. Antimicrob. Agents, 23*(6), 631-633.
[http://dx.doi.org/10.1016/j.ijantimicag.2003.11.010] [PMID: 15194136]

Srygley, F.D., Gerardo, C.J., Tran, T., Fisher, D.A. (2012). Does this patient have a severe upper gastrointestinal bleed? *JAMA, 307*(10), 1072-1079.
[http://dx.doi.org/10.1001/jama.2012.253] [PMID: 22416103]

Stanley, S.L., Jr (2003). Amoebiasis. *Lancet, 361*(9362), 1025-1034.
[http://dx.doi.org/10.1016/S0140-6736(03)12830-9] [PMID: 12660071]

Stern, E., Sugumar, K., Journey, J.D. (2022). Peptic Ulcer Perforated 2021. *StatPearls [Internet]. Treasure Island (FL): StatPearls Publishing.*
[PMID: 30855910]

Strand, D.S., Kim, D., Peura, D.A. (2017). 25 Years of Proton Pump Inhibitors: A Comprehensive Review. *Gut Liver, 11*(1), 27-37.
[http://dx.doi.org/10.5009/gnl15502] [PMID: 27840364]

Szajewska, H., Horvath, A., Piwowarczyk, A. (2010). Meta-analysis: the effects of Saccharomyces boulardii supplementation on Helicobacter pylori eradication rates and side effects during treatment. *Aliment. Pharmacol. Ther., 32*(9), 1069-1079.
[http://dx.doi.org/10.1111/j.1365-2036.2010.04457.x] [PMID: 21039671]

Takeuchi, T., Furuta, T., Fujiwara, Y., Sugimoto, M., Kasugai, K., Kusano, M., Okada, H., Suzuki, T., Higuchi, T., Kagami, T., Uotani, T., Yamade, M., Sawada, A., Tanaka, F., Harada, S., Ota, K., Kojima, Y., Murata, M., Tamura, Y., Funaki, Y., Kawamura, O., Okamoto, Y., Fujimoto, K., Higuchi, K. (2020).

Randomised trial of acid inhibition by vonoprazan 10/20 mg once daily vs rabeprazole 10/20 mg twice daily in healthy Japanese volunteers (SAMURAI pH study). *Aliment. Pharmacol. Ther., 51*(5), 534-543. [http://dx.doi.org/10.1111/apt.15641] [PMID: 31990424]

Talarico, V., Aloe, M., Monzani, A., Miniero, R., Bona, G. (2016). Hemolytic uremic syndrome in children. *Minerva Pediatr., 68*(6), 441-455. [PMID: 27768015]

Tanaka, J., Yamashita, M., Yamashita, M., Kajigaya, H. (1999). Effects of tap water on esophageal burns in dogs from button lithium batteries. *Vet. Hum. Toxicol., 41*(5), 279-282. [PMID: 10509426]

Terés, J., Planas, R., Panes, J., Salmeron, J.M., Mas, A., Bosch, J., Llorente, C., Viver, J., Feu, F., Rodés, J. (1990). Vasopressin/nitroglycerin infusion vs. esophageal tamponade in the treatment of acute variceal bleeding: a randomized controlled trial. *Hepatology, 11*(6), 964-968. [http://dx.doi.org/10.1002/hep.1840110609] [PMID: 2114350]

Thomas, D.E., Elliott, E.J. (2013). Interventions for preventing diarrhea-associated hemolytic uremic syndrome: systematic review. *BMC Public Health, 13*(1), 799. [http://dx.doi.org/10.1186/1471-2458-13-799] [PMID: 24007265]

Tiryaki, Ö. (2005). *İshal yakınmasıyla acil servise başvuran hastalara yaklaşım ve antibiyoterapinin değerlendirilmesi. Dokuz Eylül Üniversitesi. Acil tıp.*. Tez Çalışması.

Tsuchiya, M., Imamura, L., Park, J.B., Kobashi, K. (1995). Helicobacter pylori urease inhibition by rabeprazole, a proton pump inhibitor. *Biol. Pharm. Bull., 18*(8), 1053-1056. [http://dx.doi.org/10.1248/bpb.18.1053] [PMID: 8535394]

Tsutsui, N., Taneike, I., Ohara, T., Goshi, S., Kojio, S., Iwakura, N., Matsumaru, H., Wakisaka-Saito, N., Zhang, H.M., Yamamoto, T. (2000). A novel action of the proton pump inhibitor rabeprazole and its thioether derivative against the motility of Helicobacter pylori. *Antimicrob. Agents Chemother., 44*(11), 3069-3073. [http://dx.doi.org/10.1128/AAC.44.11.3069-3073.2000] [PMID: 11036024]

Uhlich, G.A., Sinclair, J.R., Warren, N.G., Chmielecki, W.A., Fratamico, P. (2008). Characterization of Shiga toxin-producing Escherichia coli isolates associated with two multistate food-borne outbreaks that occurred in 2006. *Appl. Environ. Microbiol., 74*(4), 1268-1272. [http://dx.doi.org/10.1128/AEM.01618-07] [PMID: 18083883]

Uyar, Y., Taylan Ozkan, A. (2009). [Antigen detection methods in diagnosis of amebiasis, giardiasis and cryptosporidiosis]. *Turkiye Parazitol. Derg., 33*(2), 140-150. [PMID: 19598091]

Wada, Y., Matsui, T., Matake, H., Sakurai, T., Yamamoto, J., Kikuchi, Y., Yorioka, M., Tsuda, S., Yao, T., Yao, S., Haraoka, S., Iwashita, A. (2003). Intractable ulcerative colitis caused by cytomegalovirus infection: a prospective study on prevalence, diagnosis, and treatment. *Dis. Colon Rectum, 46*(10) (Suppl.), S59-S65. [PMID: 14530660]

Wang, H., Kanthan, R. (2020). Multiple colonic and ileal perforations due to unsuspected intestinal amoebiasis-Case report and review. *Pathol. Res. Pract., 216*(1), 152608. [http://dx.doi.org/10.1016/j.prp.2019.152608] [PMID: 31564573]

Wang, Z., Du, Z., Zhou, X., Chen, T., Li, C. (2020). Misdiagnosis of peripheral abscess caused by duodenal foreign body: a case report and literature review. *BMC Gastroenterol., 20*(1), 236. [http://dx.doi.org/10.1186/s12876-020-01335-7] [PMID: 32703254]

Webb, W.A. (1995). Management of foreign bodies of the upper gastrointestinal tract: update. *Gastrointest. Endosc., 41*(1), 39-51. [http://dx.doi.org/10.1016/S0016-5107(95)70274-1] [PMID: 7698623]

Whelan, K., Myers, C.E. (2010). Safety of probiotics in patients receiving nutritional support: a systematic review of case reports, randomized controlled trials, and nonrandomized trials. *Am. J. Clin. Nutr., 91*(3), 687-703.

[http://dx.doi.org/10.3945/ajcn.2009.28759] [PMID: 20089732]

World Health Organization. The World Health Report 2018: Turkey Household Health Research: Noncontagious Diseases Prevalence of Risk Factors, 2017: World Health Organization. (2017). https://www.who.int/ncds/surveillance/steps/WHO_Turkey_Risk_Factors_A4_ TR_19.06.2018.pdf

Xie, Y., Zhu, Z., Wang, J., Zhang, L., Zhang, Z., Lu, H., Zeng, Z., Chen, S., Liu, D., Lv, N. (2018). Ten-Day Quadruple Therapy Comprising Low-Dose Rabeprazole, Bismuth, Amoxicillin, and Tetracycline Is an Effective and Safe First-Line Treatment for Helicobacter pylori Infection in a Population with High Antibiotic Resistance: a Prospective, Multicenter, Randomized, Parallel-Controlled Clinical Trial in China. *Antimicrob. Agents Chemother., 62*(9), e00432-e18.
[http://dx.doi.org/10.1128/AAC.00432-18] [PMID: 29914954]

Xu, X.Y., Ding, H.G., Li, W.G., Jia, J.D., Wei, L., Duan, Z.P., Liu, Y.L., Ling-Hu, E.Q., Zhuang, H., Hepatology, C.S.O., Association, C.M. (2019). Chinese guidelines on management of hepatic encephalopathy in cirrhosis. *World J. Gastroenterol., 25*(36), 5403-5422.
[http://dx.doi.org/10.3748/wjg.v25.i36.5403] [PMID: 31576089]

Yang, H., Pan, C., Liu, Q., Wang, Y., Liu, Z., Cao, X., Lei, J. (2020). Correlation between the Glasgow-Blatchford score, shock index, and Forrest classification in patients with peptic ulcer bleeding. *Turk. J. Med. Sci., 50*(4), 706-712.
[http://dx.doi.org/10.3906/sag-1906-154] [PMID: 32041384]

Yilmaz, S., Karcioglu, O., Dikme, O. (2021). Pre- and post-training changes in the test-ordering behavior of the emergency physicians in the management of adults with acute gastroenteritis. *Signa Vitae, 17*(6), 37-42.
[http://dx.doi.org/10.22514/sv.2021.091]

Zhang, H., Yang, Z., Ni, Z., Shi, Y. (2017). A Meta-Analysis and Systematic Review of the Efficacy of Twice Daily PPIs *versus* Once Daily for Treatment of Gastroesophageal Reflux Disease. *Gastroenterol. Res. Pract., 2017*, 9865963.
[http://dx.doi.org/10.1155/2017/9865963] [PMID: 28912807]

Zou, D., Goh, K.L. (2017). East Asian perspective on the interaction between proton pump inhibitors and clopidogrel. *J. Gastroenterol. Hepatol., 32*(6), 1152-1159.
[http://dx.doi.org/10.1111/jgh.13712] [PMID: 28024166]

Zulfiqar, H., Mathew, G., Horrall, S. Amebiasis 2022. *StatPearls [Internet]. Treasure Island (FL): StatPearls Publishing; 2022.*
[PMID: 30137820]

CHAPTER 5

Specific Diagnoses and Management Principles of the Intestines and Lower Digestive Canal

Abstract: Acute appendicitis, visceral perforations, diverticulitis (including bleeding and abscesses) acute calculous cholecystitis, acute ischemic bowel, mesenteric artery ischemia and infarction can cause acute abdominal conditions which prompt emergency interventions. Inflammatory bowel diseases (ulcerative colitis and Crohn's disease) may be followed up in some time without remarkable complications, although at some point with abscesses, hemorrhagic diarrhea and acute abdominal syndromes. However, the differential diagnosis (DD) of patients presenting with acute abdominal pain is much broader than this, including many benign conditions as well. Some etiologies of abdominal pain such as cholangitis strangulated hernias, colonic diverticulitis, perianal/ perirectal abscesses and fistulas may progress and turn into life-threatening conditions like abdominal sepsis without proper management.

Keywords: Acute abdominal pain, Anal abscess, Anal fistula, Acute appendicitis, Colonic diverticulitis, Surgical abdomen, Visceral perforation.

ACUTE APPENDICITIS (AAP)

(Information is also Provided in the Introductory Chapters)

It is one of the most common causes of acute AP and undoubtedly the most common etiology of surgical acute abdominal syndromes. Diagnosis becomes difficult at the extremes of age and during pregnancy. There are certain diagnostic misdiagnosis rates at all ages. It can be confused with many entities, causing missed or delayed diagnoses. PID in women and ureteral stones in men are the most common misdiagnoses.

History: AP with severe, colicky pain in the middle of the abdomen often accompanied by nausea and vomiting is the classic history of onset. Pain that migrates to the right iliac fossa, a.k.a. McBurney point after a certain period is typical, although not the rule.

Ozgur KARCIOGLU, Selman YENİOCAK, Mandana HOSSEINZADEH & Seckin Bahar SEZGIN

A substantial proportion of atypical presentations are recorded. Some patients present with diarrhea or dysuria/pollakiuria. The location of appendix affects this situation (retrocecal 74%; pelvic 21%; paracecal 2%; others 3%).

EXAMINATION

While there may be few or subtle findings in the early stage in AAp, a patient with a poor general condition, septic shock or generalized peritonitis may be encountered in the advanced stage. In patients between these two extremes, fever, tachycardia, decreased/loss of appetite, guarding in the right lower quadrant, Rovsing sign, tenderness in the rectal exam in the right and proximal (close to the appendix) part can be noted. It should be known that the findings will not be apparent and definite in cases with plastron appendicitis. Especially in elderly patients, ambiguous findings, subfebrile temperature, moderate pain, and palpable mass may be noted (Table **1**).

Table 1. The predictive values (pooled likelihood ratios) of the findings in the history and examination in diagnosing appendicitis (Andersson, 2004).

Signs/symptoms	Positive likelihood ratio (LR+)	95% confidence interval	Negative likelihood ratio (LR-)	95% confidence interval
Age>= 20	1.25	(1.10–1.42)	0.74	(0.62–0.89)
Male sex	1.62	(1.49–1.76)	0.62	(0.57–0.68)
Vomiting	1.63	(1.45–1.84)	0.75	(0.69–0.80)
Migratory pain	2.06	(1.63–2.60)	0.52	(0.40–0.69)
Indirect tenderness (Rovsing)	2.47	(1.38–4.43)	0.71	(0.65–0.77)
Rectal tenderness	1.03	(0.83–1.27)	0.96	(0.85–1.08)
Psoas sign	2.31	(1.36–3.91)	0.85	(0.76–0.95)
Rebound tenderness	1.99	(1.61–2.45)	0.39	(0.32–0.48)
Percussion tenderness	2.86	(1.95–4.21)	0.49	(0.37–0.63)
Guarding	2.48	(1.60–3.84)	0.57	(0.48–0.68)

The probability of diagnosis of AA can be predicted significantly using the Alvarado score (Table **2**).

Table 2. Alvarado score is a tool recommended to be used in the preliminary diagnosis of appendicitis.

Migrating pain	1 point
Loss of appetite	1 point

(Table 2) cont.....

Nausea or vomiting	1 point
Tenderness in the right iliac fossa	2 point
Indirect tenderness	1 poin
Fever (>37.3C)	1 point
Leukocyte count>10,000/mm3	2 point
Left shift > 75% PNL	1 point
TOTAL	10 point

Descriptions and notes: Eight points and above obtained from Alvarado score indicates AAp in 96%. A score of 0 to 4 excludes AAp. Of note, scoring changes during pregnancy (see the relevant section).

Elderly: 1/3 of operated AAp in the elderly patient is already perforated at the time of diagnosis (Yeo, 2006). Mortality is higher compared to young people, mainly due to delays in treatment resulting from time losses until diagnosis. Pain localization to the right lower quadrant occurs as a late finding in the elderly. Distention mimicking small bowel obstruction is common. Elderly patients have also a higher likelihood to deteriorate due to missed or delayed diagnosis and succumb to sepsis and/or septic shock more commonly.

WORK UP

The presumptive diagnosis of AAp is made by clinical picture and follow-up, and the definitive diagnosis is made by pathological examination. Urine test and pregnancy test must be taken, but USG and CT may be ordered in accord with the patient's condition. Although an increase in leukocytes is usually expected, a diagnosis cannot be made based solely on this, since it will also ensue in other diagnoses such as intra-abdominal abscess or PID. Since leukocyturia may also occur in patients with AAp, a patient with suspected AAp who has not been diagnosed with urinary tract infection (UTI) and whose pain has not resolved should not be discharged.

AAp and CT: MDCT is viewed as the diagnostic modality of choice to diagnose most acute abdominal diseases including AAp. Satisfactory figures of sensitivity (91% to 94%) and specificity (90% to 95%) as a diagnostic study for AAp were achieved, respectively.

How can I Diagnose AAp? Established Criteria are as Follows

An enlarged appendix (greater than 6 mm in diameter)

Wall thickening over 2 mm,

Wall enhancement

Surrounding inflammation evidenced by periappendiceal fat stranding or free fluid.

The presence of an obstructing fecalith may also be present though its absence does not preclude the diagnosis.

There is an ongoing debate on whether the diagnostic cut-off of greater than 6 mm diameter is too small to prevent negative appendectomies. This cut-off may be a suitable value for children; however, many adult patients have normal appendix diameters between 6 to 7 mm. It can be postulated that using a cut-off value of over 7 mm (8.4 mm in one study) can increase the accuracy of CT.

USG exam is undertaken with graded compression and evaluates several factors:

diameter (over 6 mm),

surrounding pericaecal fatty tissues,

periappendiceal inflammation,

free fluid,

reactive lymph nodes,

mural hyperplasia.

Surrounding inflammation is often the most reliable sign of AAp on USG, and the lack of its presence is a robust indicator to rule it out.

A common mimic of AAp on USG is lymphoid hyperplasia, which is a benign condition causing enlargement of the appendiceal diameter, specifically in the lamina propria. The lamina propria can be seen as a hypoechoic later in the innermost of the appendix. If thickened by more than 0.8mm, that is diagnostic of lymphoid hyperplasia, even in the setting of an overall enlarged appendix. This condition is non-operative and typically associated with inflammatory diseases such as viral enteritis.

Second-line USG or CT for AAp? Some studies have reported that around 40% of pediatric cases with suspected AAp underwent a nondiagnostic screening USG and that 15% of this group had been diagnosed with AAp eventually (Schuh 2011, Sulowski 2011, Schuh 2015). Accordingly, some authors advocated that a second-line USG will be a noninvasive, radiation-free, practical and repeatable approach to enhance the diagnostic strength in the emergency setting.

In a meta-analytic study, pooled sensitivities and specificities of second-line US for diagnosis of AAp in children were 91.3% (95% CI: 83.8%, 95.5%) and 95.2% (91.8%-97.3%), respectively; and in adults, the pooled sensitivities and specificities were 83.1% (70.3% - 91.1%) and 90.9% (59.3% - 98.6%), respectively (Eng, 2018).

Regarding second-line CT in children, the pooled sensitivities and specificities were 96.2% (95% CI: 93.2%, 97.8%) and 94.6% (95% CI: 92.8%, 95.9%); and in adults, the pooled sensitivities and specificities were 89.9% (95% CI: 85.4%, 93.2%) and 93.6% (95% CI: 91.2%, 95.3%), respectively.

How to distinguish a tumor in the appendiceal tissue? CT has a diagnostic sensitivity of 95% in symptomatic patients with neoplasms. The use of contrast media, (IV + oral) can help identification and staging tumors. The diagnostic criterion is an enlarged appendix greater than 15 mm in diameter, characteristics of cystic dilatation, or a soft tissue mass (Kim, 2018). Specifically, if a neuroendocrine tumor is suspected, one would look for a very small (less than 1 cm) submucosal mass in the distal appendix, which enhances significantly with or without calcifications.

When investigating for neoplasm, mucoceles may also be visible on ultrasound. They appear as an ovoid cystic mass with variable echogenicity. Typically, they will have concentric echogenic layers ("onion skin"), acoustic shadowing from mural calcifications, and the appendix will be pear-shaped (Jones, 2021). They can also demonstrate regional adenopathy, fat stranding, and free fluid (Kim, 2018).

Case presentation. Forty-year-old woman presented to the ED due to right-lower quadrant pain, nausea and fever lasting for five days (Fig. **1**).

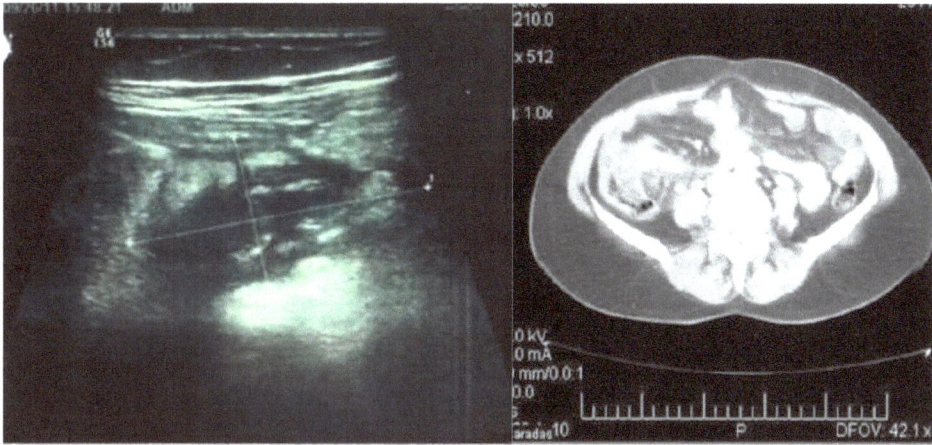

Fig. (1). A. Abdominal USG image depicts pericecal fluid accumulation surrounding with omentum. B. Axial tomographic image demonstrates pericecal fat tissue and fecal inflammatory changes.

Can we use MRI for AAp? Regarding second-line MRI in children, pooled sensitivities and specificities were 97.4% (95% CI: 85.8%, 100%) and 97.1% (95% CI: 92.1%, 99.0%); and in adults, the pooled sensitivities and specificities were 89.9% (95% CI: 84.8%, 93.5%) and 93.6% (95% CI: 90.9%, 95.5%), respectively (Eng, 2018).

It appears that second-line USG, CT, and MRI have comparable and high accuracy in helping to diagnose AAp in both children and adults, including pregnant women.

In a recent study, Repplinger *et al*. analyzed and compared the sensitivity and specificity of MRI and CT in establishing a diagnosis of AAp in adolescents and adults (>12 years) ((Repplinger, 2018). Likelihood of AAp was scored on a five-point scale for imaging *via* both CT and MR.

Five-point Scale

1 = definitely not,

2 = probably not,

3 = not sure/possibly,

4 = probably,

5 = definitely

The figures were 96.9% and 81.3% for MRI and 98.4% and 89.6% for CT, respectively, when a cutoff point of 3 or higher was used. The positive and negative likelihood ratios were 5.2 and 0.04 for MR imaging and 9.4 and 0.02 for CT, respectively. Analysis revealed that the optimal cutoff point to maximize accuracy was 4 or higher, at which point there was no difference between MR imaging and CT (Repplinger, 2018).

MRI is commonly used for the pregnant and pediatric populations due to the lack of ionizing radiation. The study is typically accomplished without contrast. It has a sensitivity of 96% to 86% and specificity of 96% to 97% in evaluating for AAp, though it has been shown to be slightly more effective in identifying the appendix in adults versus children (Jones, 2021).

In brief, the **diagnostic accuracy** of MRI was similar to that of CT for the diagnosis of AAp, although the decisions as to which one should be prioritized need to be based on individual characteristics, institutional capabilities, cost-effectiveness, radiation and other factors.

Differential Diagnosis

There is a wide list of DD from UTI to PID, from diverticulitis to biliary tract diseases and complications of pregnancy. When history and examination are meticulously done, we narrow this list and request laboratory investigations accordingly. It is most easily diagnosed in young men. Difficulty increases in women, pregnant women, elderly, and immunosuppressed individuals.

AAp is best masqueraded as caecal diverticulitis (CDiv) without doubt. CDiv is a rare condition that can easily be misdiagnosed as AAp due to similar signs and symptoms (Uhe, 2021). The most frequent symptoms of CDiv were noted as right iliac fossa pain (93.2%), nausea and/or vomiting (35.4%) and fever (26.9%) which can easily be mixed up with AAp. The entity can result in unnecessary surgical exploration.

Stump appendicitis (SApp) can be encountered following laparoscopic appendectomy. It can result in high morbidity due to delayed diagnosis. A systematic review revealed that most SA (98.7%) underwent surgery: 52% by laparoscopic approach and 36% through an open approach. Stump appendectomy was performed in 94.4% of cases with SApp and an extended resection in 5.6% (Casas, 2021).

Treatment

Although it varies according to the center it has been studied, 10% to 15% (-) appendectomy rate, that is, the percentage of reporting pathologically normal appendices is expected. With proper use of CT, this rate drops to around 5% but never zero. The recurrence rate is 5% to 10% in non-operative management protocols.

- Since most of the patients are dehydrated, IV fluids should be given.
- Administer IV opioids and antiemetics (*e.g.* ondansetron 8 mg for the whole group, or slow IV metoclopramide 10 mg if decreased bowel sound/paralytic ileus is suspected).
- If AAp is suspected, discontinue oral intake and consult the patient with surgery. Pre-operative broad-spectrum antibiotics can be administered should the benign entities be ruled out or the operation is pending.

Non-operative management of AAp (NOMAAp) was evaluated in studies before and during COVID-19 era. They concluded that NOMAAp'in the setting of COVID-19 is viewed as a safe temporary strategy instead of operative interventions with acceptable failure rates and complications (Emile, 2021).

ANTIBIOTICS FOR AAP: A REAL REMEDY?

Studies suggested that localized AAp can be managed successfully with appropriate antibiotic regimens in a controlled environment. In a systematic review, including nearly 3000 patients by Talan *et al.* pointed out that patients with AAp between 5 and 50 years of age without evidence of abscess, phlegmon, or tumor have been treated with antibiotic regimens consistent with intra-abdominal infection treatment guidelines for 7 to 10 days (Talan, 2019). Initial response rates were higher than 90% and most participants improved by 24 to 48 hours, without any recorded severe sepsis or deaths.

Which antibiotics are best to manage AAp? A meta-analysis disclosed that surgery significantly increased one-year treatment success, compared with cephalosporins [OR: 16.79; 95% credible interval: 3.8-127.64] or β-lactam/--lactamase inhibitor combinations (OR: 19.99; 95% credible interval: 4.87-187.57), but not carbapenems (OR: 3.50, 95% credible interval: 0.55-38.63) (Wang, 2021). In contrast, carbapenems were associated with fewer treatment-related complications compared with surgery (OR: 0.12; 95% credible interval: 0.01-0.85). In conclusion, carbapenems can be recommended as the initial antibiotic regimen for the non-operative management of adult patients with AAp.

Acute Epiploic Appendagitis (AEA)

AEA is a benign condition of the epiploic appendix that is often self-limiting. Adipose tissue and blood vessels are the main frames of the structure. It is a pedunculated, paracolic fatty lesion. There are hundreds of epiploic appendages at the antimesenteric colonic border, and primary inflammation of any can present with acute abdomen.

On the other hand, "intraperitoneal focal fat infarction" (IFFI) defines various benign conditions precipitated by focal fatty tissue necrosis. Most patients with IFFI involve torsion or infarction of the greater omentum or the epiploic appendages (Lazaridou, 2021). IFFI clinically may mimic other pathologies, such as AAp or diverticulitis.

AEA mostly presents with sudden onset pain in the left lower quadrant of the abdomen. The diagnosis is made at the age of 40, on average. The most common localization is the proximity of the sigmoid colon.

The patient is usually non-febrile and the leukocyte count may be normal. It is most often diagnosed at laparotomy, but typical findings can be noticed if CT is performed first.

In the DD, most attention should be paid to omental torsion, acute diverticulitis and AAp.

USG and CT have a high sensitivity and specificity for the diagnosis of AEA and IFFI. Contrast-enhanced CT is the most sensitive tool for diagnosis (Fig. **2**). The structure next to the colon with fatty attenuation called the "ring sign", is the typical appearance. If ultrasound is performed, a *hypoechoic* halo may be observed around the small oval, uncompressed *hyperechoic* structure, but it is not a rule.

Treatment is often conservative. In most cases, the clinical evolution is self-limiting, thus helping to reduce the need for unnecessary surgeries.

Omental Infarct (OI)

Although primary OI is not a common cause of AP, it is an emergency situation that causes significant morbidity. Since the first case was reported in 1899, more than 300 cases have been published (Charieg, 2016).

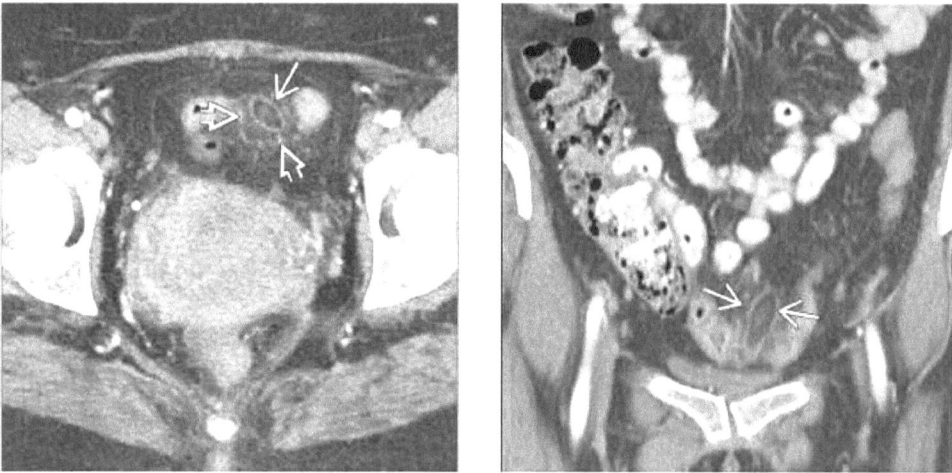

Fig. (2). A. Axial contrast-enhanced CT section shows a well-circumscribed fatty mass with soft tissue attenuation adjacent to the sigmoid colon (arrow). There are also fatty streaks in the surrounding adipose tissues (hollow thick arrows). **B.** Coronal contrast-enhanced CT section of the same patient shows a well-defined longitudinal fatty mass with soft tissue attenuation adjacent to the sigmoid colon (arrows).

It develops as a result of decreased blood flow to the omentum. It should be noted that OI is also in the DD list of other acute AP etiologies. With the widespread use of CT, intra-abdominal AEA, fat infarction, or segmental OI are increasingly being diagnosed. The male/female ratio for OI is around 3.5.

Most cases are among obese and male people between 30 and 50 years old (Vagholkar, 2016).

OI may emerge primarily, as well as secondary to causes such as hernia, hypercoagulation, and vascular pathologies. The etiology of primary OI remains unknown. However, obesity, post-meal venous congestion, trauma and hypercoagulability are among the risk factors. OI may also accompany torsion of the omentum.

Two different pathological mechanisms have been pointed out for OI: (1) vascular pedicle torsion on its own axis, and (2) thrombotic processes due to hypercoagulable states or circulatory stasis. Both situations lead to a vascular compromise of the omental tissues, producing haemorrhagic extravasation, with bloody fluid, necrosis and adhesions (Breunung, 2009).

The presentation is usually on the right side (lower+-upper quadrant), with a sudden onset, localized, progressively worsening acute AP. Nausea and vomiting are not usually seen.

Examination findings vary. Tenderness and rebound tenderness is mostly noted in the right upper/lower quadrants. If there is a torsion involving a large segment of the right omental tissues, there may be a palpable mass. Mild fever and leukocytosis may occur but are not the rule.

Since most cases with OI are started at the right side of the omentum, OI can be confused with AAp, cholecystitis, diverticulitis, Meckel's diverticulum (MD) and urolithiasis. The diagnosis is often established during the operation in patients who are operated on with the suspicion of AAp. USG and CT findings are distinctive (Figs. **3** and **4**). On USG, a hyperechoic solid mass lesion can be detected beneath the abdominal wall. The disadvantage of USG is its low sensitivity, for the fatty lesion in the omentum can easily be confused with the intra-abdominal adipose tissue.

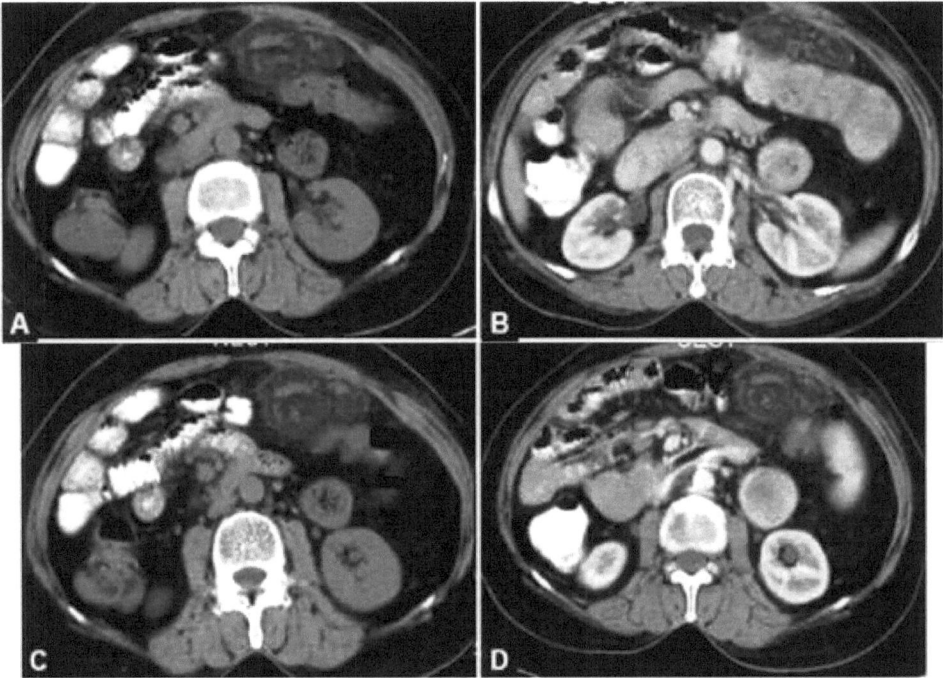

Fig. (3). It is noteworthy that in non-contrast (**A**, **C**) and contrast enhanced (**B**, **D**) axial abdominal CT scans, oval-shaped, non-enhancing fat density is visualized on the left periumbilical region with a size of 5.5x3 cm (arrow). It is also noted that fatty streaks increase in neighboring structures.

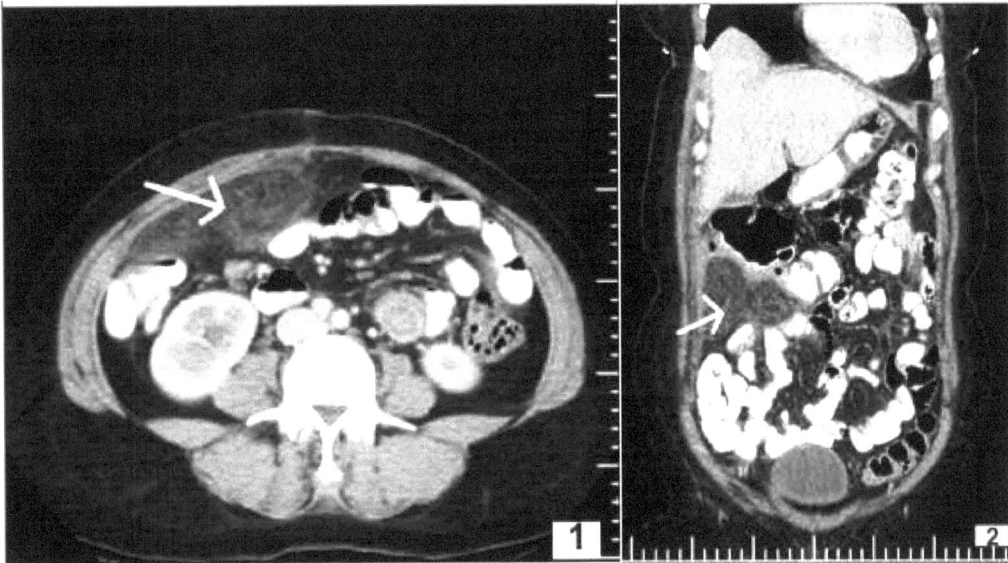

Fig. (4). Omental infarct image on axial and coronal sections in IV + oral contrast-enhanced tomography.

Treatment includes analgesia and general supportive care. Since OI is self-limited, conservative treatment is primarily recommended. Unnecessary operations should be avoided with an early and accurate diagnosis by performing appropriate imaging studies in patients with suspected OI.

In a recent systematic review, Medina-Gallardo *et al.* analysed 90 articles including 146 patients diagnosed with OI following CT evaluation (Medina-Gallardo *et al*, 2020). A majority (73.3%) of the patients received conservative treatment with a failure rate of 15.9% (patients needing surgery) and 26.7% underwent surgery at the initial phase. The mean length of stay in the hospital was significantly longer for the conservative treatment group compared to the surgery group (5.1 *vs.* 2.5 days, p = 0.00). Younger age and leukocytosis ($\geq$12000/μl) predicted the failure of the conservative treatment arm.

It can be postulated that surgery appears to have advantages in regard to the length of stay in the hospital.

INTESTINAL OBSTRUCTION, ILEUS

It can be mechanical or paralytic/functional.

Paralytic ileus comes to the ED more rarely than mechanical bowel obstruction (MBO). **Postoperative ileus** and electrolyte disturbances such as hypokalemia are common causes of paralytic ileus. MBO occurs 80% in the small intestine (SBO) and 20% in the colon. A majority of colonic obstructions are due to cancer (70%) and recurrent diverticulitis (10%).

Mortality is around 10% in intestinal obstruction, but it increases to 30% with ischemia-perforation (Reddy, 2017). The severity of the obstruction is determined by the level of obstruction and the physiological reserves of the patient.

MBO Basically Develops in Three Ways

- external pressure (adhesions and hernias),
- Bowel wall-related causes (tumor, inflammation, edema, infection),
- intraluminal obstruction (stones, fecalomas, intussusception)

Causes of Mechanical Obstruction

- Brids and adhesions
- Obstructed hernias: inguinal, femoral, paraumbilical, incisional.
- Cancer.
- Volvulus (most common: sigmoid)
- Inflammatory mass (diverticular disease, Crohn's disease).
- Peptic ulcer disease.
- Gallstone ileus.
- Intussusception.

Adhesions: Congenital or acquired, incomplete or complete, and single-band or matted adhesions can cause SBO. Congenital adhesions which are mostly asymptomatic and present as an incidental finding in all ages (Liakakos, 2001). These form during organogenesis are rarely encountered (3%) (Bruggmann, 2010).

Single-band adhesions (SBA) are <1 cm long and >1 cm in diameter and compress the bowel externally to develop SBO.

SBA causes bowel ischemia (BI) and complete ileus much more commonly than matted-bands. Matted adhesions are multiple, dense, and tangled, and cause SBO through intestinal kinking or torsion (Tong, 2020). This type of adhesions conveys an augmented risk of perforation, and earlier recurrence (Delabrousse, 2009). Two points along a segment of the bowel can be obstructed at a single point which is known as closed-loop obstruction which is accompanied by higher risks of strangulation and infarction with a mortality risk between 10% and 35% (Pothiawala, 2012, Hellebrekers 2011).

Abdominopelvic surgery constitutes a majority (85%) of peritoneal injuries causing local inflammation which eventually results in intraabdominal adhesions, followed by peritonitis, endometriosis, and radiation (Tong, 2020). Partial ileus a.k.a. incomplete obstruction allows passage of fluid and gas to some extent which produces milder signs and symptoms when compared to complete ileus which gives no way to fluid or gas to the distal parts of the bowels (Osada, 2012) (Fig. **5**).

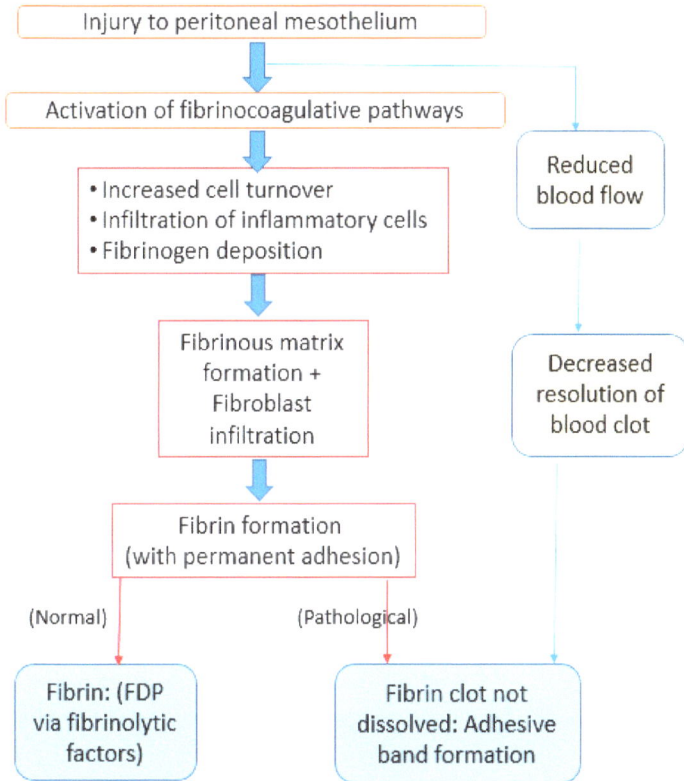

Fig. (5). Pathogenesis of acquired adhesions in the small bowel.

Ogilvie's syndrome defines acute colonic pseudo-obstruction (ACPOOS) in which bowel transition time is prolonged without apparent mechanical obstruction. The main etiology is decreased or uncoordinated colonic muscle contractions. Marked dilatations can be recorded in colon and/or small bowel. Various risk factors have been cited in the literature (Table **3**).

Table 3. A patient with ACPOOS always has one or more of the following risk factors.

• Antikinetic drugs (calcium channel blockers, anticholinergics, phenothiazines, anti-Parkinsonian agents);
• Severe electrolyte disturbances;
• C-reactive protein >75 mg/L
• Neurological diseases: Parkinsonism, diabetic neuropathy:
• Thyroid disease;
• Major acute medical illnesses (coronary artery disease, major operations)

Clinical condition of the patients with intestinal obstruction are generally worse off than those with ACPOOS. The transition point is not visible. Intestinal obstruction can be differentiated from ACPOOS by the predominance of small bowel dilatation and the absence of rectal air image.

Examination and Evaluation in a Patient Suspected to have MBO

In the typical patient, crampy AP, distention, vomiting, and inability to pass gas and stool are expected. If the pain is continuous and progressive rather than cramping/colicky, ischemia and perforation should be considered first. The localization of the obstruction determines the severity of complaints and findings. The more proximal occlusion, the earlier symptoms appear. In the colonic obstruction, except for volvulus, the findings develop more slowly. More severe pain than expected suggests vascular pathology, *e.g.*, ischemia (such as strangulated hernia). Fecaloid vomiting occurs in distal obstruction.

Fever and dehydration should be noted. Fever is a poor prognostic finding. Some patients may present with hypovolemic or septic shock. Operation scars should be searched for. Peritoneal findings are not expected. If there is evidence of peritonitis / guarding/ rigidity, it becomes clear that there is a "surgical" abdomen.

There may be markedly increased bowel sounds in mechanical obstructions, especially in the initial phase, while there may be no bowel sounds in paralytic ileus. It should be known that this finding is nonspecific and does not lead to a specific etiological diagnosis. For example, after orthopedic injuries and operations, hypoperistalsis may develop with being bedridden.

Areas of tympanism or dullness on examination should be noted. Although tenderness is common, the involved area does not correlate with the location of the obstruction. The rectum may be empty on exam, but the reverse does not exclude the diagnosis. Fecal impaction and obstruction with fecaloma is common in elderly patients and should be evacuated if such a situation exists.

Cancer patients present special challenges because even the distinction between mechanical and paralytic ileus can be difficult. Findings suggestive of malignancy such as palpable abdominal mass(es) and hepatomegaly should be sought. Lymphadenopathies such as, Virchow's nodule (right supraclavicular LAP) are also clues for malignancy. In addition, LAP should be sought in periumbilical, inguinal and other areas, even if without a complaint.

When perforation occurs as a result of obstruction or for another reason (Crohn's disease, malignancy, *etc.*), findings indicative of peritonitis such as widespread guarding and rigidity will ensue.

X-ray: Chest X-ray (CXR) and supine/decubitus abdominal X-ray can be an inexpensive and practical first test to screen for obstruction. It should be known that the findings will not be sensitive and specific. Direct CT may also be requested, since further examination will be performed in almost every patient with suspected obstruction. Enlargement of the intestinal loops and multiple large air-fluid levels are typical on radiographs. The appearance of air (pneumobilia) in the biliary tree is a non-negotiable operative indication. Intestinal passage radiograph taken with oral iodinated contrast (Gastrografin) is an approach that can have both diagnostic and therapeutic uses (Branco, 2010).

Abdominal USG can reveal the presence of both free fluid and incarcerated hernia performed as POCUS at the bedside or radiology unit. Aerial images of the distended abdomen make it difficult to examine well, however, with specific findings such as a blizzard image, it may increase the likelihood the diagnosis of ileus (Table **4**). Various signs have been suggested to indicate increased likelihood of SBO (Fig. **6**) (Rosano, 2021). Nevertheless, tomographic images will be ordered as a diagnostic test before admission in almost all cases.

Table 4. USG criteria to consider small bowel obstruction (SBO).

-	Simple	Decompensated	Complicated
Bowel Loop Diameter	Increased	Increased	Increased
Parietal Thickness	Normal	Normal or increased	Increased
Valvulae Conniventes	Not thickened	Not thickened	Thickened
Peristalsis	Present and/or Hyperkinetic	Decreased	Absent
Free Fluid	Absent	Present	Present

Abdominal CT: Oral Gastrographin + IV contrast-enhanced CT has high sensitivity and specificity in revealing the etiology of ileus (Table **5**) (Figs. **7 - 9**).

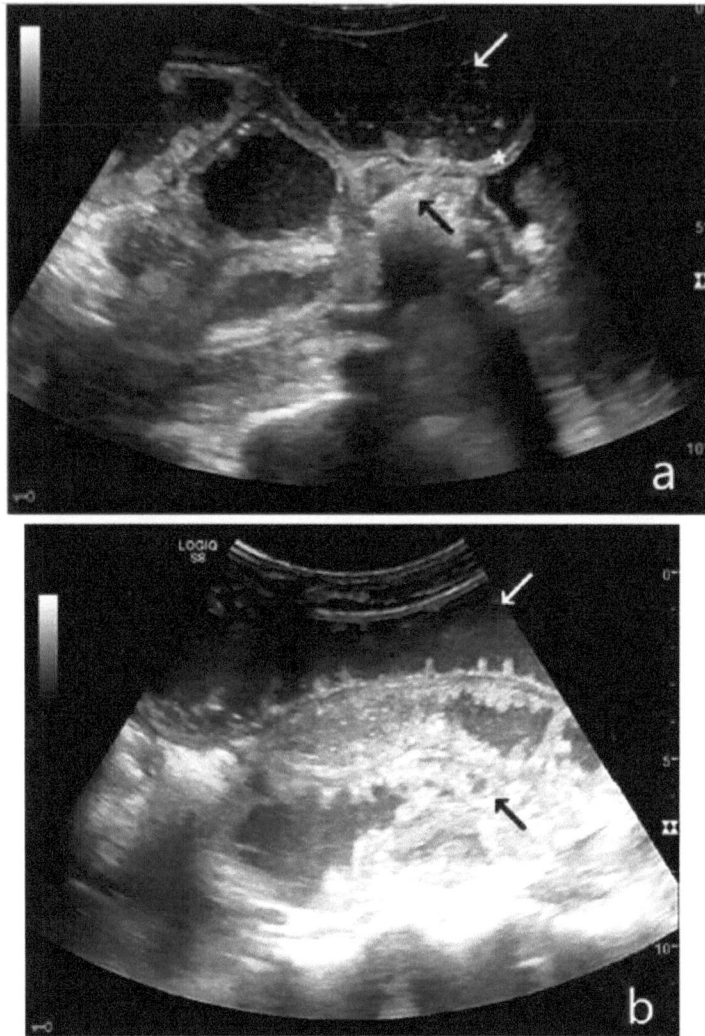

Fig. (6). A patient with severe clinical findings compatible with SBO, exhibiting fluid-filled, dilated intestinal loops with enhanced wall thickening (*) **(a)** and free fluid between bowel loops **(a)**. 'Caliber jump' is a marked increase in caliber between the swollen loops seen proximally (white arrows) **(a,b)** and the collapsed loops distal of the obstruction (black arrows) **(a,b)**.

Whirl sign: Mesenteric vessels and intestinal loops rotate around each other. Therefore, the "beak" appearance emerges. It is a finding suggestive of intestinal volvulus (see relevant section). Patients with this finding undergo operation 25 times more frequently than those without (Duda, 2008).

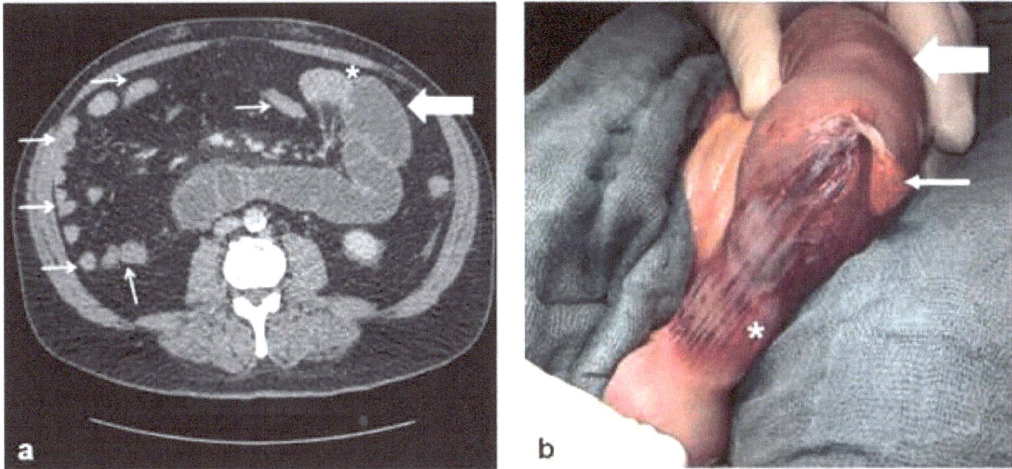

Fig. (7). CT images and intraoperative findings in a patient with mechanical intestinal obstruction: **a)** Prestenotic dilatation (thick arrow) on CT section, sharp diameter change (*), "hungry bowel" distal to stenosis (thin arrows). **b)** The intraoperative view of the same patient, proximally dilated small intestine (thick arrow), adhesion (thin arrow), and the slowly healing bowel segment (*), still hypoperfused due to strangulation due to adhesion.

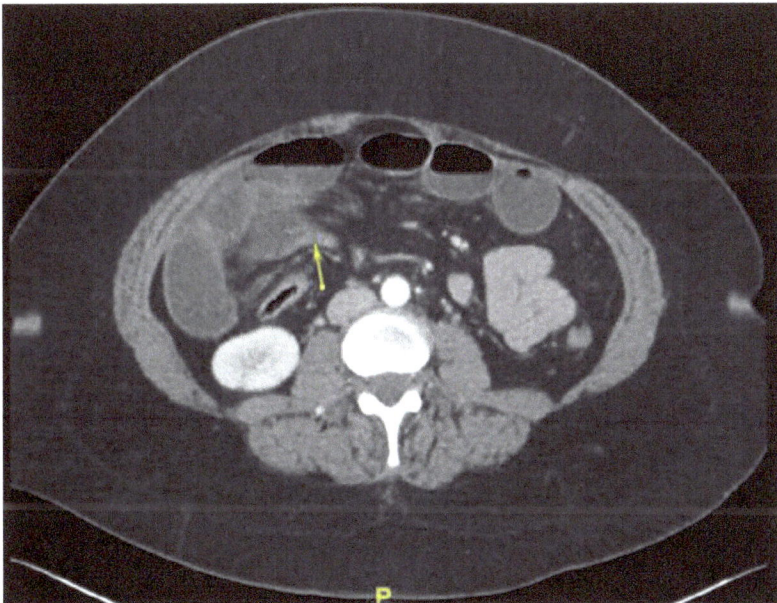

Fig. (8). A woman who had undergone tubal ligation performed more than ten years ago showed signs of small bowel obstruction. The computed tomography scan shows dilated distal jejunal loop with abrupt transition, suggestive of small bowel obstruction. Yellow arrow shows the transition point. (Adapted from Tong 2020).

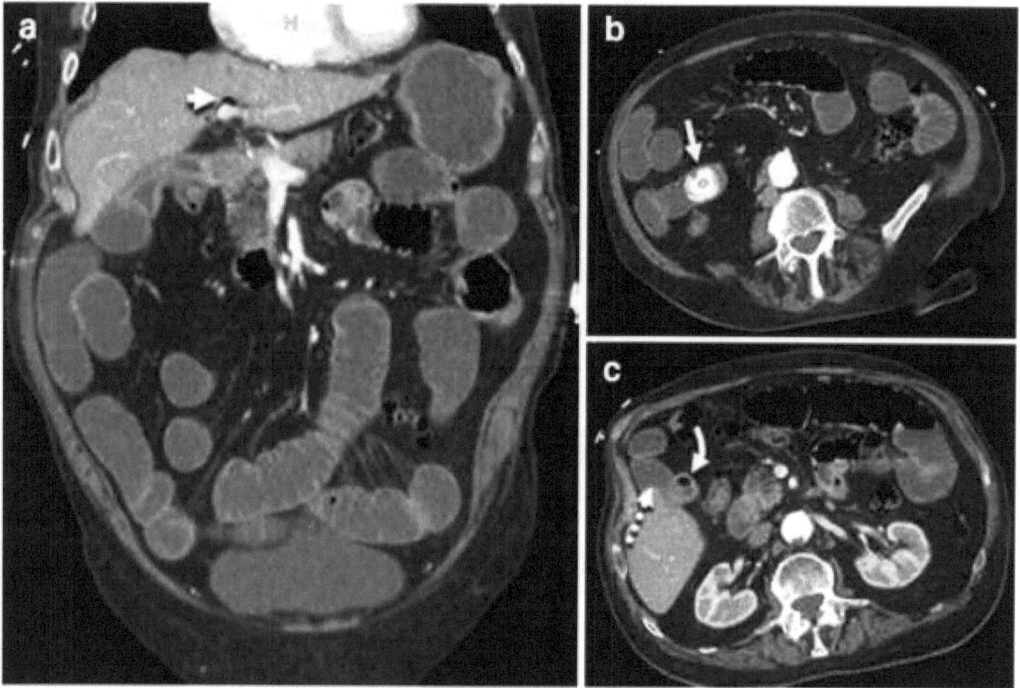

Fig. (9). A 78-year-old man presents with small bowel obstruction caused by gallstones. Contrast-enhanced CT coronal reformatted images **(a)** show fluid-filled small bowel loops and a small image of pneumobilia (arrowhead). Axial contrast-enhanced CT **(b)** high attenuating round intraluminal mass (arrow) in the distal small intestine. A large gallstone is observed in the lumen at the small bowel obstruction transition point. On axial contrast-enhanced CT **(c)**, intraluminal gas in the gallbladder (curved arrow), difficult to discern from the adjacent small intestine (dashed arrow), is consistent with cholecystoenteric fistula. Note: For invagination and intussusception, see. The Chapter "Abdominal pain in children".

Table 5. Tomographic findings suggestive of intestinal ischemia.

1. Mural thickening (>3 mm)
2. Mesenteric edema
3. Fluid in the mesentery and/or peritoneal cavity
4. Marked change in the contrast enhancement in the bowel wall
5. Mesenteric vessel occlusion
6. Mesenteric vein filling
7. Whirl sign
8. Closed-circuit obstruction or volvulus
9. Pneumatosis intestinalis
10. Mesenteric venous gas image
11. Portal venous gas

Laboratory: There is no specific finding suggestive of bowel obstruction. ECG is a *sine qua non* in middle-aged and older patients and ABG should be seen in patients with poor general condition. pH and lactate levels provide information about metabolic acidosis and the severity of the disease. Acidosis and hyperlactatemia also indicate organ hypoperfusion.

Procalcitonin is the most useful test. Values above 0.57 ng/mL predict ischemic bowel in 83% of the instances, while values below this cut-off value exclude the entity in 91% (Cosse C, 2013).

Diagnostic paracentesis should be performed in patients with apparent ascites which can exclude peritonitis. When peritonitis develops with perforation, the neutrophil count in the ascitic fluid becomes >250/mm3, protein > 1 g/dL, and glucose <50 mg/dL (Cappell, 2008).

Hypokalemia suggests functional ileus.

The triad of hypokalemia, hyponatremia, and acidosis is a precursor to ischemic bowel and perforation. BUN and creatinine should be checked. Prerenal and/or renal failure may ensue due to fluid loss and absence of intake. Beta-HCG should be analyzed quantitatively in every female patient of childbearing age presenting with AP.

Table **6** depicts risk factors for strangulation in patients with ileus to be evaluated preoperatively.

Functional/paralytic ileus (FPI): It is the end-product of insufficiency in smooth muscle contraction. Post-op ileus, intra-abdominal or retroperitoneal lesions (tumor, bleeding, infection), opioid or neuroleptic drug use, metabolic ileus (hypokalaemia or diabetes mellitus, vascular ileus (intestinal hypoperfusion) can lead to FPI.

Table 6. Risk factors for strangulation in ileus patients who will undergo surgery (Schwenter, 2010)*.

• AP lasting longer than 4 days
• Peritoneal findings
• C-reactive protein >75 mg/L
• Leukocytes >10,500 μL
• >500 mL free fluid
• Diminished mural contrast-enhancing

*One point is given for each positive criterion in the patient. Scores of 3 and above are 70% sensitive and higher than 90% specific for the presence of strangulation. Therefore, it is considered an indication for emergency surgery (level of evidence: IIa).

Cancer and ileus: Especially cancers of the GIS and female genital organs cause ileus by spreading to the peritoneum. Opiates used for analgesia also pave the way to ileus by slowing bowel movement significantly. In these patients there is a substantial likelihood to develop both paralytic and mechanical ileus. These conditions should be ruled out in every patient with ileus, because paralytic ileus is not an operative indication. Patients should be scanned with contrast-enhanced CT to rule out ischemia, strangulation, perforation, which may be an emergency surgical indication. CT can also delineate the tumor burden at the same timeframe. In cases of proximal stenosis, PEG will be appropriate for drainage, and if there is distal stenosis, dilatation + stent will be appropriate (Laval, 2014).

Management

- Principles in management are fluid resuscitation, correction of electrolyte balance, antibiotic therapy, cessation of oral intake, NG drainage.
- Give O2 and IV fluids (crystalloids) in patients with poor general condition, dehydrated and prone to shock. Attach a Foley catheter and record the urinary output +GI losses with vomiting.
- IV saline infusion is the rule, while lactated Ringer's can be alternative.
- Decompress the stomach with the NG tube which will also prevent aspiration.
- As a bridging treatment in patients with distal stenosis, drainage with a decompressive tube or stent is the best strategy before the last stop-definitive surgery. This approach prevents prestenotic dilatation and may also alleviate ischemia.
- MBOs are often treated surgically, while those with paralytic ileus are rarely operative.
- Although it is thought that surgery is required as early as possible in mechanical ileus, conservative treatment is now an option, especially in small bowel obstructions. It has been reported that ¾ of patients with SBO due to adhesions are treated conservatively (Keenan, 2014).
- Administer IV opioids (morphine/fentanyl) for analgesia and antiemetic agents against vomiting (*e.g.* ondansetron 8 mg or H1 blocker).
- Notify the surgeon. In selected moribund patients, it may be considered to consult the ICU first.

Elective non-operative management has a success rate of 70–90% in patients with brid ileus (Richard, 2013).

Surgical intervention is prompted in individuals with signs and symptoms supported by laboratory and radiological evidence attributed to ischemia, strangulation, perforation, peritonitis, or unfavorable follow-up after non-operative management (ten Broek, 2018).

> **A brief motto on the entity can be: "a sun should not both rise and set on an established case of strangulation."**

Management options for patients with adhesive intestinal obstruction were summarized in Table 7.

Table 7. Management options for patients with adhesive intestinal obstruction and their pluses and minuses (Adapted from Tong, 2020).

A. Non-operative management versus operative management.

Benefits	Risks
Accurately predicts need for surgery (98%)	Delay in surgical treatment
Shorter time to resolution	↓Disease-free interval
Shorter length of stay	↑Readmission rate
No effect on need for surgery/ morbidity/ mortality/ recurrence rate	↑Risk of recurrence

B. Laparoscopic adhesiolysis (LAL) versus midline laparotomy with adhesiolysis.

Potential benefits of LAL	Disadvantages of LAL
↓Morbidity, mortality ↓Duration of surgery (by 50%) ↓Postoperative length of stay ↓Adhesion reformation ↓Post-operative complications: pain, wound infection, incisional hernia, pleuropulmonary/ cardiac complications, venous thromboembolism ↓Intraoperative injury to bowel ↓Time to recovery of GI function ↓Overall complications	Difficulty handling bowel loops Higher costs Poor visibility of the cause of obstruction

FACTORS IN FAVOR OF COLOSTOMY

- Dilated prestenotic bowel segment
- Elderly patient with comorbidities
- Surgeon's inadequacy or lack of experience for definitive surgery
- Risks of anastomotic failure
- Prior incontinence
- Peritonitis with perforation
- Sepsis
- End stage/ metastatic cancer
- Those receiving chemotherapy or immunosuppressive therapy
- Rectal stenosis

VOLVULUS

It involves the cecum or sigmoid and is responsible for 1/10 of large bowel obstructions.

Sigmoid volvulus presents with intermittent cramps in the elderly patient. Lower abdominal pain and distension gradually increase without interruption. While some patients are relieved by spontaneous gas and stool passage, other patients progress to strangulation with complete obstruction. Abdominal radiographs typically show a single large and closed loop in the lower left side of the abdomen, so-called 'bent inner tube'.

Notify the surgeon. It can be treated in the early phase with sigmoidoscopy without progression to strangulation. If strangulated, there is no other way than surgery.

Cecal volvulus is mostly seen between 25 and 35 years of age. It mostly presents with complaints suggesting small bowel obstruction.

Abdominal radiographs show a single dilated colon segment close to the midline, accompanied by distention of the small intestines (Fig. **10**). An empty appearance is detected in the distal colon.

Inflammatory Bowel Diseases (IBD)

Ulcerative colitis (UC) is a chronic inflammatory condition characterized by recurrent inflammation limited to the mucosal layer of the colon. It involves the rectum in all patients, but may involve the proximal part of the colon in the ongoing process. It may also present as chest pain, nausea and dyspepsia. Its findings may also resemble those of IBS in the initial stage. It develops most commonly between the ages of 15 and 30.

Crohn's Disease is characterized by transmural inflammation of the bowel walls causing fibrosis and obstruction, resulting in microperforation and sinus tracts that may progress to fistula formation. Crohn's disease most commonly involves the ileum and proximal colon, whilst it can involve anywhere from the mouth to the perianal region.

In patients with IBD, physical examination is often normal, but mild abdominal tenderness and increased bowel sounds may be noted. In patients with constipation, especially in patients who complain of dyssynergic defecation and incomplete emptying, rectal examination should be performed.

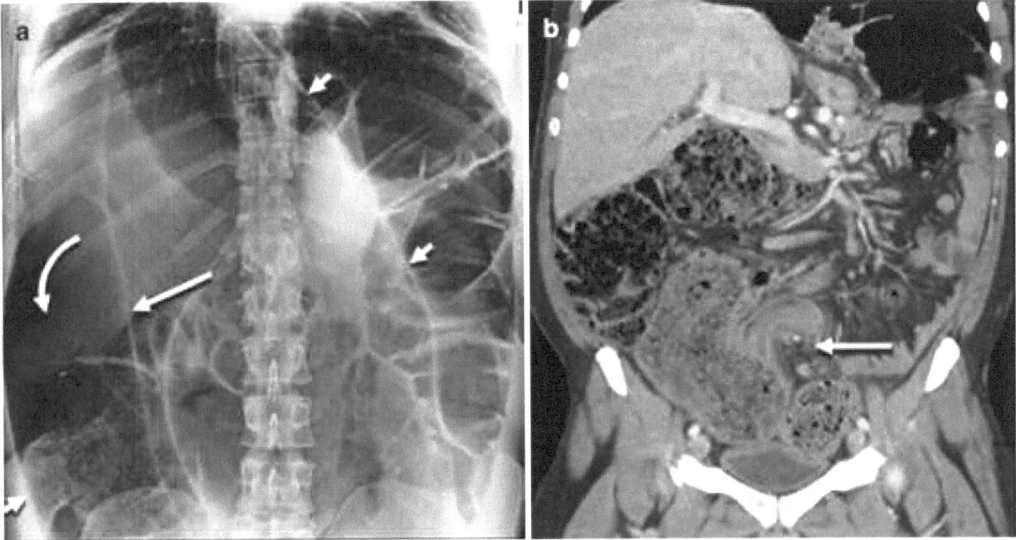

Fig. (10). Sigmoid volvulus in a 68-year-old man. Upright abdominal X-ray **(a)** shows markedly dilated colon shadows in the right upper quadrant in an inverted "U" configuration. The "coffee bean sign" is apparent, the medial walls of the dilated sigmoid colon volvulus form the central cleft (arrow), as the lateral walls of the sigmoid colon make the outer contours of the "coffee bean" (short arrows). Gallstones are visualized in the right part of the abdomen (curved arrow). Contrast-enhanced CT coronal reformat images show **(b)** "beak sign" which is a mesenteric vortex finding in the volvulus region of the mesentery (arrow).

Diagnostic Tests

Serum Markers: Systemic inflammation is investigated with CRP and sedimentation. In the absence of other causes to cause abnormal levels of inflammation markers (infection, rheumatoid arthritis, *etc.*), such a finding indicates intestinal inflammation in patients with IBD associated with AP. However, normal values do not rule out active inflammation.

Fecal Markers of Inflammation: Fecal calprotectin is measured to evaluate intestinal inflammation. Values below 50 mcg/g generally indicate improvement. If above the reference range, ileocolonoscopy or advanced imaging of small bowels are recommended.

Other Stool Studies: In case of acute diarrhea, microbiological stool studies (Clostridium, stool culture *etc.*) are performed. In chronic diarrhea, stool studies for chronic infectious pathogens (Giardia duodenalis, *etc.*) and studies on the risk factors of the patient can be performed (*e.g.*, amebiasis if there is a recent travel history, parasites, *etc.*).

Imaging: Small bowel imaging is performed in patients with Crohn's disease who are suspected to have active small bowel inflammation, if the process cannot be evidenced by ileocolonoscopy and biopsy. Colonic shortening is typical in chronic UC. Although the diagnostic sensitivity of X-ray images is low, specific findings such as the "lead pipe scene" are highly valuable and reliable (Fig. **11**). Inflammation is common in the distal 5 to 25 cm of the ileum (backwash ileitis).

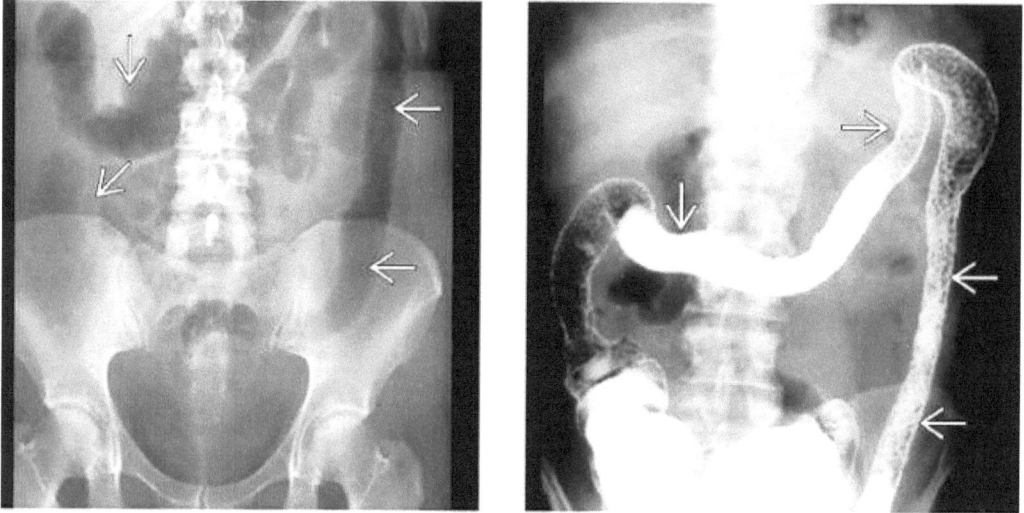

Fig. (11). "The lead pipe appearance". **A.** On plain abdominal X-ray, gas content of the narrowed colon is seen without any indentations and haustral signs (arrow). This finding is called the "lead pipe scene" suggestive of UC. **B.** abdominal X-ray after ingestion of Barium enema shows a narrowed colon without haustral signs and indentations (arrow). Small filling defects are seen (pseudopolyps and granular mucosa).

In the UC, proctitis is defined by a thickness of rectal valve exceeding 6.5 mm or its absence in double-contrast enema studies.

Diffuse colonic thickening and a wall thickness of <10 mm on abdominal CT are typical for UC.

Colorectal Narrowing: Presacral Distance > 1.5 cm is also an Important Finding for UC.

Contrast-enhanced CT: Target or Halo Sign: Inner mucosa is enhanced, middle ring of the submucosa layer is not enhanced, outer ring of the muscularis propria is enhanced.

CT enterography, MRI enterography, capsule endoscopy, or USG are other imaging options. MRI is superior to CT as it does not contain radiation and details stenotic lesions. It can also be performed in pregnant women. Abdominal USG is more acceptable to the patient and does not require preparation, however it is limited due to user dependency and low sensitivity in certain conditions.

MR: Colonic wall thickening (4.7-9.8 mm) is typical and indicates severity.

Ileocolonoscopy is performed together with biopsy. In patients with distal colitis, flexible sigmoidoscopy can be employed instead of colonoscopy.

Tests for constipation-predominant diseases: Plain abdominal X-ray, gastrointestinal USG are used to investigate stool load, especially in patients with UC.

Differential Diagnosis

Celiac Disease: Often bloodless diarrhea, malabsorption findings such as iron deficiency

Infectious diarrhea: History of travel to endemic areas

Lactose malabsorption: Respiratory hydrogen test

Small bowel bacterial overcolonization: Intestinal hypomotility, previous surgery

Bile acid diarrhea: diarrhea after cholecystectomy

Pancreatic exocrine insufficiency: Fecal elastase test

IBD as a Manifestation of "HLA B27 Syndromes"

IBD may be a harbinger of a *de novo* enteropathic arthritis or occur later in the disease course. Attention is necessary to any changes in bowel habits and hematochezia. Additionally, many patients may experience subtle inflammation of the bowels, hard to distinguish in the early phases. In addition, patients may develop non-radiographic axial spondyloarthritis, with symptom severity equal to radiographically evident disease. The presence of inflammatory features, including an elevated C reactive protein and abnormal MRI short tau inversion recovery (STIR) imaging, is used to detect inflammatory changes, particularly in patients with non-diagnostic plain film imaging (Parameswaran, 2021). A traditional finding on late presenters is a "bamboo" spine with advanced spinal fusion.

Treatment

The essential aim of the treatment is to relieve the complaints. Lifestyle change is important. Mild to moderate exercise improves well-being in these patients. In persistent cases who do not benefit from these former interventions, pharmacotherapy is employed to relieve their complaints. A fiber diet is recommended in patients with symptoms of constipation. A lactose-restricted diet is recommended for those with complaints related to lactose-containing foods.

In remission IBD with functional complaints, a diet low in slowly absorbed, indigestible short-chain carbohydrates, fermented oligosaccharides, disaccharides, monosaccharides and polyols (low-FODMAP) is recommended (Staudacher, 2017).

While antidiarrheal agents (*e.g.*, loperamide 6-8 mg/day) can be used in patients with diarrhea, it is not used in patients with active mucosal inflammation or apparent infection. Antispasmodics (eg dicyclomine, hyoscyamine) and tricyclic antidepressants (imipramine 10-25 mg/day or amitriptyline 10-25 mg/day) can be used in patients with diarrhea- predominant complaints accompanied by AP.

Management in Pediatric IBD: Current therapies in pediatric Inflammatory Bowel Diseases (IBD) target the immune system and often fail to sustain long-term remission. A systematic review of antibiotic use in children highlight the lack of evidence in pediatric IBD. In mild-to-moderate Crohn's disease, azithromycin+metronidazole compared to metronidazole alone did not induce a significantly different response (Verburgt, 2021). More evidence must be elicited before drawing firm conclusions in routine practice.

Probiotics: It has been reported that the administration of *Saccharomyces boulardii* as an adjunct to the diet is beneficial against diarrhea seen in Crohn's and UC cases and in preventing and delaying the recurrence of the disease and alleviates the symptoms (Floch *et al.* 2008).

In a randomized controlled study conducted in patients with Crohn's disease, it was found that the colonic permeability of patients receiving Saccharomyces boulardii improved positively and as a result, the risk of bacterial translocation was reduced (Garcia *et al.* 2008).

Antispasmodics can be used in patients without constipation. Low-dose tricyclic antidepressants (amitriptyline 10-25 mg/day, titrated to effect) or selective serotonin reuptake inhibitors (SSRIs) can be used for patients who are not relieved by these. Gabapentin can be used in patients with chronic AP that is not relieved by antidepressants. Opioids should be avoided in patients with IBD because of their effects leading to constipation.

ADMISSION AND DISCHARGE

Patients who are not yet being followed up in the outpatient clinic and newly diagnosed with IBD should be hospitalized or discharged only in accord with the recommendation of a consultant.

Patients with the following criteria should be hospitalized (not to be discharged until thorough evaluation and exclusion of serious conditions):

- Presence of active complaints,
- Unresponsiveness to medication,
- Diarrhea associated with dehydration,
- Bloody diarrhea,
- Fever,
- Poor oral intake,
- Severe abdominal pain and failure of ruling out acute abdomen

Meckel's Diverticulum (MD)

MD is the most common congenital anomaly of the small intestine. MD, the remnant of the vitelline duct from the embryonic life, is a true diverticulum that structurally includes all layers of the small intestine. It can be found in 2 to 3% of the population. It occurs resulting from the failure of the omphalomesenteric duct to close in the intrauterine period, located between 40 to 100 cm proximal to the ileocecal valve and on the antimesenteric surface of the ileum, containing all layers of the intestinal wall, and blooded by the remnant of the vitelline artery. MD is more common in childhood. Most often, male toddlers under the age of two are admitted to the hospital. The presentation can vary from country to country. For example, in a large series from Istanbul, the mean age at presentation was reported as 3.8 years (Çelebi, 2016). Of note, peptic ulcers most commonly occur in the stomach and duodenum though they can occasionally be found in MD (Stern, 2021).

Acid secretion from the ectopic gastric mucosa within the diverticulum can result in GI bleeding associated with AP in patients with MD (An, 2021).

Presentation: MD is often asymptomatic, and when it presents, a complication such as acute diverticulitis, GI bleeding, ileus, bowel perforation must have ensued. It has been reported that only 1 out of 6 MD cases in the USA gives symptoms (Park, 2005). In summary, acute abdomen syndrome is often evident in symptomatic cases. Acute AP in the right lower quadrant and sometimes painless rectal bleeding are the most common presentation forms. If the diagnosis is not established in the early period, serious complications may occur.

Ileal mucosa is often found in MD, but heterotopic gastric, pancreatic, duodenal, and colonic mucosa can also be found. If there is ectopic gastric mucosa in the MD content and the length of MD exceeds 2 cm, the risk of complications is estimated to be high (Groebli, 2001). Ileus and/or invagination due to MD can occur in various forms and is the second most common finding in children after bleeding. Therefore, the physician should rule out these entities in a symptomatic child with manifest findings associated with severe acute AP (Table **8**).

Table 8. The rule of 2s is an important adjunct to remember the main characteristics.

• 2% of the population: prevalence of Meckel diverticulum
• 2% are symptomatic,
• 2 years old or younger,
• 2X females' incidence = males' incidence
• 2 feet (60 cm) proximal to the ileocecal valve,
• 2 inches (5 cm) long or less
• 2 types of the mucosal lining can be found

Diagnosis: Recognition of MD on USG or CT becomes easier after complications develop. Preoperative diagnosis is rare. Images in USG/POCUS can reveal fluid-laden enlarged, non-compressible tubular structure located far from the cecum, pelvic abscess, thickening of the diverticulum wall, and intussusception which expedite the diagnosis. However, in clinical practice, only the presence of intussusception on USG or the presence of MD on scintigraphy obtained after a previous attack has practical significance. Tc-99m pertechnetate scintigraphy is very useful in demonstrating MD including gastric mucosa, but false (+) and (-) results may occur.

MD in adults is more difficult to diagnose. Pre-op diagnosis is extremely difficult and unlikely. Diagnosis and treatment are mostly intraoperative. Abdominal USG and CT often show secondary changes (Figs. **12** and **13**).

In particular, MD is confused with AAp and is identified in patients who underwent laparotomy with this preliminary diagnosis. In a series reported from south-east Turkey, the mean age was 30.7 years (Korkmaz, 2008). The female/male ratio was found to be around 1. The mean length of the diverticulum was 2.9 ± 0.7 cm and no ectopic tissue was found in the histopathological examination. The overall morbidity and mortality rates were 18.5% and 3.7%, respectively.

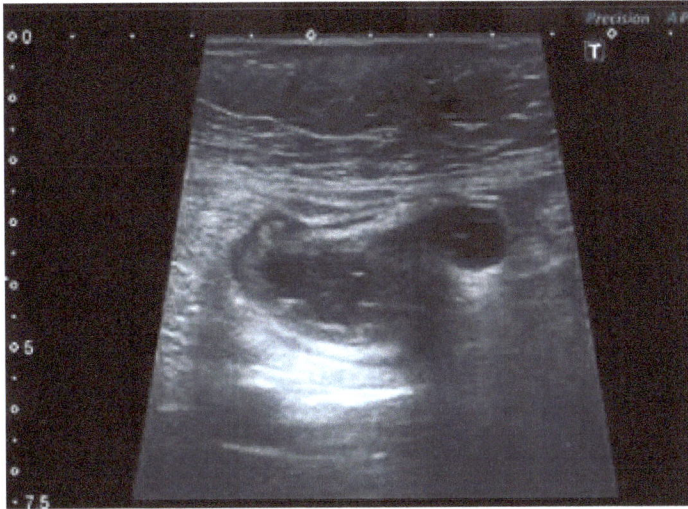

Fig. (12). 60-year-old female patient presents with severe acute right lower quadrant pain. Serial USG images show inflamed ileal segments, Meckel's diverticulum, and intestinal edema. There is minimal fluid between the bowel segments.

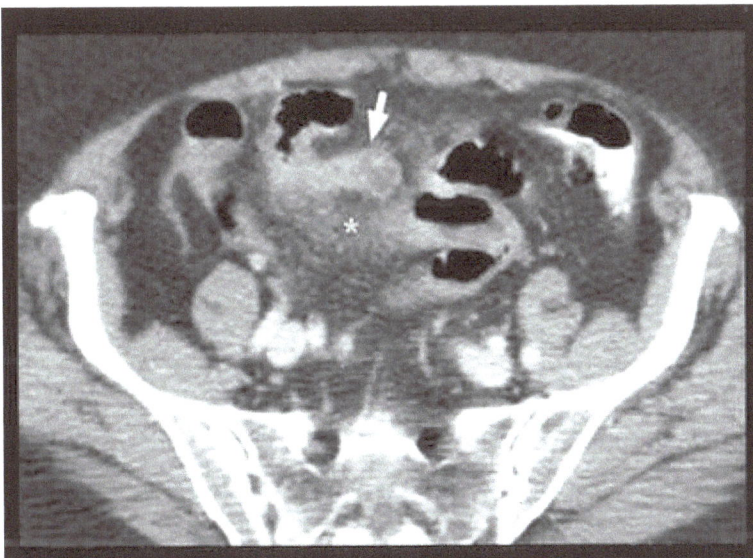

Fig. (13). A case of MD confirmed at surgery. In a 76-year-old patient, MD is visualized as a fluid-filled, blunt-ended structure on IV contrast-enhanced CT (arrow). Peridiverticular mesenteric fatty streaks (asterisk) suggest inflammation.

What is the Most Important Distinction between MD and Appendicitis?

It is the absence of a clear connection or relationship with the cecum in MD.

Complications of MD: The most common complication of MD in children is rectal bleeding resulting in anemia (St-Vil 1991). The most common complication in adults is a small bowel obstruction (Dumper, 2006).

Acute Diverticulitis (AD)

A colonic diverticulum is an outward bulging or pocketing in the colon wall. When there are no symptoms, it is called diverticulosis, which is very common over the age of 50. AD is one of the most frequent emergency conditions of the bowels presenting with acute abdomen. AD constitutes 3.8% of causes of abdominal pain in patients presented to the emergency departments (Sebbane, 2011). AD is associated with male gender, obesity, smoking, sedentary life, and NSAID use.

The inflammation and perforation due to AD may be limited to the serosa layer of the colon wall. If AD is left untreated, it can lead to abscess or bowel obstruction. It may also be fistulized into the bladder or other intestinal structures. Pericolic abscess develops when perforated AD remains localized, and generalized peritonitis develops when spilled into the peritoneum. Findings on examination reflect this: Localized tenderness or generalized rigidity may be evident in the lower abdomen. Sometimes there may be mild fever and a palpable mass in the lower abdomen. In the very old, debilitated, and immunosuppressed patients with AD, the findings are subtler than expected.

Work up can be initiated with abdominal radiographs which typically show non-specific changes. It serves to exclude DD such as ileus. An upright plain chest X-ray may show an image of subdiaphragmatic free air in the presence of perforation.

MDCT is essential for the primary diagnosis of the acute diverticulitis and its complications. The best examination method is CT with oral+IV contrast (Fig. **14-16**).

Management: Analgesia and IV fluids are the musts. Stop oral intake, consult with general surgeon. Mild diverticulitis is treated with antibiotics. Start broad spectrum antibiotics. Surgery is needed in complicated patients who have no signs of relief in the first days despite appropriate treatment.

COMPLICATIONS

• **Perforation:** It may be localized, may evolve to abscesses and/or generalized (rigidity).

• **Massive hematochezia.**

• **Fistulization** to adjacent structures: fistula may develop in the small intestine, uterus, vagina, bladder.

• **Adhesions** after AD.

• **Intestinal obstruction**: May lead to colonic or intestinal obstruction.

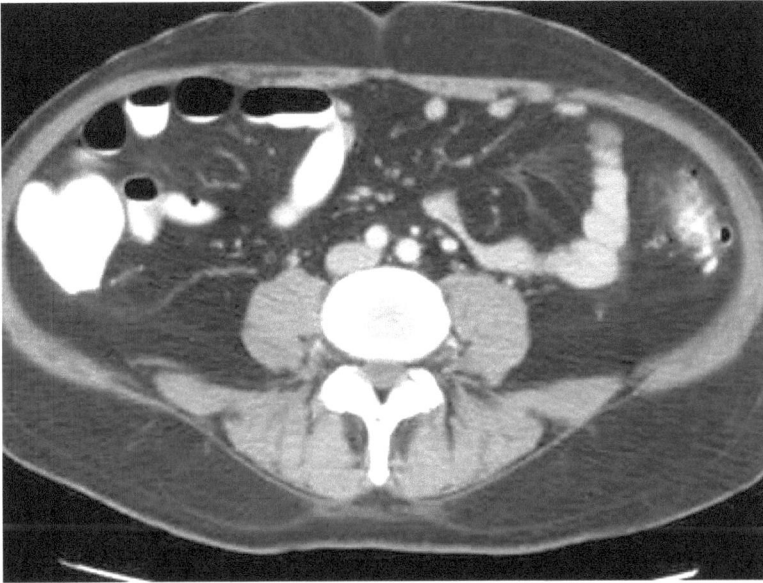

Fig. (14). A case of mild diverticulitis in the descending colon with contamination in pericolic adipose tissue, wall thickening, divericular image, and contrasting pattern.

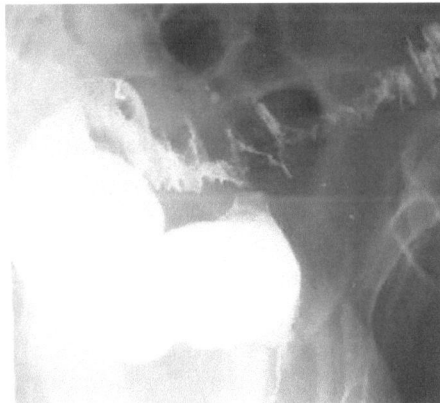

Fig. (15). Mild sigmoid diverticulitis with thickening of the mucosal folds and luminal narrowing in a barium enema study.

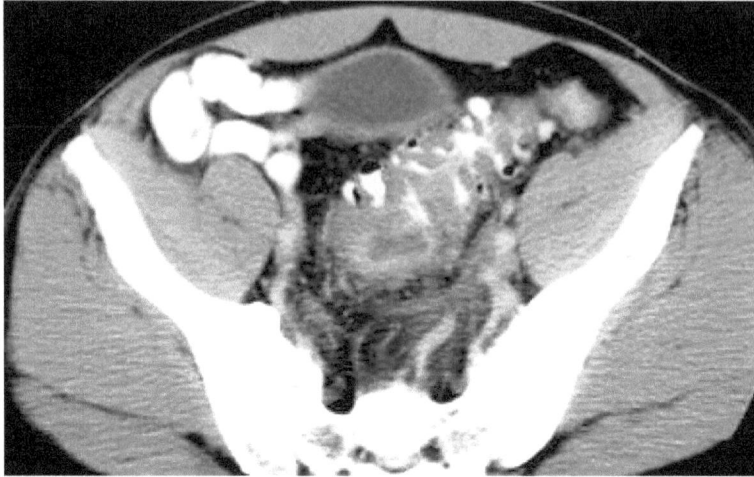

Fig. (16). CT image of the patient with diverticulitis depicts an intramural abscess in the sigmoid colon and a contrast-filled abscess adjacent to the rectosigmoid colon.

Complete ileusoccurs rarely in patients with AD; however, sub-ileus or partial bowel obstruction secondary to inflammation and mucosal edema or abscess formation may ensue. Intramuscular fibrosis encountered in the chronic phase may also result in obstruction in 10% to 20% of the cases (Shen, 2005).

Additionally, pylephlebitis, perforation, and abscess formation are among the rarely seen complications (Onur, 2017).

Prevention

A high fiber diet, exercise and drinking lots of water are effective in prevention.

Perforation of AD is due to severe inflammation of bowel wall layers with subsequent necrosis and loss of intestinal wall integrity. Perforation from colonic diverticulitis almost always occurs on the left side (Puylaert, 2012). Well-contained perforations manifest as small and self-limited; however, non-contained perforations which occur in 1%–2% of patients with AD may lead to local abscess and fistula formation (Stoker, 2009).

CASE PRESENTATION: PERFORATED AD

A man in his 38 with a well-contained perforation of AD. Axial contrast-enhanced CT demonstrates edema and thickening of the sigmoid colon wall with multiple diverticulums (Fig. **17**).

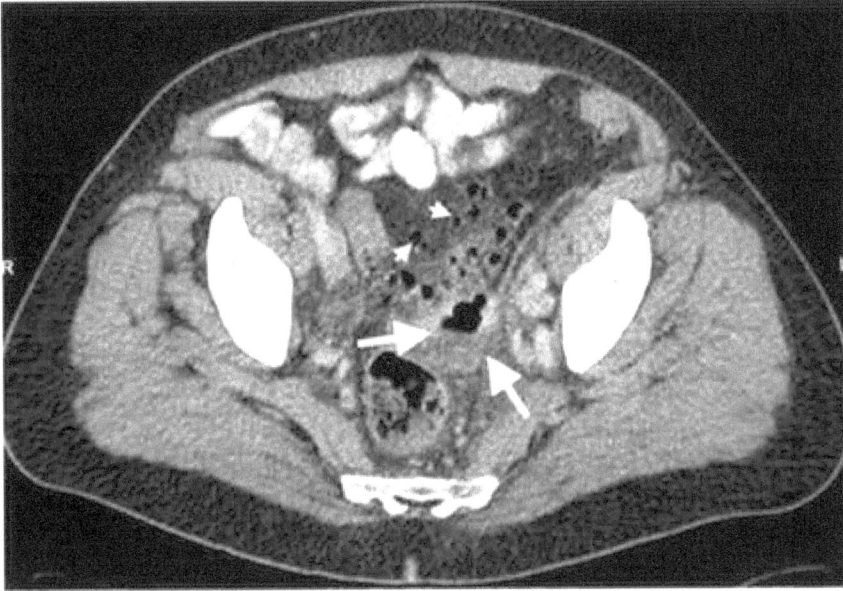

Fig. (17). A fluid collection adjacent to the sigmoid colon (*arrows*) is an abscess caused by perforation of the diverticulitis. Free air pockets (*arrowhead*) confined to the pericolonic region are noted.

HERNIAS

In terms of anatomical origin and onset, hernias can be classified as external (*e.g*, inguinal and femoral) and internal (*e.g*, paraduodenal) hernias.

Inguinal hernias (IH) are mostly seen in the indirect form (IIH). For IIH, herniation occurs from the patent processus vaginalis lateral to the inferior epigastric artery. IIH are viewed as an acquired pathology, not congenital, due to weakening of the inner inguinal ring. In contrast, direct hernias (DIH) occur due to weakness of the transverse fascia and are localized medial to the inferior epigastric vessels.

Femoral hernias (FH) are encountered less commonly than IH. It is attributed to a defect in the adhesion of the transverse fascia to the pubis. It is located medial to the femoral vein, and posterior to the inguinal ligament. On the other hand, the rate of incarceration (and the need for emergency operation) in FH is much higher than the other common types.

Ventral hernias, abdominal wall hernias (AWH) is an aponeurotic defect which allows an organ protrude from its original cavity (Reza Zahiri, 2018). Umbilical, epigastric, and hypogastric hernias are midline defects which comprise the most common surgical conditions (Fig. **18**). It occurs *via* congenital defects in children, acquired defects in adults due to pregnancies, ascites, and obesity.

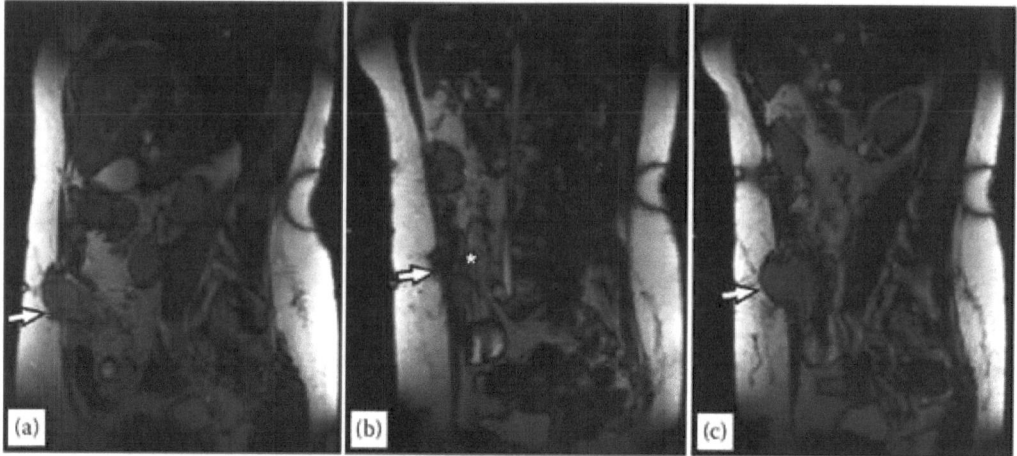

Fig. (18). Functional cine-MRI of the 45-year-old man, evaluated due to suspicion of incidental hernia. A hernia in the ventral abdominal wall is seen in images **(a, c)** in the sagittal plane during the Valsalva maneuver (arrow). In the intestinal segment entering the hernia sac; the orifice is visible at rest **(b)**, the absence of excursion and separation movements of the abdominal wall and intestinal loops (asterisk).

Lateral defects of the abdominal wall: The most common are Spigelian hernias, which develop from a defect in the linea semilunaris. They are characterized by protrusion of the omentum and small bowel segments after aponeurosis or acquired weakness in the surgical incision. incarceration rate is high (Miller, 1995).

Incisional hernias are caused by a defect in the abdominal wall following a laparotomy and their reported incidence is as high as 22.4% at 3 years after surgery, with some reports as high as 36% (Yang, 2017). Delayed complications of abdomino-pelvic surgery, which occur mostly in the first months, are evaluated in this group. It is more common in vertical incisions than in transverse ones. Age, obesity, postoperative wound infection, and ascites are typical risk factors.

Incarcerated hernia is a common condition in acute setting, with a rate of emergency operation of about 10–15% (Birindelli, 2017, Beadles, 2015). In umbilical hernias, the rate of incarceration and strangulation is high and spontaneous reduction is not expected (Fig. **19**). It is characterised by the inability of reduction of the content during examination, due to a narrow opening in the abdominal wall or to adhesions between the content and the hernia sac (Nazeeruddin, 2021).

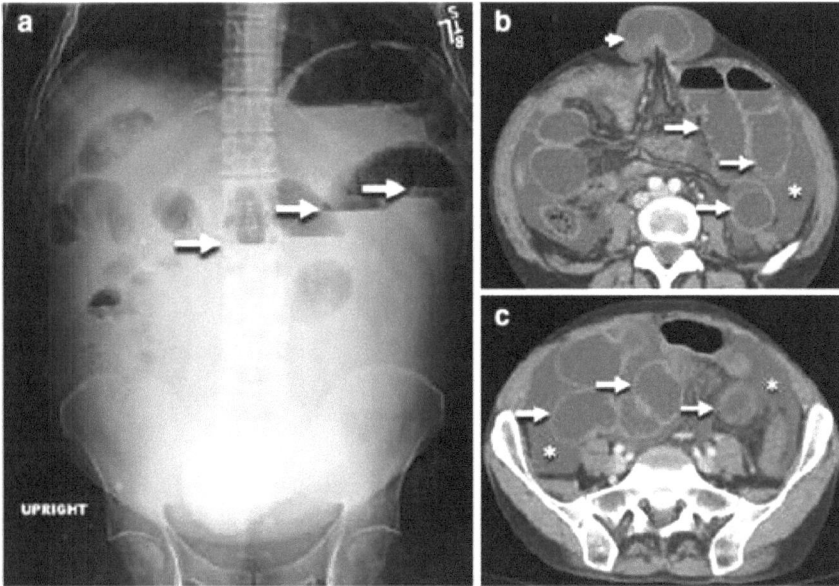

Fig. (19). A male patient in his 47 is diagnosed with an incarcerated umbilical hernia. In the upright abdominal X-ray **(a)**, enlarged intestinal loops and air-fluid levels are visualized (arrows). The round area with increased opacity in the pelvis is parallel to the palpable swelling in the midline on physical examination. Axial contrast-enhanced CT images show a fluid-filled small bowel segment (arrowhead) in the midline umbilical hernia. Proximal to this, dilated small bowel loops and air-fluid levels draw attention (arrows). Presence of ascites also indicate the underlying cirrhotic process (asterisk).

Case Presentation

A man in his 57 is referred to the ED due to repetitive vomiting and periumbilical pain for three days. He has a history of multiple laparotomies. A strangulated incisional para-umbilical hernia with local cellulitis and tenderness in the right flank is remarkable on examination. Abdominal CT scan revealed strangulated hernia (Fig. **20**).

Benign Anorectal Diseases

They are important diseases that are more common than is thought in the community and are underrepresented in the health statistics. Among these, hemorrhoids, anal fissures, fistulas, and anorectal abscesses are the most common entities. Although we can recognize most diseases in this group with the history and examination, more advanced techniques may be required in cases in between. While some diseases such as acute anal fissures can be discharged from the ED with a prescription, anorectal abscesses and fistulas, chronic complicated anal fissures must be resolved with surgical consultation.

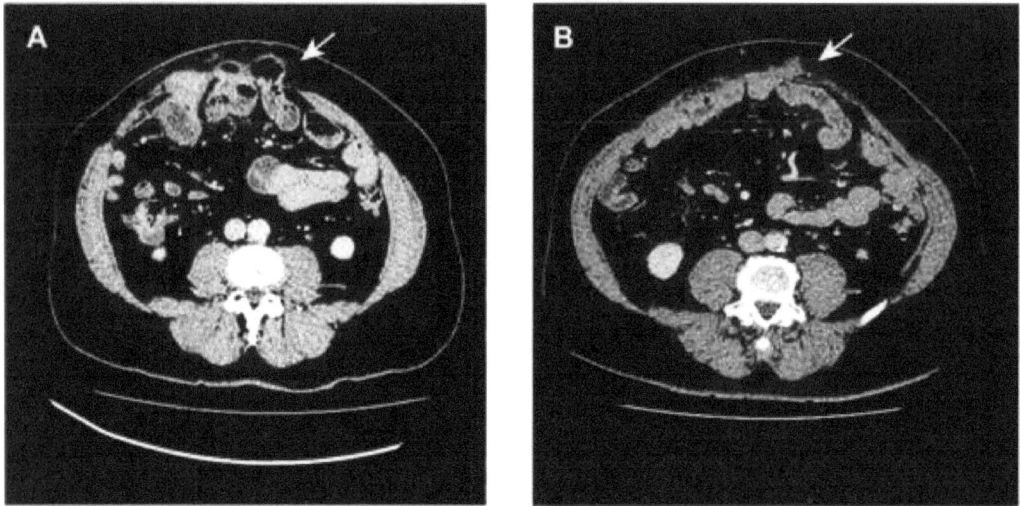

Fig. (20). Abdominal CT scan of the strangulated hernia (arrow) in axial view in the ED and at one-year follow up.

Digital rectal examination will reveal various pathological findings indicative of different diagnoses (Mott, 2018) (Table **9**).

Table 9. Patients with rectal pain, bleeding, or mass are evaluated and differentiated with regard to presumptive diagnoses.

Diagnosis	History	Physical Examination
Abscess	Gradual onset of pain	Tender fluctuant mass
Cancer	Pain, bleeding, changes in bowel movements, weight loss	Ulcerating, indurated lesion
Condyloma	Possible bleeding; anal intercourse	Verrucous lesions
Fissure	Tearing pain with bowel movements	Visible tender fissure
Fistula	Soiling, itching	Visible opening of fistula
Inflammatory bowel disease	Bloody diarrhea, abdominal pain, family history	Possible fistula; colitis on anoscopy
Polyps	Painless bleeding	Polyps on endoscopy
Proctalgia fugax	Painful rectum, no bleeding	Normal examination; diagnosis of exclusion
Proctitis	Painful rectum, bleeding	Tenderness on digital rectal examination
Rectal prolapse	Mass with Valsalva maneuver	Prolapse of rectal mucosa
Skin tags	History of hemorrhoids, no bleeding	Tags covered with normal skin

Hemorrhoids

Hemorrhoids are engorged fibrovascular cushions lining the anal canal. Hemorrhoidal size, thrombosis, and location (*i.e.*, proximal or distal to the dentate line) determine the extent of pain or discomfort (Mott, 2018). Predisposing factors include chronic constipation, increased intra-abdominal pressure, and prolonged straining. Around 5% of Americans and almost one-half of those above 50-yea--old experience symptomatic hemorrhoids (Fox, 2014).

Diagnosis is mostly established *via* systemic examination and an elaborate history. Internal hemorrhoids (IH) most commonly present with painless bleeding +- prolapse after defecation. Mild faecal incontinence, mucous drainage, perianal fullness sensation, and painful skin irritation with or without ulcers may occur resulting from prolapse. Thrombosed external hemorrhoids (TEH) are more painful and present with a palpable tender perianal mass. If the lesion ulcerates, it may bleed. It would be wrong to accept the patient presenting with rectal bleeding as IH without a full examination, because rectal cancers can be overlooked (Fig. **21**). Anoscopy is necessary for imaging IHs. If anoscopy is found to be normal in painless rectal bleeding, diagnostic colonoscopy is indicated urgently.

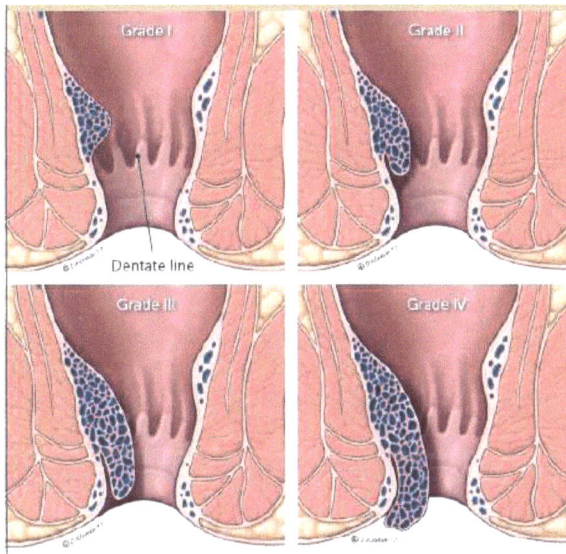

Fig. (21). Grading of internal hemorrhoids. (Patients may experience painless bleeding with any grade). Grade I = asymptomatic outgrowth of anal mucosa caused by engorgement of underlying venous plexus and connective tissue; grade II = hemorrhoid prolapses but spontaneously reduces; grade III = hemorrhoid prolapses and must be manually reduced; often accompanied by pruritus and soilage; grade IV = hemorrhoid prolapse that cannot be reduced; often accompanied by chronic local inflammatory changes.

Symptomatic hemorrhoids are often self-limited and respond to conservative medical therapy.

Most hemorrhoids and anal fissures are relatively benign and do not require imaging for diagnosis or management.

Rubber band ligation is the most common procedure for grades II and III IHs. It provides treatment by causing tissue necrosis. Not applicable in EHs and in patients using anticoagulants.

Acute hemorrhoidal crisis is a rare but important entity. On examination, typical red ulcerated or necrotic IHs are observed. This lesion occurs when incarceration develops as a result of sphincter spasm in addition to the IH+ prolapse. The entity prompts hospitalization.

The treatment of acute hemorrhoid crisis mostly consists of prevention of constipation, sitz baths and pain treatment. Prolapsed and strangulated hemorrhoids are managed with stool softeners, analgesics, rest, warm soaks, and ice packs until recovery; residual hemorrhoids are banded or excised later (Fox, 2014). Necrotic hemorrhoids and perineal sepsis require exploration and excisional biopsy.

Open or conventional excisional hemorrhoidectomy results in greater surgical success rates but also incurs more pain and a prolonged recovery than office-based procedures; therefore, hemorrhoidectomy should be reserved for recurrent or higher-grade disease (Mott, 2018).

Surgical intervention is more appropriate for Grade III and IV IHs and those with persistent symptoms. In the case of TEH, surgical intervention should be performed no later than the first 48 hours.

Incision-drainage is ineffective, as the entire hemorrhoidal tissue must be removed along with the skin (Table **10**).

Table 10. Comparison of outcomes between different surgical procedures for treatment of hemorrhoids (Jacobs 2014, MacRae 1995, Wald 2014, Picchio 2015).

Procedure	Resolution of symptoms	Reduction of prolapsing tissue (mucopexy)	Likelihood of recurrence	Amount of postsurgical pain	Longer recovery time
Banding (*i.e.*, rubber band ligation)	++	+	++	++	+
Infrared photocoagulation	+	Not applicable	+++	+	+

(Table 10) cont.....

Procedure	Resolution of symptoms	Reduction of prolapsing tissue (mucopexy)	Likelihood of recurrence	Amount of postsurgical pain	Longer recovery time
Open hemorrhoidectomy	+++	++	+	+++	+++
Closed hemorrhoidectomy	+++	++	+	+++	+++
Stapled hemorrhoidopexy	++	+++	++	++	++
Hemorrhoidal artery ligation (without mucopexy)	++	Not applicable	++	+	+
Hemorrhoidal artery ligation (with mucopexy)	++	++	++	++	+

+ = Outcome less likely.
++ = Outcome relatively neutral in comparison with other surgical procedures.
+++ = Outcome more likely.

Anal Fissure (AF)

AF is a linear tear in the anal mucosa. This usually extends from the dentate line to the anal entrance. Those that do not improve in 4-8 weeks are called chronic AF (Fig. **22**). It is often seen in young and healthy people. A clear association with elevated internal anal sphincter pressures and AF is established. Though hard bowel movements are implicated in fissure etiology, they are not universally present in patients with anal fissures (Beaty, 2017). Hard stool and constipation were predominant in the etiology in only 13% of the cases. High internal sphincter pressure, on the other hand, causes the acute cases to become chronic. The low content of nitric oxide in the tissue has also been reported in studies.

The most common localization is the posterior midline with 90% of the cases. Lateral fissures are rare and if found, inflammatory bowel diseases, tuberculosis, HIV, syphilis should be sought for.

Treatment: Stool softeners, increase fibrous food in diet, sitz baths, lidocaine gel for pain control provide a good start up of treatment.

Half of the patients recover with increased fiber food and sitz baths and pharmacological agents (Beaty, 2017). Lidocaine gel does not represent a radical cure, it only provides short-lasting symptomatic relief. The main aim of the treatment is to reduce the internal sphincter tone and to provide healing.

When nifedipine gel topical hydrocortisone and lidocaine were compared in well-designed studies, it was noted that nifedipine treatment achieved relief in 95% of AF cases within 21 days, and in only 50% of the control or treatment groups (Antropoli, 1999).

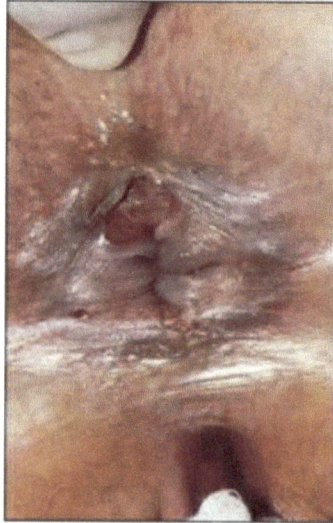

Fig. (22). Chronic anal fissure. The sphincter muscle became visible at the base of the wound.

Anorectal Abscesses and Fistulas

Infection often begins in the anal crypts and glands and spreads from there to the external and internal sphincters. It is more common in men between the ages of 20-40.

All four types of anorectal abscesses are shown in Fig. (23).

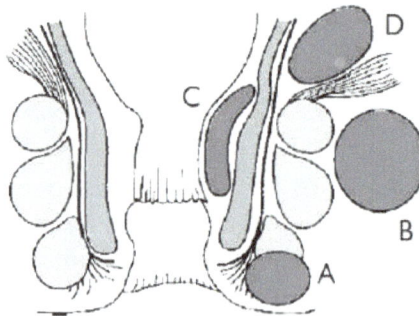

Fig. (23). Types of anorectal abscess. A. Perianal. B. Ischiorectal. C. Submucosal. D. Pelvirectal.

Perianal and ischiorectal abscesses constitute 80% of cases. Abscesses are often seen simultaneously with fistulas. Between 30% and 70% of active abscesses have a concomitant fistula (Vogel, 2016).

Images of perianal/perirectal abscesses on axial CT scans and MRI were exemplified on (Figs. **24** and **25**).

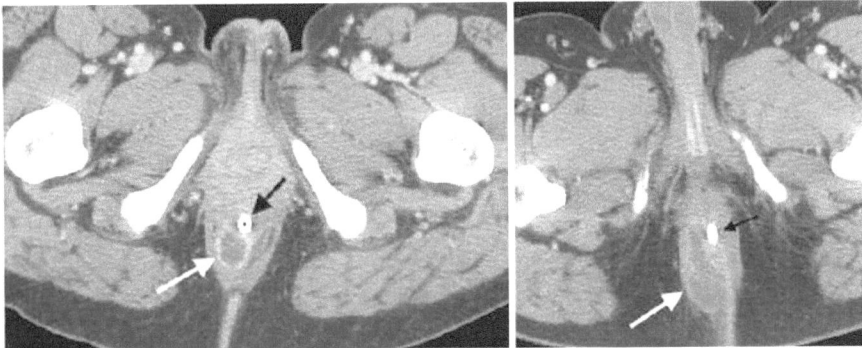

Fig. (24). Perianal/perirectal abscesses on axial CT scans. **A.** Right intersphincteric abscess in section at the level of the anus (white arrows). The rectal tube can also be seen in the lumen (black arrow). **B.** Perianal abscess (white arrow) on the right extends inferiorly to the perianal skin. The rectal tube can also be seen in the lumen (black arrow).

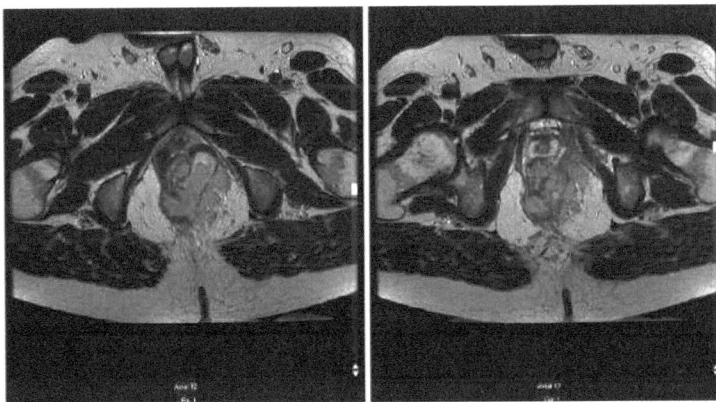

Fig. (25). Perianal abscess on MRI sections. A multilocular confluent liquid mass is observed in the ischiorectal fossa in the left perianal region. Diffusion restriction and massive perifocal inflammation are remarkable.

Findings: Pain, fever, tenderness, erythema, fluctuating mass are the prominent findings in perianal and superficial ischiorectal abscesses. There are also signs of local inflammation. The patients complain of blunt and throbbing pain. The pain increases with walking, straining and sitting, and the patient may even become unable to sit.

In deep infections, the pain progresses more slowly and is more moderate. In perianal abscess, there is tender swelling accompanied by localized fluctuant mass and erythema close to the anus. The deeper the infection, the more subtle the findings. Rectal digital exam may reveal a tender mass. Such an examination may precipitate septic spread in those with neutropenic fever, thus be cautious in these patients.

Although there are minimal findings on external examination in those with supralevator or intersphincteric abscesses, tenderness is marked on rectal exam. It is necessary to differentiate anorectal abscess from other inflammatory processes of the region, such as hidradenitis, furuncle, or pilonidal infections. Highly located abscesses such as supralevator abscesses can be visualized on IV Contrast CT.

Diagnosis is mostly made by history and examination. CT and, if necessary, MRI are helpful to delineate the extent of the disease and the operative approach.

Anal fistula is the formation of a permanent epithelialized tract extending from the anal canal to the skin.

According to the most used Parks Classification: It can be intersphincteric, transsphincteric, suprasphincteric, or extrasphincteric. Complex fistulas are highly transsphincteric (involving more than 30% of the external sphincter), extrasphincteric or suprasphincteric, and cryptoglandular ones, accompanied by a history of inflammatory bowel disease, radiation, cancer, chronic diarrhea or incontinence. 80% of fistulas are of cryptoglandular origin.

If a fistula does not fit the Parks classification, Crohn's disease must be excluded if multiple fistulas and major skin changes are present. Not every fistula will require imaging. Instead, the fistula tract can be mapped under anesthesia. If this is not successful, endorectal USG will determine the fistula map with an accuracy of 80% to 89% and rectal MRI with an accuracy of 90% (Steele, 2011).

How do we define fistula? We should mention the following features

- The location of the mucosal opening in axial sections should be determined with the help of the "anal clock".
- The distance of the mucosal defect to the perianal skin should be noted in the coronal images.
- Secondary fistulas or abscesses should be recorded.

CT is an effective and practical diagnostic tool for assessment of the patients with the clinical suspicion of perianal abscess and/or infected fistulous tract. The diagnosis can be easy if the fistulous tract or abscess is visible on inspection of the perianal skin (Khati, 2015).

On the other hand, MRI is an advantageous modality to identify and visualize complex fistulous tracts (Fig. **26**).

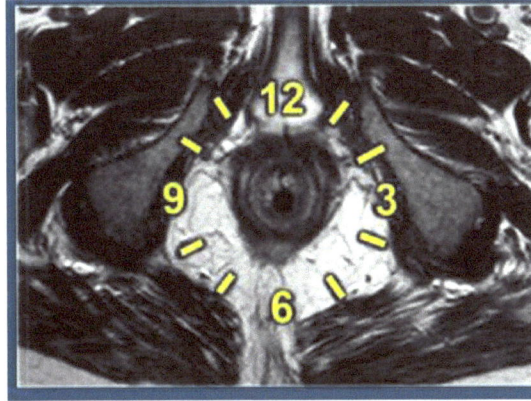

Fig. (26). In the drawing, the way the physician sees the perianal region when the patient is in the lithotomy position is depicted with the concept of "Anal clock". This scheme corresponds to the orientation of axial MR images in the perianal region.

The main treatment is surgery, but procedures vary: *e.g.* fistulotomy +-seton application, fibrin glue, endorectal flap, and "ligation of intersphincteric fistula tract" (LIFT).

Analgesia should be provided and the patient should be referred with surgical consultation. Incision and drainage are performed under general anesthesia.

Proctitis is diagnosed *via* detection of consistent signs and symptoms. It is an inflammation involving the anus and the distal part of the rectum, frequently diagnosed in the context of inflammatory bowel diseases (IBD) (Rizza, 2020). The symptoms include anorectal itching, pain, tenesmus, bleeding episodes, constipation and discharge in and around the anal canal (de Vries. 2021). On the oter hand, the most common presenting symptoms were rectal bleeding (47,5%), anal symptoms (30%) and change in bowel habits (25%) (Bosma, 2021). Genital ulcers or inguinal buboes are also highly suggestive of Lymphogranuloma venereum (LGV). A definitive diagnosis is established with the laboratory tests. The majority of rectal chlamydia trachomatis (CT) and gonococcal infections are asymptomatic. Therefore, especially when there is a history of anal contact, anorectal infections should be ruled out as part of standard screening for STDs. Proctitis due to LGV is getting more common in HIV-negative men with a history of anal intercourse. Anorectal mycoplasma genitalium is to be searched for in patients with symptomatic proctitis, Intestinal spirochetosis can also be identified in colonic biopsies. Traumatic etiologies of proctitis should be taken into account in men and women with a history of anal penetration.

Neves *et al.* analysed more than 16.000 swabs, urine analysis and real-time PCR for CT infection (Neves, 2021). A total of 1602 of cases were attributed CT diagnoses established, from which 168 (10.5%) corresponded to LGV, with both infections showing a rising evolution, between 2016 and 2019, LGV predominantly affected men with a history of anal intercourse (97.0%). Proctitis was the main clinical presentation of LGV (76%), whilst around 15% of the cases are found to be asymptomatic. The presence of concomitant infection with HIV was dominant (73%).

Case presentation (Fig. **27**).

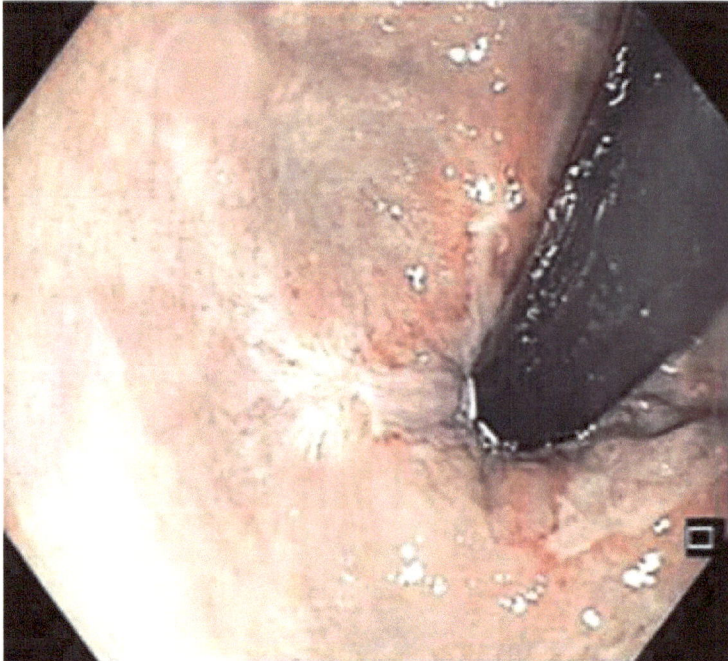

Fig. (27). A man in his fifties presented with intermittent bright red hematochezia and abdominal pain. His sexual history revealed unprotected anal intercourse. He had a near-normal hemoglobin level (12.8 g/dL) and mildly elevated CRP (3.5 mg/dL). Ulceration on the hemorrhoidal plexus in the distal rectum was in continuity with the anal verge. Treatment with doxicillin was extended to three weeks and this led to the resolution of symptoms.

MESENTERIC ARTERY ISCHEMIA (MAI) AND INFARCTION

Sudden cessation of mesenteric circulation leads to irreversible ischemia and gangrene in a short time. It may occur by thrombosis or embolization to arteries supplying blood to bowels. reported incidence rate of MAI is 12.9 per 100,000 person-years and death rate is very high (50%–70%) (Lim, 2019).

Embolization of a thrombus into superior mesenteric artery (SMA) is the widespread cause of *de novo* MAI. SMA embolisation and resultant MAI can be caused by various cardiac diseases (myocardial ischaemia/acute coronary syndromes, supraventricular tachyarrhythmias, endocarditis, ventricular aneurysms and valvular disorders, cardiomyopathies,), aortic or other arterial aneurysms, arterial atherosclerotic plaques *etc.* (Pay 2021, Janež, 2021).

In some patients, it may result from general ischemia as well as in the post-MI period (nonocclusive mesenteric ischemia, NOMI). Its mortality of the entity is quite high, despite diagnostic and therapeutic advances. The main problem is the difficulty to diagnose in the early period.

EVALUATION

Many patients are middle-aged and older patients with a history of cardiac diseases including atrial fibrillation (AF) and a history of claudication involving other vessels. Excessive AP beyond the physical findings is remarkable. The AP is usually extensive in the allover the abdomen. Slow but steady progress of the physical examination findings in the abdomen is notable. Pain on the right side and a color close to the appearance of hematochezia in the stool are typical for NOMI.

Distension, shock, absence of bowel sounds, and widespread abdominal tenderness on percussion (rigidity) are typical. AF or MI leading to a mural thrombus is present in most cases. While there are mild symptoms at the very beginning, the picture quickly becomes noisy and progresses to sepsis and septic shock.

Amylase and leukocyte count may be slightly to moderately increased in the work up.

- Severe metabolic acidosis and high lactate levels can be seen in ABG.
- AF or previous MI can be detected on ECG, although not a rule.
- Doppler USG, CT, angiography facilitate and expedite diagnostic decision making.

CASE EXAMPLE (FIG. 28)

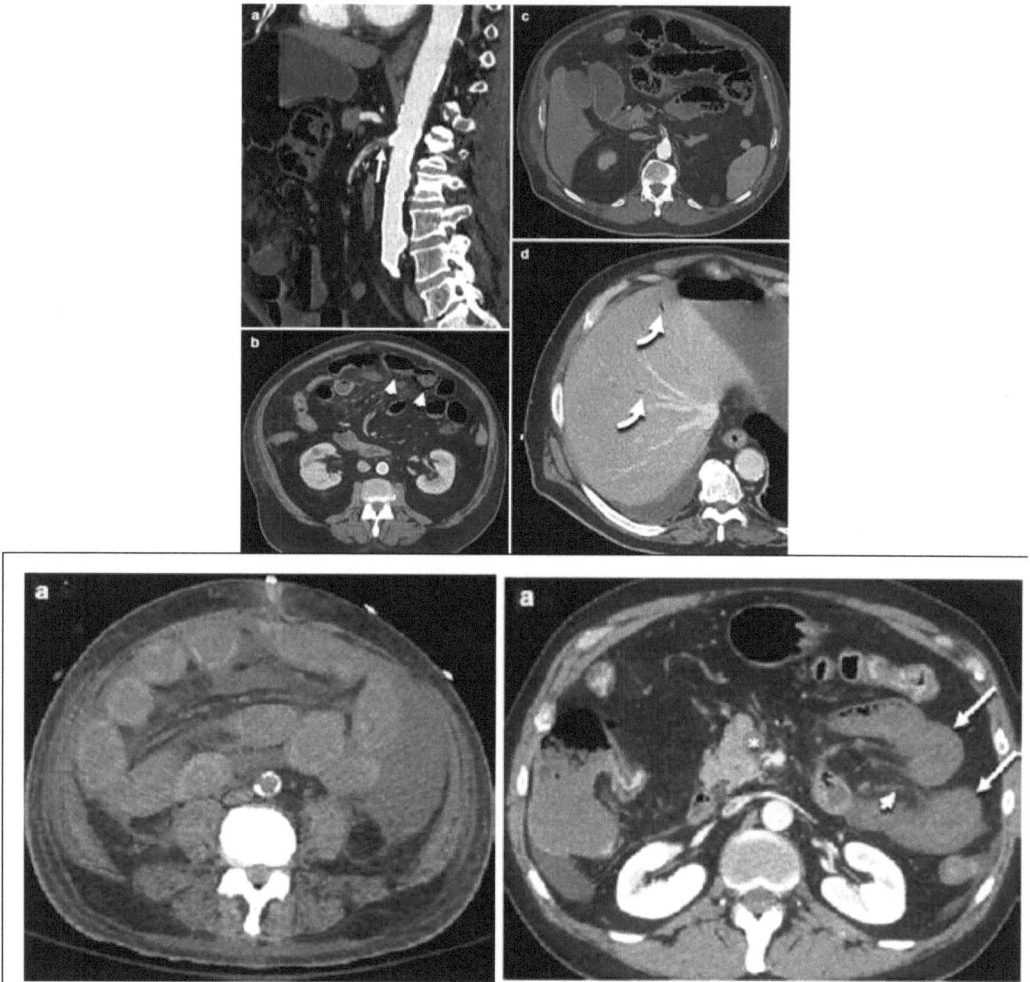

Fig. (28). Arterial occlusive mesenteric ischemia in a 74-year-old male patient. Contrast-enhanced CT sagittal reformatted images **(a)** show an occlusive thrombus (arrow) at the exit of the SMA with signs of atherosclerotic disease in the aorta and SMA. Axial contrast-enhanced CT images **(b–d)** of pneumatosis (arrowheads) and small portal venous gas in the small intestine loops are observed in the left-mid abdomen (curved arrows). We can see that small bowel ischemic segment walls are less contrast-enhanced and thinner due to ischemia.

Case Presentation

A nonagenarian man was admitted to the ED with AP on the upper belly. He was diagnosed with ST-elevated myocardial infarction associated with acute MAI. ECG and angiography revealed the cause of the thrombi and the consequent embolization (Fig. **29**).

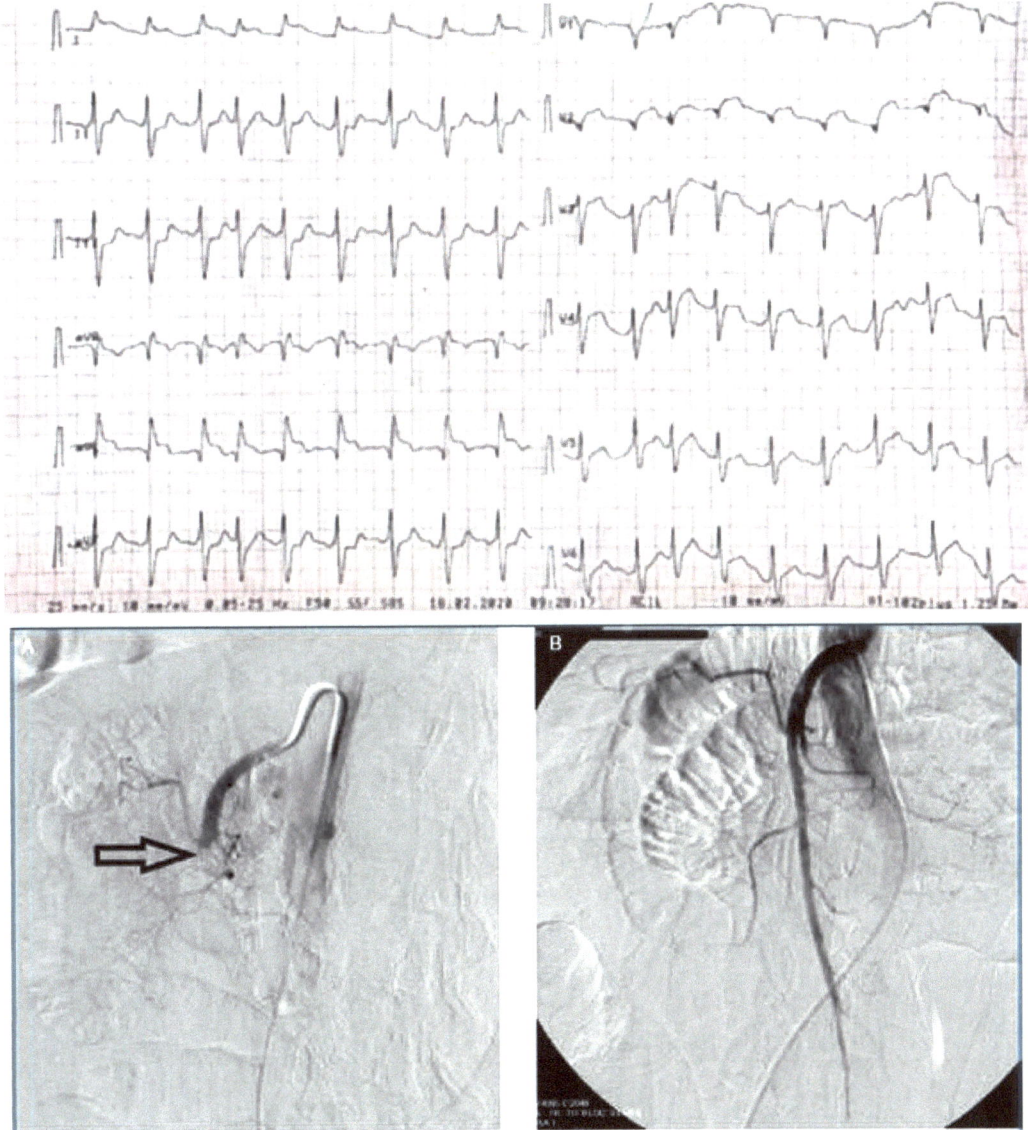

Fig. (29). ECG of the patient represents ST segment elevation in leads DI, aVL, V2, V3, and V4 and reciprocal ST segment depression in leads DII, DIII, and aVF. The rhythm is atrial fibrillation. Complete SMA occlusion (arrow) is visualized *via* angiography. Blood flow was restored following balloon angioplasty of the SMA.

Of note, an etiology of aortic thrombosis could be pandemic infection. Even though, as acute MAI usually occurs in elderly patients with ischaemic heart disease and AF, younger patients with acute MAI need to be evaluated carefully in regard to COVID-19 (Janez, 2021). D-dimer levels can serve as a useful guide in distinguishing patients with high likelihood of thromboembolism.

Management

Initiate treatment of the suspected patient without waiting for the definitive diagnosis. Notify the surgeon. In selected patients, it may be considered to inform the intensive care unit first.

- IV saline infusion is the first choice.
- Give O2 and IV fluids in patients with the poor general condition and prone to shock. Attach a Foley catheter and monitor the urinary output.
- Administer IV opioids (morphine/fentanyl) and antiemetics (*e.g* ondansetron 8 mg or H1 blocker).
- Decompress the stomach with the NG tube. It will also prevent aspiration.

Initiate combined antibiotherapy with broad-spectrum antianaerobic action.

ISCHEMIC COLITIS AND ISCHEMIC BOWEL SYNDROMES

CI (colonic ischemia) is the form of mesenteric ischemia in which it manifests itself with circulatory insufficiency of the large intestines. It is the most common disease of the colon in patients over 65 years of age and consists of various clinical syndromes resulting from colonic ischemia and necrosis for different reasons (Table **11**).

Table 11. Subgroups of patients with ischemic colitis.

• -**Reversible colopathy:** Only ischemia and submucosal or intramural hemorrhage without necrosis.
• Transient colitis: ischemia/necrosis limited to the mucosa and submucosa.
• Acute hemorrhagic erosive gastritis
• Chronic segmental colitis
• Stricture
• Gangrene
• Fulminant colitis: ischemia is transmural, progressing to necrosis

The most severe form, fulminant colitis, occurs as a result of superior mesenteric artery (SMA) embolism or non-occlusive mesenteric ischemia (NOMI). Shock may ensue and mortality is more than 50% (see relevant section).

IC most commonly involves the descending colon or sigmoid, transverse colon, and splenic flexure region.

Chronic arterial insufficiency in the intestinal circulation typically affects the mucosa and submucosa around the splenic flexure on the left. This region is the intersection of SMA and IMA regions of blood flow. It presents with pain, mostly in the left iliac fossa. Melena/hematochezia-like defecation may occur. Rectal blood, mild fever and tachycardia may be seen on a digital rectal exam. Bleeding rarely reaches levels that would prompt transfusion. There is no pain in ¼ of the cases, the most prominent complaint/finding in this group may be abdominal distention or GIB.

Postoperative Ischemic Colitis: It is a more frequent and severe disease than previously thought. Particular care should be taken after surgeries involving the aorta.

GI ischemia in coronavirus disease 2019 (COVID-19): Keshavarz *et al*. performed a systematic review in 2020 including keywords related to GI ischemia in association with COVID-19 (Keshavarz, 2021). They reported that macrovascular arterial/venous thrombosis is recorded in almost half of COVID-19 patients with bowel ischemia. Two-thirds of patients required laparotomy and bowel resection. Overall mortality in COVID-19 patients with GI ischemia and mesenteric thrombotic occlusion was 38.7% and 40%.

Colonoscopy is Performed within a Few Days in Any of the Following Cases

- After surgery for ruptured AAA
- If the cross-clamp time is too long
- Intact flow in IMA in preoperative aortography
- Detection of nonpulsatile flow in per-op hypogastric arteries
- Development of postoperative diarrhea

Upright Direct Abdominal X-ray: Shows only non-specific bowel dilatation and air-filled bowel loops. It may be helpful in excluding causes of acute AP, such as perforation and ileus. Fingerprint sign ("thumbprint") can be detected most frequently around the splenic flexure in half of the cases (Fig. **30**). This is a sign of submucosal colonic edema.

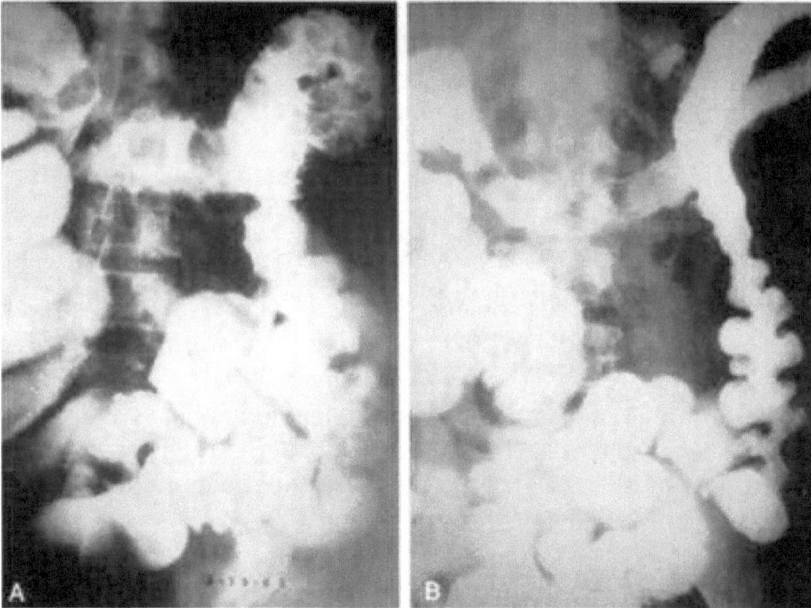

Fig. (30). Findings of IC in colon and splenic flexure. **A:** "fingerprint" findings in the ischemic colon segment. **B:** After 7 days, the "fingerprint" findings disappeared and segmental colitis developed.

Management principles: Notify the surgeon. IV saline infusion is the rule. Attach a Foley catheter and monitor the output. Administer IV opioid (morphine/fentanyl) and antiemetic (*e.g* ondansetron 8 mg or H1 blocker). Caution should be exercised since the narcotic analgesics may exacerbate abdominal distention *via* hypoperistaltism.

Indications for surgical intervention are listed in Table **12**.

Table 12. Indications for surgery in a case of IC.

• Peritoneal irritation signs
• Detection of pneumoperitoneum in radiology
• Colonic gangrene findings on colonoscopy
• Persistent sepsis unresponsive to medical therapy
• Persistent (esp. Bloody) diarrhea
• Long-term symptomatic strictures
• Prolonged or recurrent symptomatic colitis

Abdominal Compartment Syndrome (ACoS) is defined as a sustained raised level of intra-abdominal pressure (IAP) more than 20 mmHg with or without abdominal perfusion pressure less than 60 mmHg and the development of new end-organ failure (Usuda, 2020). intra-abdominal hypertension (IAH) is referred to as a permanent elevation of IAP above 12 mmHg. The risk factors of ACoS reported to date were included in the Table **13** (Keohane 2019, Ho, 2018).

Table 13. Risk factors for ACoS and causes of IAH include many different entities.

ACS	Primary cause of IAH	Secondary cause of IAH
surgical interventions on the abdomen, multiple trauma, volvulus and bowel obstruction, distended abdomen, fecal impaction, acute pancreatitis, hepatic disorders, sepsis, shock states, high body mass index advanced age.	Diseases of the abdominopelvic region trauma Abdominal surgery pancreatitis	Sepsis Extra-abdominal causes Burns

If untreated, ACS can lead to multisystem organ deficiency and death, with nearly 100% mortality (Maluso, 2016).

Management: Critically ill patients with raised IAP should be emergently treated in order to prevent organ failures and to avoid progression to ACS (De Keulenaer, 2015). Critical level of IAP which warrants treatment is around 15 mmHg, and especially if pressures reach 20 mmHg or greater with new-onset organ failure (Malbrain, 2015). Therapy for IAH/ACS consists of five treatment "columns": intraluminal evacuation, intra-abdominal evacuation, improvement of abdominal wall compliance, fluid management, and improved organ perfusion (Hecker, 2016). The key to optimizing outcome is early abdominal closure within 7 days (Ho, 2018).

CONCLUSION

As acute abdominal pain is the primary presenting complaint of patients with many conditions, differential diagnosis and specific clues of each condition are of paramount importance. Evaluation of acute abdominal pain needs to rule out life-threatening conditions of the lower GI system which can lead to abdominal sepsis and other catastrophes, such as acute appendicitis, intraabdominal abscesses and mesenteric artery infarction.

Acute appendicitis is the most common abdominal emergency and affects almost every age, causing major morbidity throughout the world. Visceral perforations, diverticulitis (including bleeding and abscesses) acute cholecystitis, acute ischemic bowel, mesenteric artery ischemia and infarction are acute abdominal conditions triggering emergency interventions. Inflammatory bowel disease comprises distinct conditions (Crohn's disease and ulcerative colitis) that are characterized by chronic inflammation of the gastrointestinal (GI) tract with major morbidities such as abscesses and hemorrhagic diarrhea.

Although hernias are mostly diagnosed with a thorough physical examination, imaging may be required for DD and while planning the operation. Obesity and the presence of scarring on the abdominal skin pose a high risk in this regard. In emergencies, USG and CT are highly helpful, MRI is also an option, although more time-consuming and expensive.

REFERENCES

An, J., Zabbo, C.P. Meckel Diverticulum. 2021 May 10. In: StatPearls [Internet]. Treasure Island (FL): StatPearls Publishing; 2021.

Andersson, R.E.B. (2004). Meta-analysis of the clinical and laboratory diagnosis of appendicitis. *Br. J. Surg., 91*(1), 28-37.
[http://dx.doi.org/10.1002/bjs.4464] [PMID: 14716790]

Antropoli, C., Perrotti, P., Rubino, M., Martino, A., De Stefano, G., Migliore, G., Antropoli, M., Piazza, P. (1999). Nifedipine for local use in conservative treatment of anal fissures: preliminary results of a multicenter study. *Dis. Colon Rectum, 42*(8), 1011-1015.
[http://dx.doi.org/10.1007/BF02236693] [PMID: 10458123]

Batke, M., Cappell, M.S. (2008). Adynamic ileus and acute colonic pseudo-obstruction. *Med. Clin. North Am., 92*(3), 649-670, ix.
[http://dx.doi.org/10.1016/j.mcna.2008.01.002] [PMID: 18387380]

Beadles, C.A., Meagher, A.D., Charles, A.G. (2015). Trends in emergent hernia repair in the United States. *JAMA Surg., 150*(3), 194-200.
[http://dx.doi.org/10.1001/jamasurg.2014.1242] [PMID: 25564946]

Beaty, J.S., Shashidharan, M. (2016). Anal Fissure. *Clin. Colon Rectal Surg., 29*(1), 30-37.
[http://dx.doi.org/10.1055/s-0035-1570390] [PMID: 26929749]

Bhangu, A., Søreide, K., Di Saverio, S., Assarsson, J.H., Drake, F.T. (2015). Acute appendicitis: modern understanding of pathogenesis, diagnosis, and management. *Lancet, 386*(10000), 1278-1287.
[http://dx.doi.org/10.1016/S0140-6736(15)00275-5] [PMID: 26460662]

Birindelli, A., Sartelli, M., Di Saverio, S., Coccolini, F., Ansaloni, L., van Ramshorst, G.H., Campanelli, G., Khokha, V., Moore, E.E., Peitzman, A., Velmahos, G., Moore, F.A., Leppaniemi, A., Burlew, C.C., Biffl, W.L., Koike, K., Kluger, Y., Fraga, G.P., Ordonez, C.A., Novello, M., Agresta, F., Sakakushev, B., Gerych, I., Wani, I., Kelly, M.D., Gomes, C.A., Faro, M.P., Jr, Tarasconi, A., Demetrashvili, Z., Lee, J.G., Vettoretto, N., Guercioni, G., Persiani, R., Tranà, C., Cui, Y., Kok, K.Y.Y., Ghnnam, W.M., Abbas, A.E., Sato, N., Marwah, S., Rangarajan, M., Ben-Ishay, O., Adesunkanmi, A.R.K., Lohse, H.A.S., Kenig, J., Mandalà, S., Coimbra, R., Bhangu, A., Suggett, N., Biondi, A., Portolani, N., Baiocchi, G., Kirkpatrick, A.W., Scibé, R., Sugrue, M., Chiara, O., Catena, F. (2017). 2017 update of the WSES guidelines for emergency repair of complicated abdominal wall hernias. *World J. Emerg. Surg., 12*, 37.
[http://dx.doi.org/10.1186/s13017-017-0149-y] [PMID: 28804507]

Bosma, J.W., van Tienhoven, A.J., Thiesbrummel, H.F., de Vries, H., Veenstra, J. (2021). Delayed diagnosis of lymphogranuloma venereum in a hospital setting - a retrospective observational study. *Int. J. STD AIDS, 32*(6), 517-522.
[http://dx.doi.org/10.1177/0956462420980641] [PMID: 33496203]

Branco, B.C., Barmparas, G., Schnüriger, B., Inaba, K., Chan, L.S., Demetriades, D. (2010). Systematic review and meta-analysis of the diagnostic and therapeutic role of water-soluble contrast agent in adhesive small bowel obstruction. *Br. J. Surg., 97*(4), 470-478.
[http://dx.doi.org/10.1002/bjs.7019] [PMID: 20205228]

Breunung, N., Strauss, P. (2009). A diagnostic challenge: primary omental torsion and literature review - a case report. *World J. Emerg. Surg., 4,* 40.
[http://dx.doi.org/10.1186/1749-7922-4-40] [PMID: 19922627]

Bruggmann, D., Tchartchian, G., Wallwiener, M. (2010). *Meunstedt K, Tinneberg H-R, Hackethal A.* Intra-abdominal Adhesions. Dtsch. Aerzteblatt Online.

Buhmann-Kirchhoff, S., Lang, R., Kirchhoff, C., Steitz, H.O., Jauch, K.W., Reiser, M., Lienemann, A. (2008). Functional cine MR imaging for the detection and mapping of intraabdominal adhesions: method and surgical correlation. *Eur. Radiol., 18*(6), 1215-1223.
[http://dx.doi.org/10.1007/s00330-008-0881-5] [PMID: 18274755]

Cappell, M.S., Batke, M. (2008). Mechanical obstruction of the small bowel and colon. *Med. Clin. North Am., 92*(3), 575-597, viii.
[http://dx.doi.org/10.1016/j.mcna.2008.01.003] [PMID: 18387377]

Casas, M.A., Dreifuss, N.H., Schlottmann, F. (2021). High-volume center analysis and systematic review of stump appendicitis: solving the pending issue. *Eur. J. Trauma Emerg. Surg., 3.*
[http://dx.doi.org/10.1007/s00068-021-01707-y] [PMID: 34085112]

Çelebi, S, Özaydın, S, Başdaş, C (2016). Çocukluk çağında Meckel divertikülü: Otuz yıllık deneyim. *Çocuk Cerrahisi Dergisi, 30*(3), 128-132.

Charieg, A., Ben Ahmed, Y., Nouira, F. (2016). A diagnosis to keep in mind: primary omental torsion in children. *EC Paediatrics, 2,* 245-249.

Cosse, C., Regimbeau, J.M., Fuks, D., Mauvais, F., Scotte, M. (2013). Serum procalcitonin for predicting the failure of conservative management and the need for bowel resection in patients with small bowel obstruction. *J. Am. Coll. Surg., 216*(5), 997-1004.
[http://dx.doi.org/10.1016/j.jamcollsurg.2012.12.051] [PMID: 23522439]

De Keulenaer, B., Regli, A., De Laet, I., Roberts, D., Malbrain, M.L. (2015). What's new in medical management strategies for raised intra-abdominal pressure: evacuating intra-abdominal contents, improving abdominal wall compliance, pharmacotherapy, and continuous negative extra-abdominal pressure. *Anaesthesiol. Intensive Ther., 47*(1), 54-62.
[http://dx.doi.org/10.5603/AIT.a2014] [PMID: 25421926]

de Vries, H.J.C., Nori, A.V., Kiellberg Larsen, H., Kreuter, A., Padovese, V., Pallawela, S., Vall-Mayans, M., Ross, J. (2021). 2021 European Guideline on the management of proctitis, proctocolitis and enteritis caused by sexually transmissible pathogens. *J. Eur. Acad. Dermatol. Venereol., 35*(7), 1434-1443.
[http://dx.doi.org/10.1111/jdv.17269] [PMID: 34057249]

Delabrousse, E., Lubrano, J., Jehl, J., Morati, P., Rouget, C., Mantion, G.A., Kastler, B.A. (2009). Small-bowel obstruction from adhesive bands and matted adhesions: CT differentiation. *AJR Am. J. Roentgenol., 192*(3), 693-697.
[http://dx.doi.org/10.2214/AJR.08.1550] [PMID: 19234265]

Duda, J.B., Bhatt, S., Dogra, V.S. (2008). Utility of CT whirl sign in guiding management of small-bowel obstruction. *AJR Am. J. Roentgenol., 191*(3), 743-747.
[http://dx.doi.org/10.2214/AJR.07.3386] [PMID: 18716103]

Dumper, J., Mackenzie, S., Mitchell, P., Sutherland, F., Quan, M.L., Mew, D. (2006). Complications of Meckel's diverticula in adults. *Can. J. Surg., 49*(5), 353-357.
[PMID: 17152574]

Emile, S.H., Hamid, H.K.S., Khan, S.M., Davis, G.N. (2021). Rate of Application and Outcome of Non-operative Management of Acute Appendicitis in the Setting of COVID-19: Systematic Review and Meta-

analysis. *J. Gastrointest. Surg., 25*(7), 1905-1915.
[http://dx.doi.org/10.1007/s11605-021-04988-1] [PMID: 33772399]

Floch, M.H., Walker, W.A., Guandalini, S., Hibberd, P., Gorbach, S., Surawicz, C., Sanders, M.E., Garcia-Tsao, G., Quigley, E.M., Isolauri, E., Fedorak, R.N., Dieleman, L.A. (2008). Recommendations for probiotic use--2008. *J. Clin. Gastroenterol., 42* (Suppl. 2), S104-S108.
[http://dx.doi.org/10.1097/MCG.0b013e31816b903f] [PMID: 18542033]

Fox, A., Tietze, P.H., Ramakrishnan, K. (2014). Anorectal conditions: hemorrhoids. *FP Essent., 419*, 11-19.
[PMID: 24742083]

Garcia Vilela, E., De Lourdes De Abreu Ferrari, M., Oswaldo Da Gama Torres, H., Guerra Pinto, A., Carolina Carneiro Aguirre, A., Paiva Martins, F., Marcos Andrade Goulart, E., Sales Da Cunha, A. (2008). Influence of Saccharomyces boulardii on the intestinal permeability of patients with Crohn's disease in remission. *Scand. J. Gastroenterol., 43*(7), 842-848.
[http://dx.doi.org/10.1080/00365520801943354] [PMID: 18584523]

Gardner, I.H., Siddharthan, R.V., Tsikitis, V.L. (2020). Benign anorectal disease: hemorrhoids, fissures, and fistulas. *Ann. Gastroenterol., 33*(1), 9-18.
[PMID: 31892792]

Gibson, P. (2019). Approach to functional gastrointestinal symptoms in adults with inflammatory bowel disease. *UpToDate., 20*.

Groebli, Y., Bertin, D., Morel, P. (2001). Meckel's diverticulum in adults: retrospective analysis of 119 cases and historical review. *Eur. J. Surg., 167*(7), 518-524.
[http://dx.doi.org/10.1080/110241501316914894] [PMID: 11560387]

Hecker, A., Hecker, B., Hecker, M., Riedel, J.G., Weigand, M.A., Padberg, W. (2016). Acute abdominal compartment syndrome: current diagnostic and therapeutic options. *Langenbecks Arch. Surg., 401*(1), 15-24.
[http://dx.doi.org/10.1007/s00423-015-1353-4] [PMID: 26518567]

Hellebrekers, B.W.J., Kooistra, T. (2011). Pathogenesis of postoperative adhesion formation. *Br. J. Surg., 98*(11), 1503-1516.
[http://dx.doi.org/10.1002/bjs.7657] [PMID: 21877324]

Ho, S., Krawitz, R., Fleming, B. (2018). Massive faecal impaction leading to abdominal compartment syndrome and acute lower limb ischaemia. *BMJ Case Rep., 2018*: bcr-2018-225202.
[http://dx.doi.org/10.1136/bcr-2018-225202] [PMID: 29930170]

Jacobs, D. (2014). Clinical practice. Hemorrhoids. *N. Engl. J. Med., 371*(10), 944-951.
[http://dx.doi.org/10.1056/NEJMcp1204188] [PMID: 25184866]

Janež, J, Klen, J (2021). Multidisciplinary diagnostic and therapeutic approach to acute mesenteric ischaemia: A case report with literature review. *SAGE Open Med Case Rep, 9*, 2050313X211004804.
[http://dx.doi.org/10.1177/2050313X211004804]

Keenan, J.E., Turley, R.S., McCoy, C.C., Migaly, J., Shapiro, M.L., Scarborough, J.E. (2014). Trials of nonoperative management exceeding 3 days are associated with increased morbidity in patients undergoing surgery for uncomplicated adhesive small bowel obstruction. *J. Trauma Acute Care Surg., 76*(6), 1367-1372.
[http://dx.doi.org/10.1097/TA.0000000000000246] [PMID: 24854302]

Keohane, D, Syed, AZ, Kavanagh, EG (2019). Unwell adolescent patient presenting to the Emergency Department with distended abdomen. *Gastroenterology, 156*(6), e12-4.
[http://dx.doi.org/10.1053/j.gastro.2018.12.032]

Keshavarz, P., Rafiee, F., Kavandi, H., Goudarzi, S., Heidari, F., Gholamrezanezhad, A. (2021). Ischemic gastrointestinal complications of COVID-19: a systematic review on imaging presentation. *Clin. Imaging, 73*, 86-95.
[http://dx.doi.org/10.1016/j.clinimag.2020.11.054] [PMID: 33341452]

Khati, N.J., Sondel Lewis, N., Frazier, A.A., Obias, V., Zeman, R.K., Hill, M.C. (2015). CT of acute perianal abscesses and infected fistulae: a pictorial essay. *Emerg. Radiol., 22*(3), 329-335.

[http://dx.doi.org/10.1007/s10140-014-1284-3] [PMID: 25421387]

Korkmaz, Ö., Yılmaz, H.G., Keleş, C. (2008). Erişkinlerde Görülen Meckel Divertikül Komplikasyonları. *Dicle Tıp Dergisi, 35*(2), 91-95.

Laval, G., Marcelin-Benazech, B., Guirimand, F., Chauvenet, L., Copel, L., Durand, A., Francois, E., Gabolde, M., Mariani, P., Rebischung, C., Servois, V., Terrebonne, E., Arvieux, C. (2014). Recommendations for bowel obstruction with peritoneal carcinomatosis. *J. Pain Symptom Manage., 48*(1), 75-91.
[http://dx.doi.org/10.1016/j.jpainsymman.2013.08.022] [PMID: 24798105]

Lazaridou, E., Aslanidi, C., Mellou, V., Athanasiou, S., Exarhos, D. (2021). Intraperitoneal focal fat infarction: the great mimicker in the acute setting. *Emerg. Radiol., 28*(1), 201-207.
[http://dx.doi.org/10.1007/s10140-020-01830-0] [PMID: 32712870]

Liakakos, T., Thomakos, N., Fine, P.M., Dervenis, C., Young, R.L. (2001). Peritoneal adhesions: etiology, pathophysiology, and clinical significance. Recent advances in prevention and management. *Dig. Surg., 18*(4), 260-273.
[http://dx.doi.org/10.1159/000050149] [PMID: 11528133]

Lim, S., Halandras, P.M., Bechara, C., Aulivola, B., Crisostomo, P. (2019). Contemporary management of acute mesenteric ischemia in the endovascular era. *Vasc. Endovascular Surg., 53*(1), 42-50.
[http://dx.doi.org/10.1177/1538574418805228] [PMID: 30360689]

MacRae, H.M., McLeod, R.S. (1995). Comparison of hemorrhoidal treatment modalities. A meta-analysis. *Dis. Colon Rectum, 38*(7), 687-694.
[http://dx.doi.org/10.1007/BF02048023] [PMID: 7607026]

Malbrain, M.L., De Keulenaer, B.L., Oda, J., De Laet, I., De Waele, J.J., Roberts, D.J., Kirkpatrick, A.W., Kimball, E., Ivatury, R. (2015). Intra-abdominal hypertension and abdominal compartment syndrome in burns, obesity, pregnancy, and general medicine. *Anaesthesiol. Intensive Ther., 47*(3), 228-240.
[http://dx.doi.org/10.5603/AIT.a2015.0021] [PMID: 25973659]

Maluso, P., Olson, J., Sarani, B. (2016). Abdominal compartment hypertension and abdominal compartment syndrome. *Crit. Care Clin., 32*(2), 213-222.
[http://dx.doi.org/10.1016/j.ccc.2015.12.001] [PMID: 27016163]

Medina-Gallardo, N.A., Curbelo-Peña, Y., Stickar, T., Gardenyes, J., Fernández-Planas, S., Roura-Poch, P., Vallverdú-Cartie, H. (2020). Omental infarction: Surgical or conservative treatment? a case reports and case series systematic review. *Ann. Med. Surg. (Lond.), 56*, 186-193.
[http://dx.doi.org/10.1016/j.amsu.2020.06.031] [PMID: 32642061]

Miller, P.A., Mezwa, D.G., Feczko, P.J., Jafri, Z.H., Madrazo, B.L. (1995). Imaging of abdominal hernias. *Radiographics, 15*(2), 333-347.
[http://dx.doi.org/10.1148/radiographics.15.2.7761639] [PMID: 7761639]

Molodecky, N.A., Soon, I.S., Rabi, D.M., Ghali, W.A., Ferris, M., Chernoff, G., Benchimol, E.I., Panaccione, R., Ghosh, S., Barkema, H.W., Kaplan, G.G. (2012). Increasing incidence and prevalence of the inflammatory bowel diseases with time, based on systematic review. *Gastroenterology, 142*(1), 46-54.e42.
[http://dx.doi.org/10.1053/j.gastro.2011.10.001] [PMID: 22001864]

Mott, T., Latimer, K., Edwards, C. (2018). Hemorrhoids: Diagnosis and Treatment Options. *Am. Fam. Physician, 97*(3), 172-179.
[PMID: 29431977]

Nazeeruddin, S., Butti, F., Herren, G. (2021). Enhanced-view totally extraperitoneal approach in emergency ventral incision hernia repair: a case report. *Swiss Med. Wkly., 151*: w20423.
[http://dx.doi.org/10.4414/smw.2021.20423] [PMID: 33635536]

Neves, J.M., Ramos Pinheiro, R., Côrte-Real, R., Borrego, M.J., Rodrigues, A., Fernandes, C. (2021). Lymphogranuloma venereum: a retrospective analysis of an emerging sexually transmitted disease in a Lisbon Tertiary Center. *J. Eur. Acad. Dermatol. Venereol., 35*(8), 1712-1716.

[http://dx.doi.org/10.1111/jdv.17302] [PMID: 33896044]

Onur, M.R., Akpinar, E., Karaosmanoglu, A.D., Isayev, C., Karcaaltincaba, M. (2017). Diverticulitis: a comprehensive review with usual and unusual complications. *Insights Imaging, 8*(1), 19-27.
[http://dx.doi.org/10.1007/s13244-016-0532-3] [PMID: 27878550]

Osada, H, Watanabe, W, Ohno, H (2012). Multidetector CT appearance of adhesion-induced small bowel obstructions: Matted adhesions versus single adhesive bands. *Jpn J Radiol, 30*, 706-12.

Parameswaran, P., Lucke, M. (2021). HLA B27 Syndromes.*StatPearls..* Treasure Island, FL: StatPearls Publishing. https://www.ncbi.nlm.nih.gov/books/NBK551523/ Updated 2021 Jul 10 Internet

Park, J.J., Wolff, B.G., Tollefson, M.K., Walsh, E.E., Larson, D.R. (2005). Meckel diverticulum: the Mayo Clinic experience with 1476 patients (1950-2002). *Ann. Surg., 241*(3), 529-533.
[http://dx.doi.org/10.1097/01.sla.0000154270.14308.5f] [PMID: 15729078]

Patcharatrakul, T., Rao, S.S.C. (2018). Update on the Pathophysiology and Management of Anorectal Disorders. *Gut Liver, 12*(4), 375-384.
[http://dx.doi.org/10.5009/gnl17172] [PMID: 29050194]

Pay, L., Kolak, Z., Çakır, B., Kamber, T., Yazıcı, S. (2021). Atrial fibrillation-related acute myocardial infarction and acute mesenteric ischemia. *Turk Kardiyol. Dern. Ars., 49*(5), 410-413.
[http://dx.doi.org/10.5543/tkda.2021.96533] [PMID: 34308875]

Peppercorn, MA, Cheifetz, AS (2019). *Definitions, epidemiology, and risk factors for inflammatory bowel disease in adults.*

Picchio, M., Greco, E., Di Filippo, A., Marino, G., Stipa, F., Spaziani, E. (2015). Clinical outcome following hemorrhoid surgery: a narrative review. *Indian J. Surg., 77* (Suppl. 3), 1301-1307.
[http://dx.doi.org/10.1007/s12262-014-1087-5] [PMID: 27011555]

Pothiawala, S., Gogna, A. (2012). Early diagnosis of bowel obstruction and strangulation by computed tomography in emergency department. *World J. Emerg. Med., 3*(3), 227-231.
[http://dx.doi.org/10.5847/wjem.j.issn.1920-8642.2012.03.012] [PMID: 25215068]

Puylaert, J.B. (2012). Ultrasound of colon diverticulitis. *Dig. Dis., 30*(1), 56-59.
[http://dx.doi.org/10.1159/000336620] [PMID: 22572686]

Rami Reddy, S.R., Cappell, M.S. (2017). A Systematic Review of the Clinical Presentation, Diagnosis, and Treatment of Small Bowel Obstruction. *Curr. Gastroenterol. Rep., 19*(6), 28.
[http://dx.doi.org/10.1007/s11894-017-0566-9] [PMID: 28439845]

Repplinger, M.D., Pickhardt, P.J., Robbins, J.B., Kitchin, D.R., Ziemlewicz, T.J., Hetzel, S.J., Golden, S.K., Harringa, J.B., Reeder, S.B. (2018). Prospective Comparison of the Diagnostic Accuracy of MR Imaging versus CT for Acute Appendicitis. *Radiology, 288*(2), 467-475.
[http://dx.doi.org/10.1148/radiol.2018171838] [PMID: 29688158]

Reza Zahiri, H., Belyansky, I., Park, A. (2018). Abdominal Wall Hernia. *Curr. Probl. Surg., 55*(8), 286-317.
[http://dx.doi.org/10.1067/j.cpsurg.2018.08.005] [PMID: 30470388]

Richard, P.G., Issa, Y., Van Santbrink, E.J.P. (2013). Burden of adhesions in abdominal and pelvic surgery: Systematic review and meta-analysis. *BMJ, 347*, 1-15.

Rizza, S., Mistrangelo, M., Ribaldone, D.G., Morino, M., Astegiano, M., Saracco, G.M., Pellicano, R. (2020). Proctitis: a glance beyond inflammatory bowel diseases. *Minerva Gastroenterol. Dietol., 66*(3), 252-266.
[http://dx.doi.org/10.23736/S1121-421X.20.02670-7] [PMID: 32218425]

Rosano, N., Gallo, L., Mercogliano, G., Quassone, P., Picascia, O., Catalano, M., Pesce, A., Fiorini, V., Pelella, I., Vespere, G., Romano, M., Tammaro, P., Marra, E., Oliva, G., Lugarà, M., Scuderi, M., Tamburrini, S., Marano, I. (2021). Ultrasound of Small Bowel Obstruction: A Pictorial Review. *Diagnostics (Basel), 11*(4), 617.
[http://dx.doi.org/10.3390/diagnostics11040617] [PMID: 33808245]

Rutkow, I.M. (2003). Demographic and socioeconomic aspects of hernia repair in the United States in 2003.

Surg. Clin. North Am., 83(5), 1045-1051, v-vi.
[http://dx.doi.org/10.1016/S0039-6109(03)00132-4] [PMID: 14533902]

Schnedl, W.J., Krause, R., Tafeit, E., Tillich, M., Lipp, R.W., Wallner-Liebmann, S.J. (2011). Insights into epiploic appendagitis. *Nat. Rev. Gastroenterol. Hepatol., 8*(1), 45-49.
[http://dx.doi.org/10.1038/nrgastro.2010.189] [PMID: 21102533]

Schuh, S., Chan, K., Langer, J.C., Kulik, D., Preto-Zamperlini, M., Aswad, N.A., Man, C., Mohanta, A., Stephens, D., Doria, A.S. (2015). Properties of serial ultrasound clinical diagnostic pathway in suspected appendicitis and related computed tomography use. *Acad. Emerg. Med., 22*(4), 406-414.
[http://dx.doi.org/10.1111/acem.12631] [PMID: 25808065]

Schuh, S., Man, C., Cheng, A., Murphy, A., Mohanta, A., Moineddin, R., Tomlinson, G., Langer, J.C., Doria, A.S. (2011). Predictors of non-diagnostic ultrasound scanning in children with suspected appendicitis. *J. Pediatr., 158*(1), 112-118.
[http://dx.doi.org/10.1016/j.jpeds.2010.07.035] [PMID: 20828717]

Schwenter, F., Poletti, P.A., Platon, A., Perneger, T., Morel, P., Gervaz, P. (2010). Clinicoradiological score for predicting the risk of strangulated small bowel obstruction. *Br. J. Surg., 97*(7), 1119-1125.
[http://dx.doi.org/10.1002/bjs.7037] [PMID: 20632281]

Sebbane, M., Dumont, R., Jreige, R., Eledjam, J.J. (2011). Epidemiology of acute abdominal pain in adults in the emergency department setting.*CT of the acute abdomen.* (pp. 3-13). Berlin, Heidelberg: Springer.
[http://dx.doi.org/10.1007/174_2010_135]

Shen, SH, Chen, JD, Tiu, CM (2005). Differentiating colonic diverticulitis from colon cancer: the value of computed tomography in the emergency setting. *J Chin Med Assoc., 68*, 411-41F8.

Silva, J.C., Rodrigues, A., Carvalho, J. (2020). Infectious Proctitis due to *Chlamydia trachomatis*: Venereal Diseases in Proctology. *GE Port. J. Gastroenterol., 27*(6), 439-440.
[http://dx.doi.org/10.1159/000507205] [PMID: 33251294]

Staudacher, H.M. (2017). Nutritional, microbiological and psychosocial implications of the low FODMAP diet. *J. Gastroenterol. Hepatol., 32* (Suppl. 1), 16-19.
[http://dx.doi.org/10.1111/jgh.13688] [PMID: 28244658]

Steele, S.R., Kumar, R., Feingold, D.L., Rafferty, J.L., Buie, W.D. (2011). Practice parameters for the management of perianal abscess and fistula-in-ano. *Dis. Colon Rectum, 54*(12), 1465-1474.
[http://dx.doi.org/10.1097/DCR.0b013e31823122b3] [PMID: 22067173]

Stern, E., Sugumar, K., Journey, J.D. Peptic Ulcer Perforated. 2021 Jun 23. In: StatPearls [Internet]. Treasure Island (FL): StatPearls Publishing; 2021.

Stoker, J., van Randen, A., Laméris, W., Boermeester, M.A. (2009). Imaging patients with acute abdominal pain. *Radiology, 253*(1), 31-46.
[http://dx.doi.org/10.1148/radiol.2531090302] [PMID: 19789254]

St-Vil, D., Brandt, M.L., Panic, S., Bensoussan, A.L., Blanchard, H. (1991). Meckel's diverticulum in children: a 20-year review. *J. Pediatr. Surg., 26*(11), 1289-1292.
[http://dx.doi.org/10.1016/0022-3468(91)90601-O] [PMID: 1812259]

Sulowski, C., Doria, A.S., Langer, J.C., Man, C., Stephens, D., Schuh, S. (2011). Clinical outcomes in obese and normal-weight children undergoing ultrasound for suspected appendicitis. *Acad. Emerg. Med., 18*(2), 167-173.
[http://dx.doi.org/10.1111/j.1553-2712.2010.00993.x] [PMID: 21314776]

Talan, D.A., Saltzman, D.J., DeUgarte, D.A., Moran, G.J. (2019). Methods of conservative antibiotic treatment of acute uncomplicated appendicitis: A systematic review. *J. Trauma Acute Care Surg., 86*(4), 722-736.
[http://dx.doi.org/10.1097/TA.0000000000002137] [PMID: 30516592]

Ten Broek, R.P.G., Krielen, P., Di Saverio, S., Coccolini, F., Biffl, W.L., Ansaloni, L., Velmahos, G.C., Sartelli, M., Fraga, G.P., Kelly, M.D., Moore, F.A., Peitzman, A.B., Leppaniemi, A., Moore, E.E., Jeekel, J.,

Kluger, Y., Sugrue, M., Balogh, Z.J., Bendinelli, C., Civil, I., Coimbra, R., De Moya, M., Ferrada, P., Inaba, K., Ivatury, R., Latifi, R., Kashuk, J.L., Kirkpatrick, A.W., Maier, R., Rizoli, S., Sakakushev, B., Scalea, T., Søreide, K., Weber, D., Wani, I., Abu-Zidan, F.M., De'Angelis, N., Piscioneri, F., Galante, J.M., Catena, F., van Goor, H. (2018). Bologna guidelines for diagnosis and management of adhesive small bowel obstruction (ASBO): 2017 update of the evidence-based guidelines from the world society of emergency surgery ASBO working group. *World J. Emerg. Surg., 13*, 24.
[http://dx.doi.org/10.1186/s13017-018-0185-2] [PMID: 29946347]

Tong, J.W.V., Lingam, P., Shelat, V.G. (2020). Adhesive small bowel obstruction - an update. *Acute Med. Surg., 7*(1): e587.
[http://dx.doi.org/10.1002/ams2.587] [PMID: 33173587]

Uhe, I., Meyer, J., Viviano, M., Naiken, S., Toso, C., Ris, F., Buchs, N.C. (2021). Caecal diverticulitis can be misdiagnosed as acute appendicitis: a systematic review of the literature. *Colorectal Dis., 23*(10), 2515-2526. Epub ahead of print
[http://dx.doi.org/10.1111/codi.15818] [PMID: 34272795]

Usuda, D., Takanaga, K., Sangen, R., Higashikawa, T., Kinami, S., Saito, H., Kasamaki, Y. (2020). Abdominal compartment syndrome due to extremely elongated sigmoid colon and rectum plus fecal impaction caused by disuse syndrome and diabetic neuropathy: a case report and review of the literature. *J. Med. Case Reports, 14*(1), 219.
[http://dx.doi.org/10.1186/s13256-020-02566-8] [PMID: 33183343]

Vagholkar, K., Chougle, Q., Agrawal, P. (2016). Omental torsion: a rare cause of acute abdomen. *Int Surg J, 3*, 1711-1713.
[http://dx.doi.org/10.18203/2349-2902.isj20163196]

Verburgt, C.M., Heutink, W.P., Kuilboer, L.I.M., Dickmann, J.D., van Etten-Jamaludin, F.S., Benninga, M.A., de Jonge, W.J., Van Limbergen, J.E., Tabbers, M.M. (2021). Antibiotics in pediatric inflammatory bowel diseases: a systematic review. *Expert Rev. Gastroenterol. Hepatol., 15*(8), 891-908.
[http://dx.doi.org/10.1080/17474124.2021.1940956] [PMID: 34148466]

Vilz, T.O., Stoffels, B., Strassburg, C., Schild, H.H., Kalff, J.C. (2017). Ileus in Adults. *Dtsch. Arztebl. Int., 114*(29-30), 508-518.
[PMID: 28818187]

Vogel, J.D., Johnson, E.K., Morris, A.M., Paquette, I.M., Saclarides, T.J., Feingold, D.L., Steele, S.R. (2016). Clinical practice guideline for the management of anorectal abscess, fistula-in-ano, and rectovaginal fistula. *Dis. Colon Rectum, 59*(12), 1117-1133.
[http://dx.doi.org/10.1097/DCR.0000000000000733] [PMID: 27824697]

Wald, A., Bharucha, A.E., Cosman, B.C., Whitehead, W.E. (2014). ACG clinical guideline: management of benign anorectal disorders. *Am. J. Gastroenterol., 109*(8), 1141-1157, 1058.
[http://dx.doi.org/10.1038/ajg.2014.190] [PMID: 25022811]

Wang, C.H., Yang, C.C., Hsu, W.T., Qian, F., Ding, J., Wu, H.P., Tsai, J.J., Yang, C.J., Su, M.Y., Chen, S.C., Lee, C.C. (2021). Optimal initial antibiotic regimen for the treatment of acute appendicitis: a systematic review and network meta-analysis with surgical intervention as the common comparator. *J. Antimicrob. Chemother., 76*(7), 1666-1675.
[http://dx.doi.org/10.1093/jac/dkab074] [PMID: 33792691]

Yang, G.P.C. (2017). Laparoscopy in emergency hernia repair. *Ann. Laparosc. Endosc. Surg., 2*, 6.
http://ales.amegroups.com/article/view/4017

Specific Diagnoses and Management Principles of the Hepatobiliary and Pancreatic Diseases

Abstract: Hepatobiliary and pancreatic diseases are among common illnesses which cause major morbidity and mortality in the middle-aged and elderly patients and some specific subpopulations. Some geographic predispositions also exist for some diseases. For example, pain, fever, jaundice, and hepatomegaly can be noted in hydatic cyst disease which may cause allergic reaction and portal hypertension in the Southeast Europe and the Middle East. Of note, hepatobiliary and pancreatic diseases are commonly confused with each other, which may complicate diagnostic and therapeutic processes. A patient with biliary stones may be asymptomatic or suffer from acute or chronic cholecystitis, biliary colic, obstructive jaundice, cholangitis, mucocele, empyema, acute pancreatitis, gallstone ileus, and carcinoma. Cholecystitis and cholangitis are among diseases with high morbidity especially in the elderly and thus need to be ruled out in any patient with abdominal pain evaluated in acute and primary care setting. Some diagnostic clues are extremely helpful, such as Charcot triad which suggest severe cholecystitis (right upper quadrant AP, jaundice and fever) or cholangitis when complicated by altered mental status and hemodynamic instability. Acute pancreatitis refers to acute response to injury of the pancreas is referred to. Chronic pancreatitis, on the contrary, results from permanent damage to the endocrine and exocrine functions of the gland. Ultrasound, computed tomography and magnetic resonance imaging are among invaluable tools in diagnosing these diseases, together with specific laboratory adjuncts such as serum lipase for pancreatitis and bilirubin for obstructive jaundice. Definitive treatment encompasses surgical procedures, mostly in patients with acute abdomen due to gallstones or pancreatic necrosis.

Keywords: Acute pancreatitis, Acute cholecystitis, Biliary tract diseases, Cholangitis, Hepatobiliary diseases, Hydatic cyst disease.

LIVER DISEASES

Hydatid Cyst

It consists of the larvae of the Echinococcus parasite (E. granulosus and E. Multilocularis). Sheep carry it, and it is transmitted to humans by dogs eating the uncontrolled meat (esp. liver) of these sheep. Infection is usually acquired in childhood, and it rarely presents clinically before the fourth decade of life.

Ozgur KARCIOGLU, Selman YENİOCAK, Mandana HOSSEINZADEH & Seckin Bahar SEZGIN

Larvae → portal vein → liver (in 75% of cases)

- **In E. Granulosus,** which is more common in most parts of the World including Southeast Europe and the Middle East, hydatid cysts grow up to 1 cm in the first 6 months and grow 2 to 3 cm every year. The outcome is better than the other subspecies.
- **In E. Multilocularis,** the larvae proliferate and penetrate the surrounding tissue. They cause a diffuse and infiltrative granulomatous reaction and may mimic **malignancy**. It progresses as **necrosis → cavitation → calcification.**

Microscopic Features of Hydatid Cysts Include

- Cyst fluid: Antigenic, light yellow, neutral pH
- Endocyst: Forms daughter vesicles/capsule may detach, revealing sediments or daughter cysts.
- Ectocyst: Acellular substance secreted by the parasite
- Pericyst: granulation/fibrosis tissue layer formed by host response

Clinical Presentation

Cysts are initially asymptomatic. Symptoms appear as the size increases or infection or rupture develops.

Pain, fever, jaundice, hepatomegaly can be noted (therefore may be confused with biliary tract disease, cholecystitis/cholangitis).

May cause allergic reaction and portal hypertension.

Typical clinical profile: Middle-aged (farming) patient presents with sudden-onset right upper quadrant pain, jaundice, and palpable mass.

Diagnostic Checklist

Hydatid cysts can masquerade (or are masqueraded by) biliary cystadenoma, pyogenic liver abscess, cystic metastases, hemorrhagic/ infected cysts. Both the imaging and clinical courses of E. multilocularis mimic a solid malignant neoplasm.

Lab: - eosinophilia, boosted serological titers are detected in 80% of patients.

- İncreased levels of alkaline phosphatase (ALP) and GGT.

Presumptive diagnosis is confirmed by advanced **imaging**. First of all, USG should be performed (Fig. **1**).

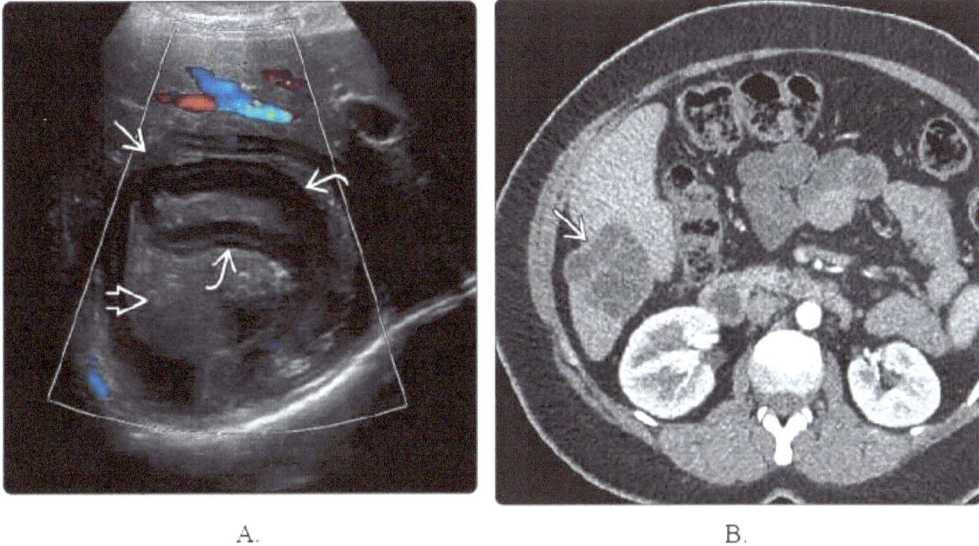

A.   B.

Fig. (1). A. Oblique abdominal color Doppler USG shows hepatic echinococcal cyst (arrow) and fine echogenic debris (hydatid sand) (hollow arrow). Separation of the endocyst membrane causes the membranes to float within the pericyst, what we call the "water lily" sign (curved arrow). **B** Axial abdominal contrast-enhanced CT shows a multiloculated cystic mass (arrow) in the right lobe of the liver.

Percutaneous cyst aspiration should be performed carefully for there is a risk of peritoneal spillage and anaphylaxis.

Tips for Radiology

Daughter cysts float inside the main cysts, and their situation changes when the patient changes his/her position.

Treatment

E. granulosus

- **Medical:** Albendazole/mebendazole
- **Direct injection** of scolicid agent
- **"PAIR"** procedure: Puncture, Aspiration, İnjection, Respiration
- **Surgery:** Segmental or lobar hepatectomy
- **E. multilocularis**

Partial hepatectomy/hepatectomy + liver transplant

Portal vein thrombosis/occlusion (PVTO) develops as a result of thrombosis, hypercoagulability, and intra-abdominal inflammation due to flow stasis. Thrombosis can develop in the main body of the portal vein or its intrahepatic branches and extends to the splenic or superior mesenteric veins. PVT frequently occurs with cirrhosis of the liver (Samant, 2021). Tumor thrombus or direct tumor invasion may also occur. Abdominal sepsis, pancreatitis, systemic lupus erythematosus, or other conditions precipitating hypercoagulable states can underlie PVTO.

The pathophysiological characteristics of PVTO comprise one or more elements of Virchow's triad.

- diminished portal blood flow,
- hypercoagulability state,
- endothelial damage on the vessels.
- **In acute thrombosis, the lumen is filled** with thrombus and thus the diameter is enlarged.
- Cavernous transformation occurs with lumen occlusion in chronic thrombosis.
  Clinical findings: The most common complaints are AP and distension. Ileus/MBO may also develop as it causes edema in the intestines. A network study revealed that non-cirrhotic non-malignant acute PVT usually presents with AP (91%), high body temperature (53%) and ascitic collection (38%) (Plessier, 2010).
  Involvement of superior mesenteric vein can trigger intestinal ischemia, bowel infarction, ileus presenting as hematochezia, fever, and sepsis and is responsible for high mortality in this subset of patients. Acute abdominal findings (guarding) may also develop as a result of bowel infarction. Besides cirrhosis, this condition can also lead to ascites, jaundice and/or variceal bleeding.
  Laboratory values: The liver functions can be normal with the exclusion of cirrhotic patients complicated by PVT. Thrombocytopenia can ensue secondary to splenomegaly and portal hypertension. Portal biliopathy may cause a rise in alkaline phosphatase and bilirubin (Samant, 2021). In addition, investigations of protein C, S, antithrombin III levels, factor V, Leiden mutation can also be ordered in consistent clinical settings.

Imaging

- **Color/spectral Doppler USG** is an investigation of choice with sensitivity and specificity ranging from 80% to 100% with an accuracy of 88% to 98%

(Samant, 2021).

It is preferred for screening and presumptive diagnosis. The absence of flow in the portal vein (PV) is suggestive of PVTO. Cavernous transformation of PV may be seen (Fig. **2**).

- Contrast-enhanced CT/MR

- **Contrast-enhanced CT/MR**

It is preferred for comprehensive evaluation. The extent of the thrombotic occlusion, collateralization, ischemic bowel or infarction can be examined *via* this modality. Damage to the adjacent organs is also visualized *via* CT or MRI. The sensitivity and specificity of MRI for detecting the main PVT are 100% and 98%, respectively (Lin, 2003).

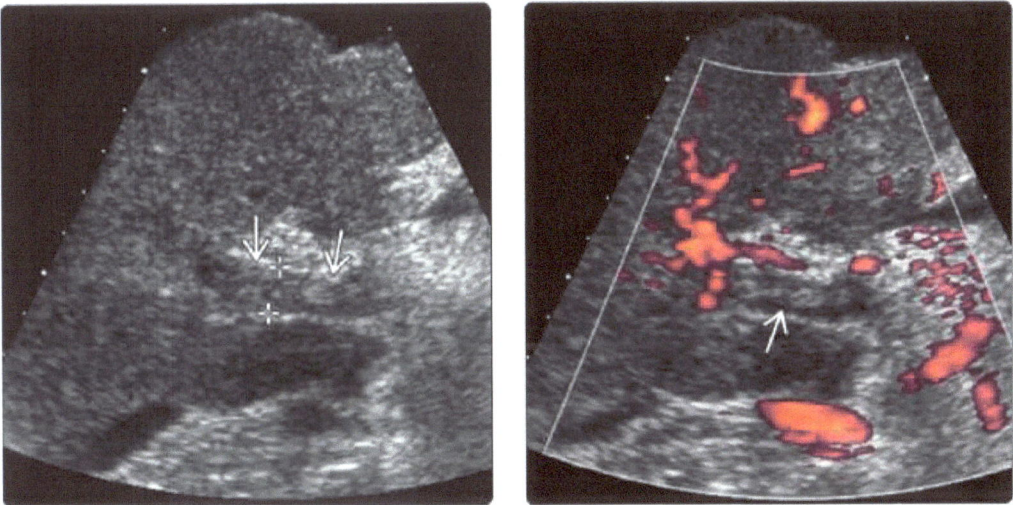

Fig. (2). A. Liver USG shows mild echogenic thrombus in the main PV (arrow). B. PVTO with Power Doppler USG confirms absence of flow (arrow). Ascites, which indicates cirrhosis, can also be visualized.

DD Include

- Budd-Chiari syndrome
- Cirrhosis
- Sarcoidosis
- Schistosomiasis
- Arsenic toxicity

Treatment

The outcome is mostly related to the severity and prevalence of the underlying disease. Besides anticoagulation and supportive treatment, TIPS + PV thrombectomy/ thrombolysis can be employed. Although challenging for radiologists, TIPS can recanalize the occluded segment by disrupting the thrombus and mechanical thrombectomy. Surgical thrombectomy or mechanical thrombectomy by percutaneous transhepatic route is associated with recurrence of thrombosis from intimal or vascular trauma to the portal vein (Rosenqvist, 2018).

B) Biliary Tract (BT) Diseases

BT diseases are mostly attributed to gallstones in the acute setting. Both cholesterol and mixed type stones are common in middle-aged and older people. Bilirubin (pigment) stones are seen in the younger group, in diseases triggering hemolysis such as malaria and hereditary spherocytosis. These stones are more numerous and smaller.

Complications of Gallstones: Acute and chronic cholecystitis, biliary colic, obstructive jaundice, cholangitis, mucocele, empyema, acute pancreatitis, gallstone ileus, and carcinoma may ensue in a patient with biliary stones.

Biliary hyperkinesia can emerge in the absence of gallstones. It is considered in patients with biliary-like pain and no evidence of gallstones on imaging modalities but who have had biliary scintigraphy scan (HIDA) that shows ejection fraction $\geq 80\%$. A meta-analytic study disclosed that patients with typical biliary colic symptoms without gallstones and markedly high ejection fraction might benefit from having cholecystectomy to alleviate their symptoms (Eltyeb, 2021).

Acute Cholecystitis (AC) defines the acutely appearing inflammation of the gallbladder. The main pathophysiology is the obstruction of the cystic duct.

Is every biliary colic cholecystitis? No. Transient blockage by sludge or stones can precipitate biliary colic.

Acute Calculous Cholecystitis (ACC) refers to cystic duct blockage with a gallstone. The term ACC should be used only after we see that the discomfort or pain is unrelieved for around six hours (Wilkins, 2017).

If no stone is identified, it is called acute acalculous cholecystitis (AAC).

Basic physiology: In a healthy human, the gallbladder takes the stimuli to empty its ingredients, namely, the bile, to the intestines through the cystic duct, following consumption of certain (types of) foods, especially fatty and spicy foods. This operation is essential in the digestion of these types of foods.

Concentrated bile is susceptible to precipitation forming stones following bile stasis, supersaturation from the liver of cholesterol and lipids, disruption in the concentration process, and cholesterol crystal nucleation (Jones, 2021). This process paves the way for the formation of ACC.

History: It manifests as nausea ± vomiting + right hypochondrial pain radiating to the right side of the back with the impaction of the stone triggering inflammation.

Examination: Fever may be present but not the rule. It is associated with Murphy's sign (Fig. **3**). A right subcostal palpable mass may be noted, which is a sign of mucocele or empyema. In the presence of empyema, the picture is aggravated with high fever, severe pain, and progression to septic shock.

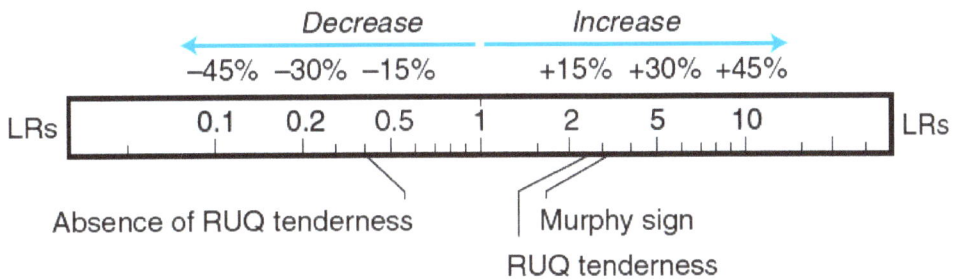

Fig. (3). Examination findings significantly increase and decrease the likelihood of acute cholecystitis. LR: Likelihood ratio, RUQ: Right upper quadrant, LUQ: Left upper quadrant.

USG findings of ACC include choledochal enlargement, visualization of stones, pericholecystic fluid collection, positive sonographic Murphy sign, wall thickness >4 mm, wall edema (target sign) and hyperemia. Of these, stone and sonographic Murphy have the most predictive power for ACC.

On the other hand, **CT** can be useful in ruling out the alternative diagnoses such as pancreatitis, pseudocyst, Bouveret's syndrome, cancer, *etc.*, and evaluating the extent of the disease. A comparison of the pros and cons of the diagnostic modalities is depicted in Table **1**.

Table 1. Comparison of CT, USG and MR in establishing a diagnosis of ACC.

• USG is ideal for stones, polyps and cholecystitis.
• USG is at the forefront as a noninvasive bedside initial test.
• USG provides an advantage with Doppler mode regarding demonstration of vascularization.
• Accuracy of USG decreases in gassy and obese patients
• CT cannot give intraluminal details.
• CT visualizes the extent of the disease, it is more advantageous in diseases such as emphysematous cholecystitis, and infiltrative cancer.

(Table 1) cont.....

• MRI shows non-calcified stones better than CT or USG.
• MRCP is superior in imaging the biliary tree and gallbladder
• MRI examinations are more expensive and slower than the other modalities.
• USG and MRI can be preferred in pregnant women safely.

Since the **Tokyo Guidelines** were introduced in 2007 (TG07) and refined in 2013 (TG13), our understanding of the diagnostic and therapeutic approaches to cholecystitis has evolved substantially (Mayumi, 2007, Yokoe, 2013). These guidelines developed a consensus methodology for assessing and describing the severity of acute cholecystitis (Escartin, 2021) (Tables **2** and **3**).

Table 2. Diagnostic criteria for acute cholecystitis in line with the Tokyo Guidelines.

A. Local signs of inflammation:
- Murphy's sign
- Right upper quadrant mass, pain or guarding
B. Signs of systemic inflammation:
- Fever> 37.5 °C
- High C-reactive protein
- Leukocytosis > $10 \times 10\,9\,/\,1$
C. Characteristic findings of acute cholecystitis:

• wall edema of > 5 mm,
    • distended gallbladder,
    • radiological Murphy's sign,
    • perivesicular fluid,
    • cholelithiasis.

Consider diagnosis: criteria A + B
Definitive diagnosis: criteria A + B + C

Table 3. Criteria for acute cholecystitis severity according to the Tokyo Guidelines.

Grade I (mild)	Grade II (intermediate)	Grade III (severe)
Does not meet any Grade II or Grade III criteria	one of the following conditions is identified:	associated with dysfunction of one of these organs or systems:

Grade I (mild)	Grade II (intermediate)	Grade III (severe)
	1) Increased white blood cell count > 18,000/mm3/ 2) Palpable soft mass in the right upper quadrant 3) Duration of symptoms > 72 hrs 4) Significant local inflammation (gangrenous cholecystitis, perivesicular abscess, liver abscess, emphysematous cholecystitis, coleperitoneum)	1) Cardiovascular: hypotension requiring treatment with dopamine ≥ 5 µg/kg/min or (independent of dose) epinephrine 2) Neurological: impaired consciousness 3) Respiration: PaO2/FiO2 <300 4) Kidney: oliguria or creatinine>2.0 mg/dL 5) Hepatic: prothrombin time, INR >1.5 6) Hematological: platelet count <100,000/mm3

Severity of ACC can be outlined *via* the detection of histopathological changes like gangrene, perforation, and empyema. Severe ACC correlates with higher morbidity and longer hospital stay. CT findings were the most important predictors of severe ACC (Khan, 2021). Patients with clinical and laboratory predictors of severe ACC should be sought using a contrast CT scan to exclude serious complications.

Management

- IV analgesia and antiemetic administration
- Leukocytes are usually high, glucose, amylase, liver enzymes/ coagulation profile is ordered. Elevations in these markers are not *sine qua non* for the diagnosis
- Chest X-ray and ECG should be obtained in every patient.
- Start antibiotics especially in the elderly, debilitated patients with comorbidities such as diabetes (you may prefer cephalosporin, eg cefazolin or cefotaxime)
- Consult the patient with the general surgeon.

Controversy Around Antibiotics After ACC

Research pointed out that extended postoperative antibiotic therapy does not improve postoperative infectious or noninfectious outcomes in patients with mild or moderate ACC undergoing emergency cholecystectomy (EC) (Hajibandeh, 2019). Postoperative antibiotics should not be routinely used and should be preserved only for selected cases.

In a randomized controlled non-inferiority trial, standard single-dose antibiotic prophylaxis (cefazolin, 2000 mg), was compared with antibiotic prophylaxis for 3 days after surgery (IV cefuroxime 750 mg plus metronidazole 500 mg, tid) patients with mild ACC (Loozen, 2017). Single-dose cefazolin administration did not lead to an increase in postoperative complications in patients with mild ACC following cholecystectomy.

In another meta-analysis including 676 patients, no significant benefit of extended antibiotic therapy in reducing surgical site infections after cholecystectomy for mild and moderate ACC (La Regina, 2018).

Which procedure to pursue? Percutaneous gallbladder drainage (PC GBD), endoscopic ultrasound-guided gallbladder drainage (EUS GBD), and endoscopic transpapillary gallbladder drainage (ET GBD) are used for patients with ACC with high surgical risk. PC GBD, EUS GBD, and ET GBD resulted in similar clinical success, adverse events, recurrent cholecystitis, reintervention, and mortality rates. PC GBD was associated with a higher success rate than EUS GBD (OR = 0.75) or ET GBD (OR = 0.73). EUS GBD was associated with the highest probability of clinical success (67.5%), and the lowest prevalences of adverse events (57.0%) and recurrent cholecystitis (60.9%). ET GBD was associated with the best reintervention outcomes (81.8%). Compared with PC GBD and ET GBD, EUS GBD appears to be preferable with respect to both safety and efficacy for the treatment of patients with ACC with high surgical risk (Lyu, 2021).

Likewise, Huang *et al.* performed a meta-analysis comparing percutaneous cholecystostomy (PC) versus EC for the treatment of ACC in high-risk surgical patients (Huang, 2021). Of note, PC was associated with increased risks of mortality (RR = 2.87; p = 0.007) and readmission rate (RR = 4.70; p < 0.00001) as compared with EC. PC was accompanied by significantly higher risks of mortality (RR = 7.47; p = 0.004), morbidity (RR = 3.71; p = 0.0005), readmission rate (RR = 7.91; p < 0.00001), when directly compared with laparoscopic cholecystectomy (LC). Therefore, EC is superior to PC for the treatment of ACC in high-risk surgical patients, and LC is the preferred surgical strategy.

Figs. (**4 - 8**) demonstrate imaging studies of case examples with gallbladder disease.

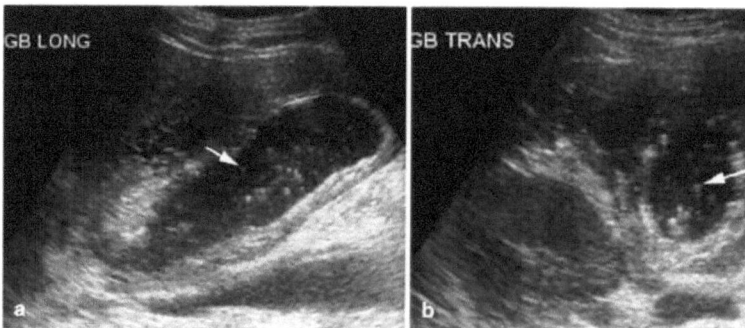

Fig. (4). 48-year old woman has a typical sludge appearance in the gallbladder. Comet-tail artifact is noted.

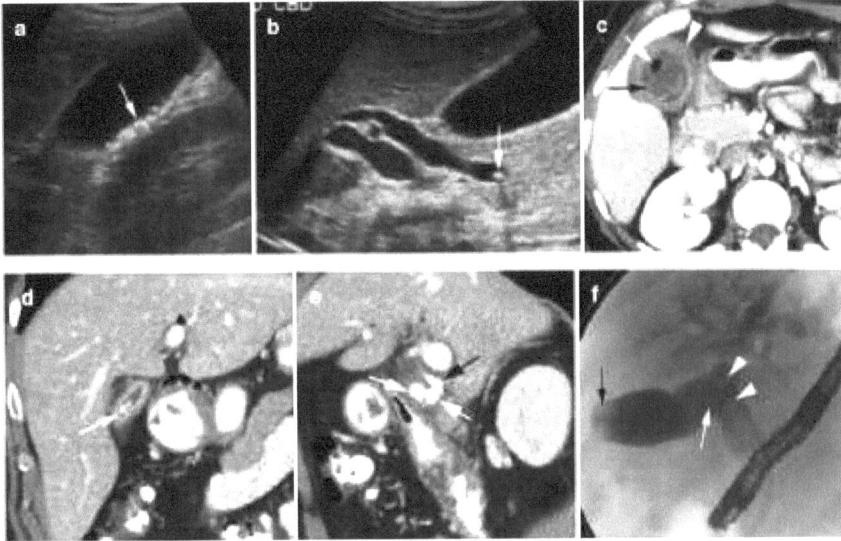

Fig. (5). Gallstones on USG and CT. **(a)** Multiple reflective echogenic foci in the gallbladder are observed on USG together with a posterior acoustic shadow (arrow). **(b)** echogenic stone visualized at the distal end of the dilated common duct (CD) with echo shadow (arrow). **(c)** Axial CT shows acute cholecystitis due to low-density stones with rim calcifications (black arrow), small gas collection in a stone (white arrow), and increased gallbladder wall thickness (arrowhead). **(d)** Coronal reformatted CT image shows multiple highly attenuated calcified stones in the contracted gallbladder (arrow). **(e)** CT sagittal reformatted image showing stones in the cystic duct (white arrows) and stent in the hepatic duct (black arrow). **(f)** Stones in the gallbladder (black arrow), cystic duct (white arrow), CD (arrowheads) visualized in ERCP.

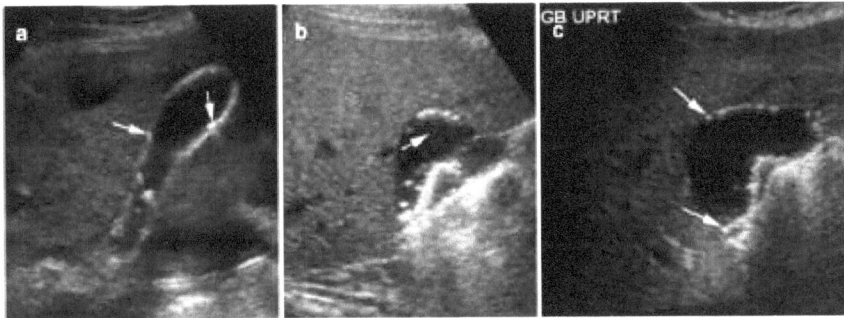

Fig. (6). Cholesterolosis. Multiple nonmobile echogenic foci in the wall of the gallbladder are seen with ring-down artifacts, and acoustic shadows are not observed. It can be localized or diffuse patchy form. Comet-tail artifact can be seen.

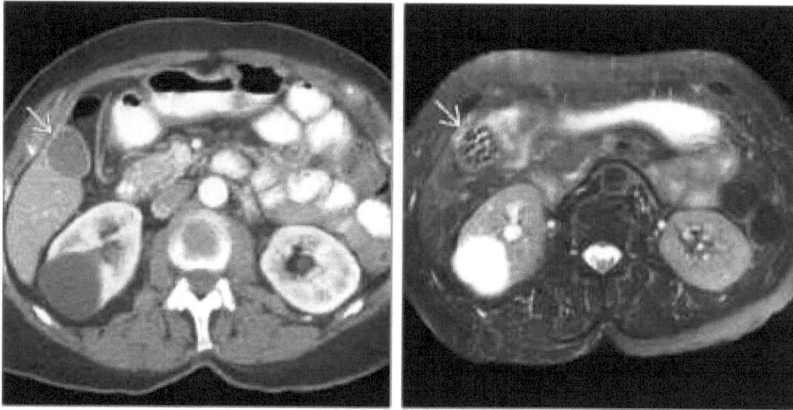

Fig. (7). Imaging in an hexagenarian woman presenting with right upper quadrant pain. **A.** Intraluminal structures appear normal on contrast-enhanced CT. **B.** In the same patient, multiple stones that could not be located in the previous CT are observed in the MRI (T2-weighted images) obtained 1 week later, and thus the patient is transferred to operation.

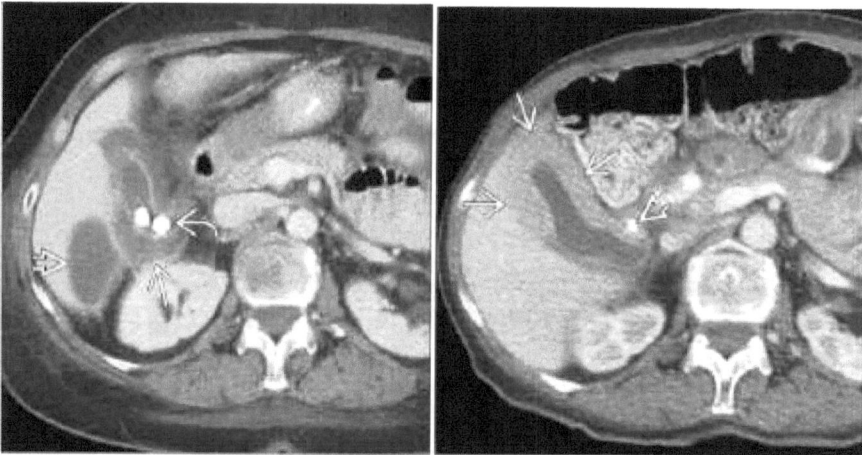

Fig. (8). Imaging in a 75-year-old female patient with signs of acute cholecystitis. **A.** Abscess and subcapsular liver abscess adjacent to gallstones and gallbladder on axial contrast-enhanced CT. Percutaneous abscess drainage was performed. **B.** In the same patient, after 3 months, gallbladder wall was massively thickened and a stone impacted the neck of the pouch. A diagnosis of xanthogranulomatous cholecystitis was established at the operation.

Acute cholangitis is a systemic disease triggered by acute inflammation and infection of the biliary tree with or without the presence of gallstones. It can result from ascending bacterial colonization and/or biliary obstruction associated with bacterial overgrowth. The entity results in substantial sequelae and death rates.

There is a predilection for females and middle-aged or elderly people, although young patients are also reported frequently. Patients with recent biliary instrumentation or previous biliary operations are at higher risk of having cholangitis.

Acute cholangitis can present in many different ways, from mild symptoms to fulminant sepsis. The case series reported that more than half of the patients belonged to a group with mild clinical severity (Grade I in Tokyo Guidelines) (Florescu, 2021). Likewise, the most common cause of acute cholangitis was shown to be obstructive lithiasis in the biliary tree (Fig. **9**).

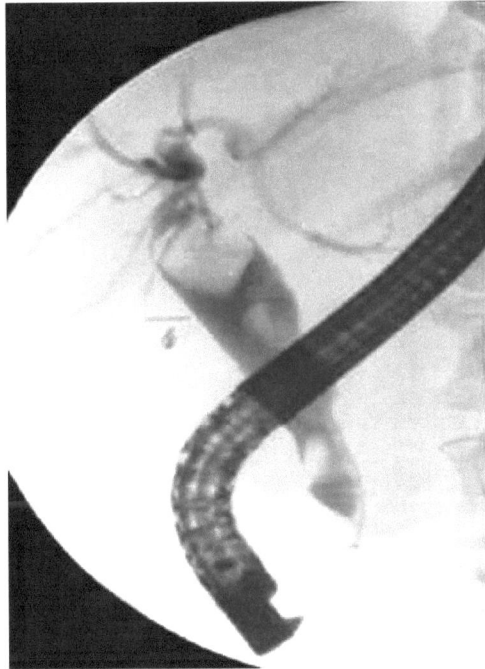

Fig. (9). Stones visualized in the biliary tree with consequent cholangitis.

Clinical findings: Biliary stasis predisposes to infection, findings known as the "Charcot triad" indicate severe cholecystitis (right upper quadrant AP + jaundice + fever) or cholangitis which also include altered mental status and hemodynamic instability.

The full triad launched by Charcot in 1877 is only seen in slightly more than half of patients. Specifically, fever is seen in over 90% of cases, pain is seen in 70% of cases, and jaundice is seen in 60% of cases (O'Connell, 2017). The addition of altered mental status and hypotension render the patient more likely to experience severe cholangitis (a.k.a. Reynold's Pentad) which is recorded in only 5%–7% of cases (Attasaranya 2008) (Table **4**).

Table 4. Reynold's Pentad is made up of five criteria.

• fever
• AP
• jaundice
• altered mentation
• low blood pressure

DD includes pyonephrosis/pyelonephritis, ACC, AAC, sepsis, septic shock, pancreatitis, and intraabdominal abscess.

On examination, there are many clinical signs that can be useful in approaching the diagnosis, including Murphys sign and Charcot's triad which show low sensitivity and limited clinical use. Therefore, some researchers sought for new methods for bedside recognition of biliary tract diseases. Indirect fist percussion of the liver (pain induced by striking the right hypochondrium with the hand in a fisted position) was suggested to have considerable diagnostic accuracy to detect hepatobiliary infection and diseases, with a higher sensitivity than Murphy's sign (Table **5**) (Ueda, 2015).

Table 5. Diagnostic accuracy of three different maneuvers for hepatobiliary infection.

	Sensitivity	Specificity	LR+	LR-
Tenderness on right upper quadrant	33 (19–49)	91 (88–94)	3.6 (2.1–6.3)	0.74 (0.60–0.92)
Murphy's sign	30 (17–47)	93 (90–96)	4.4 (2.4–8.1)	0.75 (0.61–0.92)
Indirect fist percussion of liver	60 (43–75)	85 (81–89)	4.1 (2.9–5.8)	0.47 (0.32–0.69)

The most common **causative agents** are E. coli, Klebsiella spp, and Enterococcus spp. Patients with previous biliary surgery, the elderly, and those with severe disease are more likely to have anaerobic organisms such as Clostridium or Bacteroides species, and polymicrobial infection in this population is more likely as well (Tanaka, 2007).

Diagnostic Criteria: Many authors believe that Charcot's triad has lost its validity because of low sensitivity and has been replaced with the criteria established by the Tokyo guidelines (Given in the Cholecystitis chapter). Nowadays, the diagnosis is mostly established *via* the presence of systemic inflammation, cholestasis, jaundice and biliary obstruction documented by imaging studies. The threshold for biliary duct dilation on ultrasonographic evaluation is 7 mm (DeCarlo, 2013). The presence or degree of biliary dilation does not correspond well to the severity of cholangitis; rather, severity of disease is more strongly associated with the amount of intraductal pressure (Ely, 2017).

Radiological Adjuncts

Transabdominal USG is successful to visualize around 25%–60% of the gallstones in the common bile duct. Mosler's 2011 algorithm for approach to patients with suspected cholangitis includes USG as the first choice, followed by CT (Mosler, 2011) (Fig. **10**).

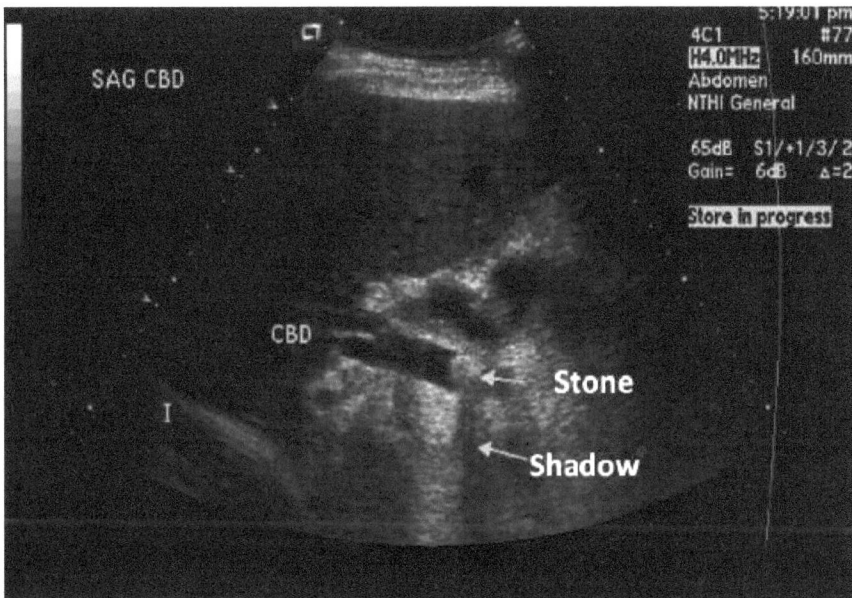

Fig. (10). Ultrasound demonstrates choledocholithiasis with dilated common bile duct.

On the other hand, multidetector contrast-enhanced CT has very high levels of sensitivity and specificity in the identification of gallstones in the common bile duct (85% - 97% and 88% - 96%, respectively) (Attasaranya 2008).

Treatment principles mostly depend on the severity of the clinical picture. The strategy varies from antibiotic therapy to emergency biliary drainage, including endoscopic retrograde cholangiopancreatography (ERCP).

Endoscopic biliary drainage in the first 24 hours after presentation resulted in a faster recovery, shortened use of antibiotics, decreased duration of hospital stay, lower morbidity and death rates compared to those that suffered the intervention more than 24 hours (Florescu, 2021). Scoring systems employed to identify patients who may tolerate a delayed approach have not been validated yet.

Appropriate recognition, early broad-spectrum antibiotics, and fluid resuscitation are paramount, and in patients with severe disease, early biliary decompression will significantly reduce mortality (Ely, 2018).

TG13 criteria request that mild disease (grade I) may be managed with a carbapenem, fluoroquinolone, penicillin with beta-lactamase inhibitor, or fourth-generation cephalosporin (Gomi, 2013).

Outcomes: The percentage of severe cases almost doubles in those with acute cholangitis (11.6%) compared with ACC (6%), and the mortality rate due to acute cholangitis is 2.7%, more than four-fold of that associated with cholecystitis (0.6%) (Kiriyama, 2012).

Case presentation: Rupture of the gallbladder (Fig. **11**).

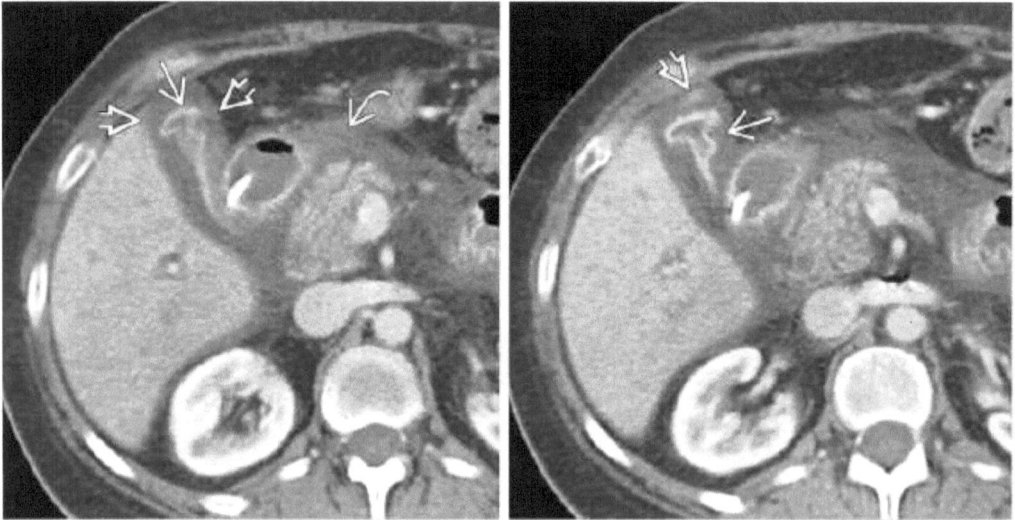

Fig. (11). Imaging of a 55-year-old male patient who had a motorcycle accident. A. Collapsed gallbladder in axial contrast-enhanced CT is remarkable with its irregular contours. The gallbladder wall is thickened and there is peripancreatic fluid. B. There is a hyperattenuated area due to hemorrhage in the thickened wall of the gallbladder.

Conditions Predisposing To Gallbladder Perforation as a Result of Trauma

Distended gallbladder,

Alcohol consumption,

Thin-walled normal gallbladder,

Inability of the abdominal muscles to guard viscera due to sudden trauma,

Contraction of the sphincter of Oddi and increased bile duct pressure.

C) ACUTE AND CHRONIC PANCREATITIS

Acute response to injury of the pancreas is referred to as acute pancreatitis. Chronic pancreatitis, on the contrary, results from permanent damage to the endocrine and exocrine functions of the pancreas which paves the way to pancreatic insufficiency.

Acute Pancreatitis

It is a common cause of AP in middle age and older. Gallstones and alcohol are common causes. There are also idiopathic ones, due to drugs or viruses, and cancer.

A majority of patients (80%) exhibit mild symptomatology and are discharged within a few days. Overall mortality is around 2% (Forsmark, 2016).

In the typical patient, ill-defined AP perceived in the mid-upper abdomen radiates to the back and is accompanied by nausea and vomiting.

The pain is mostly defined as severe sharp pain in the epigastric region and radiates to the back (Mohy-ud-din, 2021). The patient may be dehydrated and sweating cold. There may be a state of shock indicative of the need for urgent resuscitation. Although not a rule, if there is abdominal tenderness, it is mostly in the epigastric region, sometimes up to degree of guarding. The Grey-Turner sign, which is often mentioned but almost never seen, may appear days later, if any. This sign is present where there is ecchymosis in the flanks. Cullen's sign, on the other hand, is present when there is ecchymosis around the umbilicus. Both signs could indicate pancreatic necrosis leading to blood in the abdomen (Mookadam, 2005). Severe pancreatitis may also result in changes in mentation.

Work Up

- Basal metabolic values + SpO_2 should be recorded
- Serum amylase is usually $> 5 \times$ upper limit. It is recommended to be ordered together with urine amylase.
- There may be an increase in leukocytes (not a rule).
- Hyperglycemia and/or hypocalcemia may be seen and suggest more severe disease course.
- Coagulation tests.

• Chest X-ray, ECG, ABG; lactate is examined in severe patients.

CT and/or MRI are used to assess pancreatic necrosis and abscesses in patients with consistent findings. Visualization of extraluminal gas in or around pancreas is suggestive of an underlying infection (Figs. **12** and **13**).

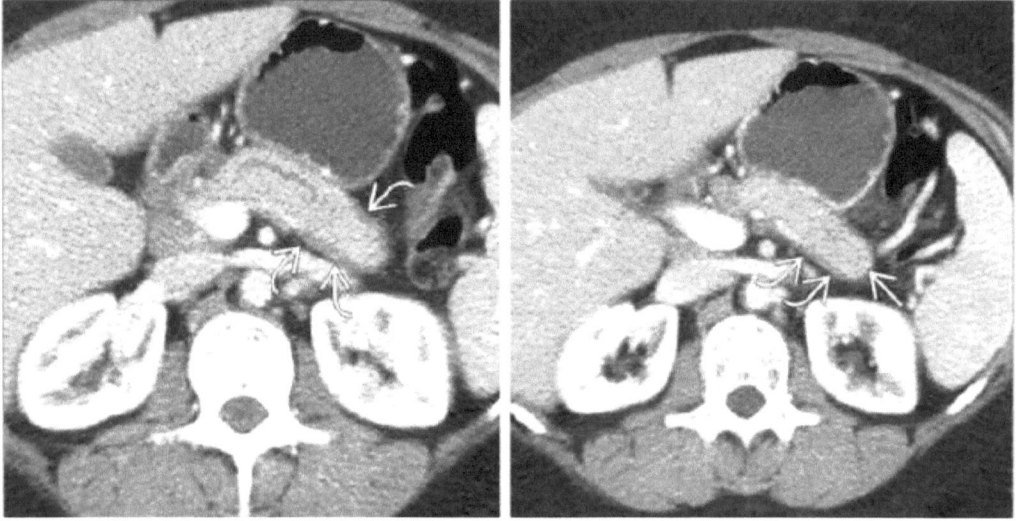

Fig. (12). "Sausage sign" in contrast-enhanced CT examination in a 55-year-old patient with pancreatitis presenting with jaundice. A. Peripheral hypoattenuation rim and minimal peripancreatic fatty streaks showing autoimmune pancreatitis on axial sections. B. Slight diffuse enlargement of the pancreas: sausage-like appearance with peripheral hypoattenuation rim. Erased lobulated contour is typical.

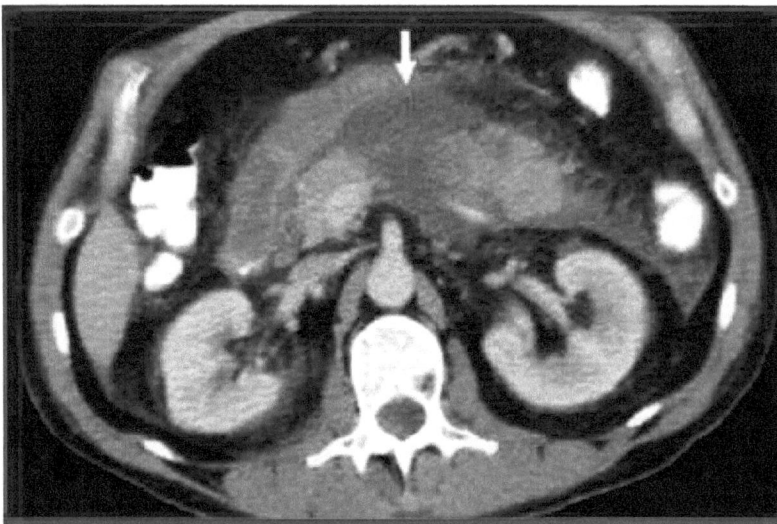

Fig. (13). The imaging findings of acute necrotizing pancreatitis.

COVID-19 and Pancreas: The pandemic disease affects almost every system and organ in the body, through overtly activated inflammatory and prothrombotic cascades (also called cytokine storm) and other abrupt changes. Some studies reported radiological findings related to COVID-19 (Goldberg-Stein, 2020, Liu, 2020, Mazrouei, 2020).

Pancreatic injury can be attributed to several factors in the pandemic disease such as drug toxicity, hyperinflammatory state, dehydration, fever, *etc.* Elevated pancreatic enzymes were noted in 13 patients, while the changes consistent with acute pancreatitis were noted radiologically in only five of these (Liu, 2020). In this study, focal enlargement of the pancreas or dilatation of the main pancreatic duct were reported without any evidence of necrosis, in those with severe COVID-19 (Liu, 2020). The good news is that most of the pancreatic radiological findings were not severe, especially in patients with severe COVID-19 (Agarwal, 2021). In addition, pancreatic ductal dilatation has been demonstrated in three patients with COVID-19 by Goldberg-Stein *et al.* (Goldberg-Stein, 2020).

Treatment

o Give O_2 (if SpO_2 is below 94%, or those with symptoms such as fever, tachycardia, agitation, ischemic-type chest pain, altered level of consciousness)

o IV fluids should be administered and titrated to beware of both pulmonary congestion and hypovolemia.

o IV analgesia (morphine/fentanyl), titrate to effect, individualize for the patient.

o Anti-emetics may be given. Ondansetron is the first choice, while H1 antagonists or metoclopramide 10 mg slow infusion is acceptable.

o **Antibiotherapy:** It should be started as early as possible in accordance with local protocols in patients who are planned to undergo an operation and in those who are thought to have sepsis/septic shock. Empirical combination therapy (ECT) is at the forefront in emergency setting, without waiting for the blood culture results. IV imipenem 500 mg IV q8h for 14 days can be preferred if cultures are positive, or "septic signs" are identified (De Campos, 2006).

- Insert NG tube.
- Monitor urine output with a Foley catheter.
- Admit in intensive care or general surgery wards, depending on the general status and scoring (APACHEII, SAPSII, Glasgow, Ranson, shock index, sepsis evaluation, NEWS).
- Methods for drainage: Abdominal paracentesis drainage and percutaneous

catheter drainage have long been employed in patients with acute pancreatitis. In a meta-analytic study, Lu *et al.* showed that early intervention with paracentesis drainage is associated with reduced mortality, treatment costs and the length of stay compared with the 'step-up' strategy of percutaneous drainage without affecting the rate of infectious complications (Lu, 2021).

Complications of Acute Pancreatitis

The short and long-term mortality rates of acute pancreatitis are quite high. Its early complications include acute renal failure, disseminated intravascular coagulation (DIC), hypocalcemia, acute respiratory distress syndrome (ARDS). Pancreatic abscess or pseudocyst may occur in the late period. Patients considered to have acute pancreatitis and did not show signs of improvement within 72 hours of appropriate management should be suspected to have an abdominal abscess, including pancreatic ones.

Pancreatic abscesses are usually complications of acute necrotizing pancreatitis and contain inflammatory material of cellular debris, pancreatic enzymes, and liquid. Infectious or non-infectious sources can progress to an abscess formation. Persistent fever, AP, and failure to improve despite appropriate treatment should suggest superimposed infection of the pancreas.

Progress to abscess formation: In the acute phase of the pancreatic inflammation, there can be an ill-defined fluid collection around the organ which is described as a peripancreatic fluid collection. After four weeks, the fluid collection becomes much more organized with a definite fibrous wall, and it is then referred to as a **pseudocyst** (Hoilat, 2021). The pseudocyst is a cyst containing pancreatic enzymes, defined by a fibrous wall but lacks an epithelial lining. If this pseudocyst gets infected, it is referred to as a pancreatic abscess (Fig. **14**).

Estimation of Risk of Death

It can be calculated based on the presence of predefined and validated prognostic indicators (Glasgow scoring system). Accordingly, if three or more of the following are present on presentation, or if they are identified within 48 hours, it will indicate the presence of severe disease (Table **6**).

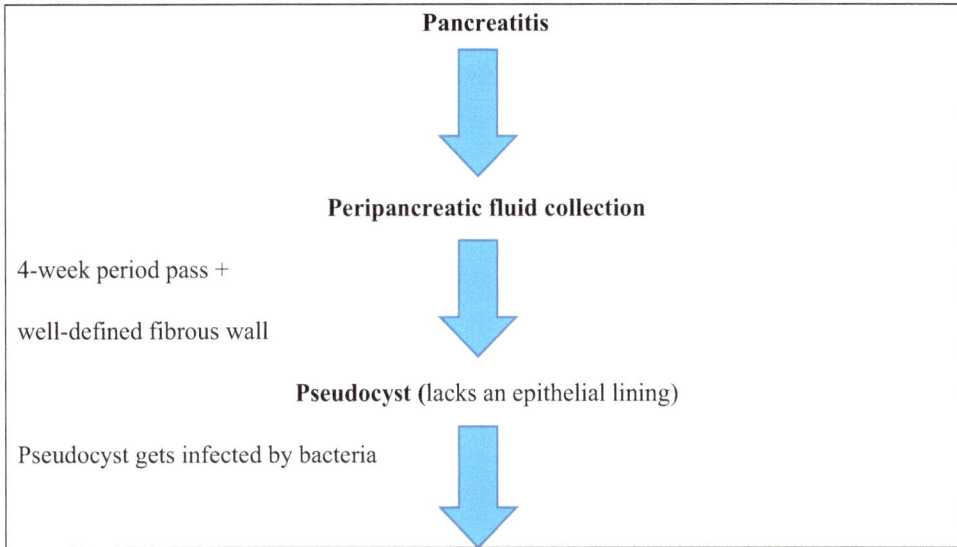

Fig. (14). "4P" Process of acute pancreatitis.

Table 6. Glasgow Scoring System is used to estimate death risk in pancreatitis.

Age > 55
WBC > 15 × 10 9 /L
Glucose (fasting) > 10 mmol/L (180 mg/dL)
Urea > 50 mg/dL
Pa O_2 < 60 mmHg
Ca_2+< 8 mg/dL
albumin < 3.2 g/dL
serum LDH > 600U/L
AST > 100U/L.

CONCLUSION

Hepatobiliary and pancreatic diseases consist of a heterogeneous group of diseases of the liver, biliary system and pancreas caused by viral, bacterial, and parasitic infections, neoplasia, toxic chemicals, alcohol consumption, poor nutrition, metabolic disorders, and cardiac failure. Population ageing causes an upward trend in the diseases of biliary tract and pancreas, in parallel with morbidity and mortality. Diagnosis requires careful physical examination with history taking which will help narrow the possible diagnostic list and ancillary laboratory and radiological tests to produce a presumptive or definite diagnosis. The evaluation of patients with known or suspected diseases of the region should include categorization of the problem into one of several clinical syndromes which will narrow the list of differential diagnoses. Hepatobiliary and pancreatic diseases are prone to overlap and misdiagnoses that complicate diagnostic and therapeutic processes. A well-organized team approach will minimize diagnostic delays and management errors in the emergency setting. For example, new horizons launched by interventional radiology procedures will ease the management of most situations in line with surgical and endoscopic techniques.

REFERENCES

Agarwal, L., Agarwal, A., Advani, S., Katiyar, V., Chaturvedi, A., Madhusudhan, K.S. (2021). The eyes see what the mind seeks: a systematic review of abdominal imaging findings in patients with COVID-19. *Br. J. Radiol., 94*(1124), 20201220.
[http://dx.doi.org/10.1259/bjr.20201220] [PMID: 34260323]

Attasaranya, S., Fogel, E.L., Lehman, G.A. (2008). Choledocholithiasis, ascending cholangitis, and gallstone pancreatitis. *Med. Clin. North Am., 92*(4), 925-960, x.
[http://dx.doi.org/10.1016/j.mcna.2008.03.001] [PMID: 18570948]

De Campos, T., Assef, J.C., Rasslan, S. (2006). Questions about the use of antibiotics in acute pancreatitis. *World J. Emerg. Surg., 1*(1), 20.
[http://dx.doi.org/10.1186/1749-7922-1-20] [PMID: 16820058]

DeCarlo, A., Mcfadden, D.W. (2013). Choledocholithiasis and cholangitis. In: Zinner, M.J., Ashley, S.W., (Eds.), *Maingot's abdominal operations.* (12th ed., pp. 1009-1028). New York: McGraw-Hill.

Eltyeb, H.A., Al-Leswas, D., Abdalla, M.O., Wayman, J. (2021). Systematic review and meta-analyses of cholecystectomy as a treatment of biliary hyperkinesia. *Clin. J. Gastroenterol., 14*(5), 1308-1317.
[http://dx.doi.org/10.1007/s12328-021-01463-x] [PMID: 34115337]

Ely, R., Long, B., Koyfman, A. (2018). The Emergency Medicine-Focused Review of Cholangitis. *J. Emerg. Med., 54*(1), 64-72.
[http://dx.doi.org/10.1016/j.jemermed.2017.06.039] [PMID: 28939398]

Escartín, A, González, M, Muriel, P, Cuello, E, Pinillos, A, Santamaría, M, Salvador, H, Olsina, JJ (2021). Litiasic acute cholecystitis: application of Tokyo Guidelines in severity grading. *Cir Cir., 89*(1), 12-21.
[http://dx.doi.org/10.24875/CIRU.19001616]

Florescu, V., Pârvuleţu, R., Ardelean, M., Angelescu, M., Angelescu, G.A., Enciu, O., Iordache, N. (2021). The Emergency Endoscopic Treatment in Acute Cholangitis. *Chirurgia (Bucur.), 116*(1), 42-50.
[http://dx.doi.org/10.21614/chirurgia.116.1.42] [PMID: 33638325]

Forsmark, C.E., Vege, S.S., Wilcox, C.M. (2016). Acute Pancreatitis. *N. Engl. J. Med., 375*(20), 1972-1981.
[http://dx.doi.org/10.1056/NEJMra1505202] [PMID: 27959604]

Goldberg-Stein, S., Fink, A., Paroder, V., Kobi, M., Yee, J., Chernyak, V. (2020). Abdominopelvic CT findings in patients with novel coronavirus disease 2019 (COVID-19). *Abdom. Radiol. (N.Y.), 45*(9), 2613-2623.
[http://dx.doi.org/10.1007/s00261-020-02669-2] [PMID: 32761402]

Gomi, H., Solomkin, J.S., Takada, T., Strasberg, S.M., Pitt, H.A., Yoshida, M., Kusachi, S., Mayumi, T., Miura, F., Kiriyama, S., Yokoe, M., Kimura, Y., Higuchi, R., Windsor, J.A., Dervenis, C., Liau, K.H., Kim, M.H. (2013). TG13 antimicrobial therapy for acute cholangitis and cholecystitis. *J. Hepatobiliary Pancreat. Sci., 20*(1), 60-70.

[http://dx.doi.org/10.1007/s00534-012-0572-0] [PMID: 23340954]

Hajibandeh, S., Popova, P., Rehman, S. (2019). Extended Postoperative Antibiotics Versus No Postoperative Antibiotics in Patients Undergoing Emergency Cholecystectomy for Acute Calculous Cholecystitis: A Systematic Review and Meta-Analysis. *Surg. Innov., 26*(4), 485-496.
[http://dx.doi.org/10.1177/1553350619835347] [PMID: 30873901]

Hoilat, G.J., Katta, S. (2021). Pancreatic Abscess. In: StatPearls [Internet]. Treasure Island (FL): StatPearls Publishing; 2022 Jan. Available from: https://www.ncbi.nlm.nih.gov/books/NBK560555/.

Huang, H., Zhang, H., Yang, D., Wang, W., Zhang, X. (2021). Percutaneous cholecystostomy *versus* emergency cholecystectomy for the treatment of acute calculous cholecystitis in high-risk surgical patients: a meta-analysis and systematic review. *Updates Surg., 73*, 481-94.
[http://dx.doi.org/10.1007/s13304-020-00894-4] [PMID: 33991327]

Jones, M.W., Genova, R., O'Rourke, M.C. (2021). Acute Cholecystitis. In: StatPearls [Internet]. Treasure Island (FL): StatPearls Publishing; 2022 Jan-. Available from: https://www.ncbi.nlm.nih.gov/books/NBK459171/.

Khan, S.M., Emile, S.H., Barsom, S.H., Naqvi, S.A.A., Khan, M.S. (2021). Accuracy of pre-operative parameters in predicting severe cholecystitis-A systematic review. *Surgeon, 19*(4), 219-225.
[http://dx.doi.org/10.1016/j.surge.2020.06.010] [PMID: 32703731]

Kiriyama, S., Takada, T., Strasberg, S.M., Solomkin, J.S., Mayumi, T., Pitt, H.A., Gouma, D.J., Garden, O.J., Büchler, M.W., Yokoe, M., Kimura, Y., Tsuyuguchi, T., Itoi, T., Yoshida, M., Miura, F., Yamashita, Y., Okamoto, K., Gabata, T., Hata, J., Higuchi, R., Windsor, J.A., Bornman, P.C., Fan, S.T., Singh, H., de Santibanes, E., Gomi, H., Kusachi, S., Murata, A., Chen, X.P., Jagannath, P., Lee, S., Padbury, R., Chen, M.F. (2012). New diagnostic criteria and severity assessment of acute cholangitis in revised Tokyo Guidelines. *J. Hepatobiliary Pancreat. Sci., 19*(5), 548-556.
[http://dx.doi.org/10.1007/s00534-012-0537-3] [PMID: 22825491]

La Regina, D., Di Giuseppe, M., Cafarotti, S., Saporito, A., Ceppi, M., Mongelli, F., Bihl, F., Balzarotti Canger, R.C., Ferrario di Tor Vajana, A. (2019). Antibiotic administration after cholecystectomy for acute mild-moderate cholecystitis: a PRISMA-compliant meta-analysis. *Surg. Endosc., 33*(2), 377-383.
[http://dx.doi.org/10.1007/s00464-018-6498-0] [PMID: 30327917]

Lin, J., Zhou, K.R., Chen, Z.W., Wang, J.H., Wu, Z.Q., Fan, J. (2003). Three-dimensional contrast-enhanced MR angiography in diagnosis of portal vein involvement by hepatic tumors. *World J. Gastroenterol., 9*(5), 1114-1118.
[http://dx.doi.org/10.3748/wjg.v9.i5.1114] [PMID: 12717869]

Liu, F., Long, X., Zhang, B., Zhang, W., Chen, X., Zhang, Z. (2020). ACE2 expression in pancreas may cause pancreatic damage after SARS-CoV-2 infection. *Clin. Gastroenterol. Hepatol., 18*(9), 2128-2130.e2.
[http://dx.doi.org/10.1016/j.cgh.2020.04.040] [PMID: 32334082]

Loozen, C.S., Kortram, K., Kornmann, V.N., van Ramshorst, B., Vlaminckx, B., Knibbe, C.A., Kelder, J.C., Donkervoort, S.C., Nieuwenhuijzen, G.A., Ponten, J.E., van Geloven, A.A., van Duijvendijk, P., Bos, W.J., Besselink, M.G., Gouma, D.J., van Santvoort, H.C., Boerma, D. (2017). Randomized clinical trial of extended versus single-dose perioperative antibiotic prophylaxis for acute calculous cholecystitis. *Br. J. Surg., 104*(2), e151-e157.
[http://dx.doi.org/10.1002/bjs.10406] [PMID: 28121041]

Lu, Z., Zhu, X., Hua, T., Zhang, J., Xiao, W., Jia, D., Yang, M. (2021). Efficacy and safety of abdominal paracentesis drainage on patients with acute pancreatitis: a systematic review and meta-analysis. *BMJ Open, 11*(8), e045031.
[http://dx.doi.org/10.1136/bmjopen-2020-045031] [PMID: 34373293]

Lyu, Y., Li, T., Wang, B., Cheng, Y., Chen, L., Zhao, S. (2021). Comparison of Three Methods of Gallbladder Drainage for Patients with Acute Cholecystitis Who Are at High Surgical Risk: A Network Meta-Analysis and Systematic Review. *J. Laparoendosc. Adv. Surg. Tech. A, 31*(11), 1295-1302.
[http://dx.doi.org/10.1089/lap.2020.0897] [PMID: 33416417]

Marrone, G., Crino', F., Caruso, S., Mamone, G., Carollo, V., Milazzo, M., Gruttadauria, S., Luca, A., Gridelli, B. (2012). Multidisciplinary imaging of liver hydatidosis. *World J. Gastroenterol., 18*(13), 1438-1447.
[http://dx.doi.org/10.3748/wjg.v18.i13.1438] [PMID: 22509075]

Maurea, S., Caleo, O., Mollica, C., Imbriaco, M., Mainenti, P.P., Palumbo, C., Mancini, M., Camera, L., Salvatore, M. (2009). Comparative diagnostic evaluation with MR cholangiopancreatography, ultrasonography and CT in patients with pancreatobiliary disease. *Radiol. Med. (Torino), 114*(3), 390-402.
[http://dx.doi.org/10.1007/s11547-009-0374-x] [PMID: 19266258]

Mayumi, T., Takada, T., Kawarada, Y., Nimura, Y., Yoshida, M., Sekimoto, M., Miura, F., Wada, K., Hirota, M., Yamashita, Y., Nagino, M., Tsuyuguchi, T., Tanaka, A., Gomi, H., Pitt, H.A. (2007). Results of the Tokyo Consensus Meeting Tokyo Guidelines. *J. Hepatobiliary Pancreat. Surg., 14*(1), 114-121.
[http://dx.doi.org/10.1007/s00534-006-1163-8] [PMID: 17252304]

Mazrouei, S.S.A., Saeed, G.A., Al Helali, A.A., Hilali, A. (2020). COVID-19-associated acute pancreatitis: a rare cause of acute abdomen. *Radiol. Case Rep., 15*(9), 1601-1603.
[http://dx.doi.org/10.1016/j.radcr.2020.06.019] [PMID: 32685078]

Mookadam, F., Cikes, M. (2005). Images in clinical medicine. Cullen's and Turner's signs. *N. Engl. J. Med., 353*(13), 1386.
[http://dx.doi.org/10.1056/NEJMicm040796] [PMID: 16192483]

Mosler, P. (2011). Diagnosis and management of acute cholangitis. *Curr. Gastroenterol. Rep., 13*(2), 166-172.
[http://dx.doi.org/10.1007/s11894-010-0171-7] [PMID: 21207254]

O'Connell, W., Shah, J., Mitchell, J., Prologo, J.D., Martin, L., Miller, M.J., Jr, Martin, J.G. (2017). Obstruction of the Biliary and Urinary System. *Tech. Vasc. Interv. Radiol., 20*(4), 288-293.
[http://dx.doi.org/10.1053/j.tvir.2017.10.010] [PMID: 29224663]

Plessier, A., Darwish-Murad, S., Hernandez-Guerra, M., Consigny, Y., Fabris, F., Trebicka, J., Heller, J., Morard, I., Lasser, L., Langlet, P., Denninger, M.H., Vidaud, D., Condat, B., Hadengue, A., Primignani, M., Garcia-Pagan, J.C., Janssen, H.L., Valla, D. (2010). Acute portal vein thrombosis unrelated to cirrhosis: a prospective multicenter follow-up study. *Hepatology, 51*(1), 210-218.
[http://dx.doi.org/10.1002/hep.23259] [PMID: 19821530]

Qian, L.J., Zhu, J., Zhuang, Z.G., Xia, Q., Liu, Q., Xu, J.R. (2013). Spectrum of multilocular cystic hepatic lesions: CT and MR imaging findings with pathologic correlation. *Radiographics, 33*(5), 1419-1433.
[http://dx.doi.org/10.1148/rg.335125063] [PMID: 24025933]

Rosenqvist, K., Ebeling Barbier, C., Rorsman, F., Sangfelt, P., Nyman, R. (2018). Treatment of acute portomesenteric venous thrombosis with thrombectomy through a transjugular intrahepatic portosystemic shunt: a single-center experience. *Acta Radiol., 59*(8), 953-958.
[http://dx.doi.org/10.1177/0284185117742683] [PMID: 29202584]

Samant, H., Asafo-Agyei, K.O., Garfield, K. (2021). Portal Vein Thrombosis. In: StatPearls [Internet]. Treasure Island (FL): StatPearls Publishing; 2022 Jan. Available from: https://www.ncbi.nlm.nih.gov/books/NBK534157/.

Tanaka, A., Takada, T., Kawarada, Y., Nimura, Y., Yoshida, M., Miura, F., Hirota, M., Wada, K., Mayumi, T., Gomi, H., Solomkin, J.S., Strasberg, S.M., Pitt, H.A., Belghiti, J., de Santibanes, E., Padbury, R., Chen, M.F., Belli, G., Ker, C.G., Hilvano, S.C., Fan, S.T., Liau, K.H. (2007). Antimicrobial therapy for acute cholangitis: Tokyo Guidelines. *J. Hepatobiliary Pancreat. Surg., 14*(1), 59-67.
[http://dx.doi.org/10.1007/s00534-006-1157-6] [PMID: 17252298]

Ueda, T., Ishida, E. (2015). Indirect Fist Percussion of the Liver Is a More Sensitive Technique for Detecting Hepatobiliary Infections than Murphy's Sign. *Curr. Gerontol. Geriatr. Res., 2015*, 431638.
[http://dx.doi.org/10.1155/2015/431638] [PMID: 26788057]

Wilkins, T., Agabin, E., Varghese, J., Talukder, A. (2017). Gallbladder Dysfunction: Cholecystitis,

Choledocholithiasis, Cholangitis, and Biliary Dyskinesia. *Prim. Care,* *44*(4), 575-597.
[http://dx.doi.org/10.1016/j.pop.2017.07.002] [PMID: 29132521]

Yokoe, M., Takada, T., Strasberg, S.M., Solomkin, J.S., Mayumi, T., Gomi, H., Pitt, H.A., Garden, O.J., Kiriyama, S., Hata, J., Gabata, T., Yoshida, M., Miura, F., Okamoto, K., Tsuyuguchi, T., Itoi, T., Yamashita, Y., Dervenis, C., Chan, A.C., Lau, W.Y., Supe, A.N., Belli, G., Hilvano, S.C., Liau, K.H., Kim, M.H., Kim, S.W., Ker, C.G. (2013). TG13 diagnostic criteria and severity grading of acute cholecystitis (with videos). *J. Hepatobiliary Pancreat. Sci.,* *20*(1), 35-46.
[http://dx.doi.org/10.1007/s00534-012-0568-9] [PMID: 23340953]

CHAPTER 7

Specific Diagnoses and Management Principles of the Urinary and Genital Tract Diseases

Abstract: Urinary tract infections (UTIs) and genital tract diseases (GTD) are among the most common infectious diseases with female predominance. On the other hand, acute epididymitis and orchitis are the most common GTDs which cause scrotal pain in adult males. Testicular torsion is a true medical emergency with vascular compromise and mandates immediate intervention to beware of serious complications. Although a majority are self-limiting diseases which can be treated easily, rapid diagnosis and management of certain UTIs and GTDs are a must to prevent grave outcomes. The infections may inflict the lower and/or the upper parts of urinary tract which also determines the severity of the disease. The urinary stone disease generally presents with ureteral colicky pain, blunt flank pain, nausea/vomiting, and hematuria with a male predominance. Most patients are managed easily in the acute setting but some are prone to deterioration with protracted urinary obstruction and resultant renal damage. The utilization of reliable, easy-to-use diagnostic tools with high accuracy is the key to expedient detection, identification and treatment. Ultrasound provides invaluable information in point-of-care diagnosis of most urinary tract diseases in both sexes. Management should be individualized in accord with the patients' signs and symptoms, general status and outcome estimations.

Keywords: Acute epididymitis, Genital tract disease, Gynecological pain, Orchitis, Ovarian torsion, Pelvic inflammatory disease, Pyelonephritis, Testicular torsion, Ureteral colic, Urinary stone disease.

ACUTE EPIDIDYMITIS AND ORCHITIS (AEO)

AEO is the most common cause of scrotal pain in adult males. Men in their third decade in life constitute nearly half of all cases. It occurs with sexual transmission under 35 years of age, or with chlamydial / gonococcal infection. If the patient is over 35 years old, it is mostly accompanied by a urinary tract infection (UTI). Escherichia coli, and Pseudomonas are mostly involved in this group. In one series, epididymitis occurred with orchitis in 58% of patients (Kaver, 1990). Rarely, it can also be triggered by trauma or autoimmune diseases.

Ozgur KARCIOGLU, Selman YENİOCAK, Mandana HOSSEINZADEH & Seckin Bahar SEZGIN

Mumps (epidemic parotitis) infection can lead to orchitis (14% to 35% of the involved patients) in postpubertal males (Azmat, 2021). When associated with mumps infection, orchitis ensues four to seven days after the emergence of parotitis (Trojian, 2009). Unaccompanied by AEO, it is almost always indicative of mumps. 1/5 to 2/3 of these patients suffer from bilateral orchitis. The dreadful complication of this appears to be **testicular atrophy.**

Orchitis is usually viral in young patients, while mumps and rubella are the most common causative agents (Kanda, 2014). In addition, coxsackievirus, varicella, echovirus, and cytomegalovirus can lead to orchitis. Bacterial orchitis can be caused by *Escherichia coli, Klebsiella pneumoniae, Pseudomonas aeruginosa*, and *Staphylococcus* and *Streptococcus* spp. (Azmat, 2021). In sexually active males *Neisseria gonorrhoeae, Chlamydia trachomatis*, and *Treponema pallidum can also be isolated.* There are also reports of orchitis caused by autoimmunity, which are classified as primary and secondary.

Acute epididymitis encompasses pain and scrotal swelling for less than 45 days, while chronic cases are symptomatic for longer than 12 weeks and are typically recognized with pain without scrotal swelling (Trojian, 2009).

Etiology varies with the patient's age and the likely pathogens. AEO is manifested as the gradual onset of posterior scrotal pain that may be accompanied by urinary symptoms such as dysuria and urinary frequency (McConaghy, 2016).

How do we Evaluate Acute Scrotal Pain (ASP) in the Emergency Setting?

DD for the patient with ASP is summarized in Table **1**. Empiric treatment with antibiotics for acute epididymitis is given in Table **2**.

Table 1. Selected differential diagnosis of acute scrotal pain (Trojian 2009, Crawford, 2014).

Diagnosis	Most Common Presentation	Signs	USG/Color Doppler (CD) Findings
Epididymitis	Slow-onset ASP on the posterior side and swelling in a few days	Scrotal swelling or inflammation and tenderness of the epididymis; Prehn sign (+) (pain relieved by scrotal elevation); cremasteric reflex spared	Hyperemia, swelling, and increased blood flow of the epididymis on CD
Testicular cancer	Some cases can present with pain	Firm and tender nodule in the involved testis	Distinct mass involving the testis on CD
Testicular torsion	Sudden onset of severe unilateral ASP	High-riding testis, absent cremasteric reflex, increased pain with scrotal elevation	Absent blood flow on CD

(Table 1) cont.....

Diagnosis	Most Common Presentation	Signs	USG/Color Doppler (CD) Findings
Torsion of testicular appendix	Sudden onset of ASP	Blue-dot sign (bluish discoloration of the scrotum, over the torsed appendage), indicating infarction or necrosis	Appendage larger than 5 mm, spherical form, or enhanced periappendiceal blood flow on CD

Table 2. Empiric antibiotic therapy for acute epididymitis (Adapted from CDC, 2015).

Population	Most likely Pathogen(s)	Antibiotic
Children younger than 24 mo	Various	Antibiotic treatment for likely underlying enteric organism and referral to a urologist
Children 2 to 14 years of age	Various, +/- anatomic abnormalities	Treatment based on urinalysis and/or urine cultures
Sexually active men younger than 35 years	Gonorrhea or chlamydia	IM ceftriaxone (single 250-mg dose) *and* Doxycycline (PO, 100 mg twice daily for 10 days)
Adults who frequently commit insertive anal intercourse	Gonorrhea or chlamydia AND an enteric organism	IM ceftriaxone (single 250-mg dose) *and* Levofloxacin PO (Levaquin; 500 mg once daily for 10 days) or ofloxacin PO (300 mg BID for 10 days)
Adults older than 35 years or who have had recent urinary tract surgery or instrumentation	Enteric organism	Levofloxacin (PO, 500 mg once daily for 10 days) *or* ofloxacin (PO 300 mg BID for 10 days)

Clinical course: Pain in the testicle(s), increases steadily over time, which is also associated with swelling in the epididymis and testicular tissues. In advanced AEO cases, there is the triad of pain+swelling+tenderness on palpation.

History of fever, dysuria and urethral discharge may be obtained. Typically, the epididymis is tender, with the testicle located well below the scrotum. Abscess formation may be seen in delayed and untreated cases. Erythema and reactive hydrocele may be noted in the scrotal wall.

A positive Prehn sign (where the passive elevation of the scrotum reduces pain) is strongly supportive of epididymitis, contrary to testicular torsion. Cremaster reflex is intact.

Elderly men (>50 years) should be evaluated for urinary tract obstruction secondary to prostatic enlargement. All patients treated for an STD should be recommended to undergo treatment with their partners (CDC, 2015).

Children (<14 years) who are treated for AEO can be referred to a urological follow-up to undergo assessment for anatomic abnormalities (Tracy, 2008).

Orchitis: Although it can be identified as primary orchitis *per se*, it often presents as epididymoorchitis, *i.e.*, in conjunction with epididymitis as a result of direct spread. Orchitis emerges by spread *via* different routes (hematogenous, lymphogenous and vas deferens). Orchitis without epididymitis occurs only with hematogenous spread.

Granulomatous orchitis, a non-specific non-infectious inflammatory process of the testicles, can sometimes be encountered in middle-aged and older men. It is an autoimmune entity that is triggered against sperm cells and progresses with a granulomatous response.

Pain and swelling in the testicles are early complaints. The pain may radiate towards the inguinal canal and may be described as groin pain. Although it varies from case to case, fever, nausea and vomiting may occur. Unlike epididymitis, waxing-and-waning symptoms with urination are not expected. On examination, the scrotal skin is hyperemic and edematous. On examination, the testicle(s) can be noted as engorged, painful and sensitive.

DD: Testicular torsion is the most prominent entity which can masquerade orchitis, especially in young men. Abscess formation, hydrocoele and epididymitis should also be ruled out or diagnosed as these can ensue concurrently with orchitis.

Work Up

Urine analysis and urethral swabs (cultures) are ordered. A "nucleic acid amplification test" (NAAT) should be obtained from the urine samples to exclude *N. gonorrhoeae* and *C. trachomatis* infections.

USG findings in patients with mumps orchitis usually subside by the seventh day (Basekim, 2000). Although not typically done, serum immunofluorescence antibody testing is useful to confirm the diagnosis of mumps orchitis.

Management

Consult with urology as early as possible. Ruling out testicular torsion takes priority.

Patients with severe pain or toxic appearance are admitted to the hospital.

If bacterial AEO is suspected, appropriate antibacterial therapy should be commenced.

Treatment consists of conservative measures and administration of interferon to prevent testicular atrophy. The way to avoid AEO secondary to mumps is through vaccination.

Quinolones (eg, ciprofloxacin), and analgesia with NSAIDs is indicated for the treatment of acute epididymitis. Cold treatment and testicular elevation before NAAT result reduce pain.

Corticosteroid use is recommended for nonspecific granulomatous orchitis in middle-aged people. Prednisolone; 1.5 mg/kg/day PO is initiated.

Empiric regimens of choice: If AEO is suspected to be due to gonorrhea or chlamydia, ceftriaxone (IM, single 250-mg dose) plus doxycycline (PO, 100 mg twice daily for 10 days) is the recommended treatment regimen (McConaghy, 2016).

In men older than 35 years with epididymitis, STD are less likely, and monotherapy with levofloxacin or ofloxacin is the empiric regimen of choice.

Complications of Orchitis

- Testicular atrophy (up to three-fifths of cases)
- Infertility or impaired fertility
- Sterility (rare)
- Epididymitis
- Reactive hydrocele

Case presentation: A 72-year-old man presented with painless swelling of the scrotum, penis and inguinal areas for 12 hours. Scrotal erythema is also noted. The findings indicated **acute idiopathic scrotal edema** (Mesquita, 2017) (Fig. **1**).

Testicular Torsion (TT)

It is a common emergency in newborns and postpubertal children. It occurs when the lower pole of the testis rotates on the spermatic cord due to weak fixation on the tunica vaginalis. The annual incidence of **TT** is estimated at 1 in 4000. This means that an estimated 1 in every 160 men will experience **spermatic cord torsion** until they are 25-year old (Velasquez, 2021). TT is identified in 25% to 50% of hospitalized patients with acute scrotal pain.

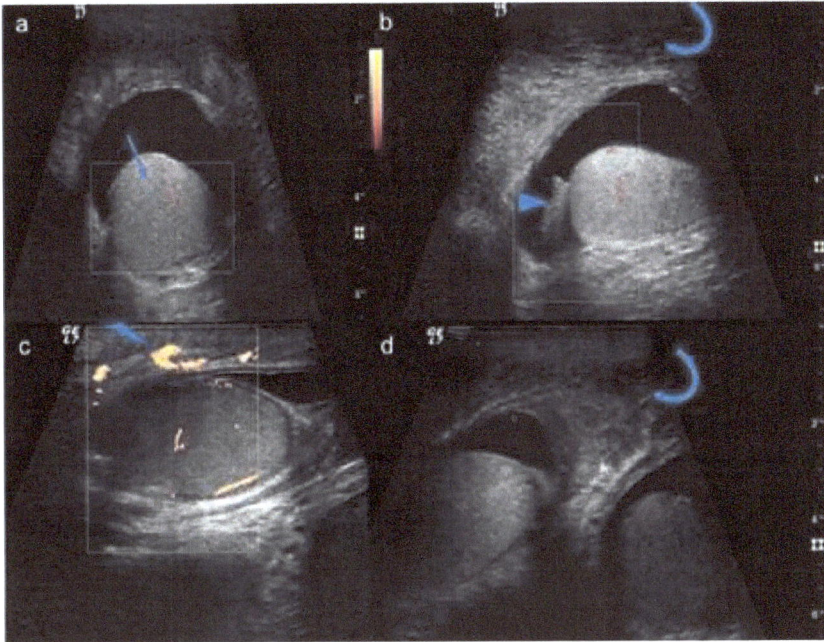

Fig. (1). Gray scale and scrotal color Doppler USG were performed. No increased vascularity in the testicles (arrow in **a**) and epididymis (arrowhead in **b**), compared with higher vascularity in the scrotal wall (lightning bolt in **c**). Scrotal wall exhibited heterogeneous striated appearance (curved arrows in **b** and **d**).

Pathophysiology: Spermatic cord torsion may be intravaginal or extravaginal. Extravaginal torsion is seen almost exclusively in neonates. On the other hand, intravaginal torsion, is most commonly accompanies the "bell clapper deformity", causes twisting of the spermatic cord itself, which ultimately blocks the arterial circulation of the involved testicle resulting in ischemia and infarction (Velasquez, 2021) (Fig. **2**). Severity and degree of TT may vary from patient to patient. Venous occlusion and congestion appear in the early stage.

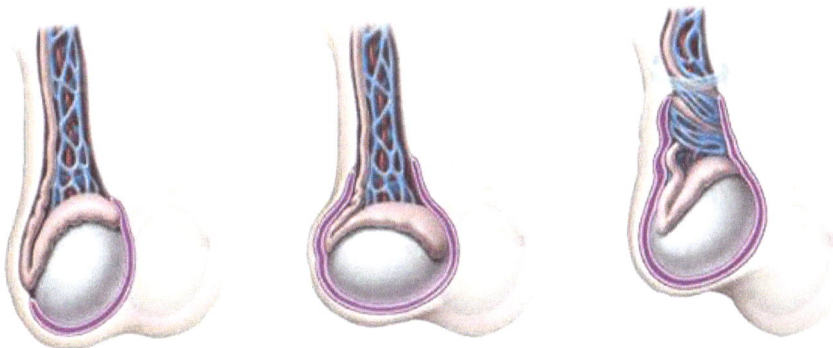

Fig. (2). The bell-clapper deformity with abnormal fixation of the tunica vaginalis to the testicle.

Course: After 8 hours of ischemia, the involved testicle is considered nonviable. It can lead to infertility. Therefore, the clinician should be alert to every child and youngsters with lower AP to rule out this entity.

Findings: The constellation of acute onset testicular pain, swelling, severe diffuse tenderness, negative cremasteric reflex are typical. Nausea/vomiting and lower AP may ensue. Nocturnal exacerbation of symptoms is also typical. Reactive hydrocele may occur within 12-24 hours.

The most important findings in evaluation of acute TT is "high-riding" asymmetrical testicle and absence of ipsilateral cremasteric reflex (Sheth, 2016).

Researchers launched TWIST (Testicular Workup for Ischemia and Suspected Torsion) score to assess the risk of TT. Included variables comprise:

• testicular swelling	(2 points)
• hardened testis	(2 points)
• absent cremasteric reflex	(1 points)
• nausea/vomiting	(1 points)
• high riding testis	(1 points)

Sheth *et al.* pointed out that TWIST score assessments recorded by nonurologists (emergency physicians, paediatricians, general surgeons or technicians) are generally accurate with a positive predictive value of 93.5% and a negative predictive value of 100% (Sheth, 2016). Patients with low risk may not be sent to USG unit to rule out TT. High risk patients can proceed directly to surgery, with more than 50% avoiding USG.

Superb Microvascular Imaging (SMI) is a recently developed Doppler modality which assesses microvascular blood flow and addresses the challenges associated with standard Doppler USG (Hata, 2014). It has the ability to evaluate low-velocity flow with less tissue movement artefacts and signals (Fig. **3**) (Karaca, 2016).

Scrotal CT is rarely indicated in cases with an acute scrotum. However, it is the choice investigation in the assessment of scrotal hernia involving the ureters, Fournier's gangrene, acute trauma and cancer staging. CT is also of value in detecting a perfusion insult in indeterminate cases.

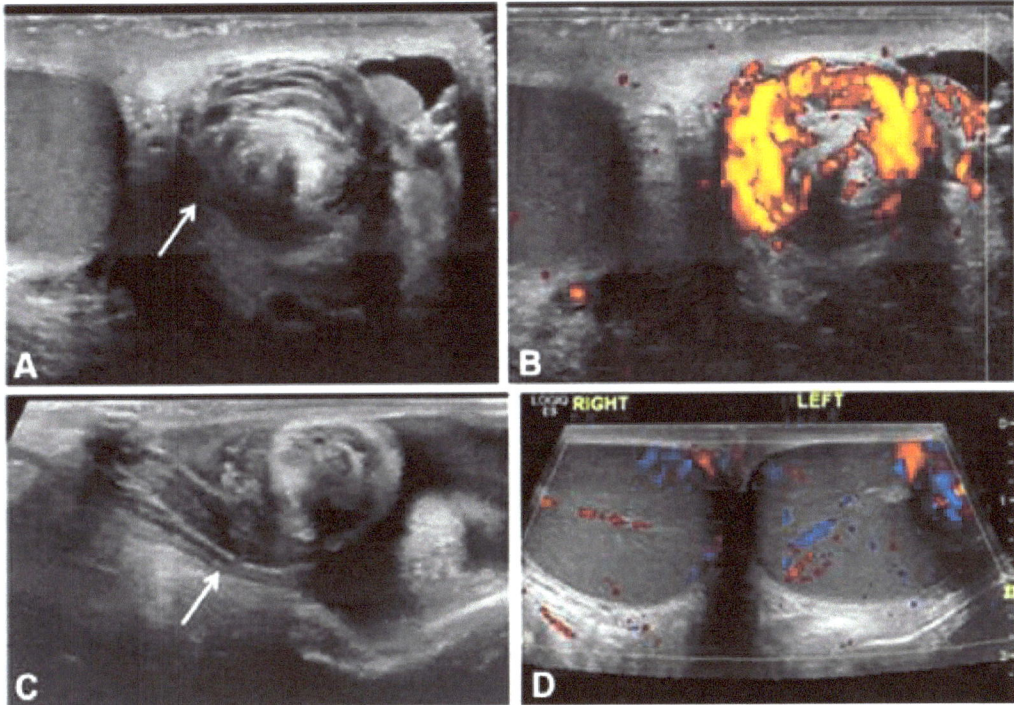

Fig. (3). "Whirlpool sign" of the spermatic cord. (**A**) Gray-scale transverse US image of upper left scrotal sac shows an eddy swirl (arrow) of the spermatic cord suggesting torsion of the cord. This 12-year-old boy woke with acute left testicular pain and experienced nausea and vomiting along with the pain. (**B**) Power Doppler US image of the same twisted cord shows a concentric pattern of preserved flow in the vessels of the twisted cord. The flow in the left testis (not shown) was minimally decreased compared to the right side and bilateral bell clapper deformity was found during orchiopexy along with complete torsion of the left testis with 360° twist. (**C**) Gray-scale longitudinal US image of the left scrotum in a 13-year-old boy with 1 day of left-side pain shows abrupt spiral twisting of the spermatic cord (arrow) at the external inguinal ring, creating a whirlpool sign. (**D**) Color Doppler transverse image of the testes in the same boy as in (**C**) shows preserved and symmetrical flow bilaterally. After manual detorsion in the emergency room, he underwent orchiopexy and was diagnosed with intermittent torsion. (Image obtained from Bandarkar AN, Blask AR. Testicular torsion with preserved flow: key sonographic features and value-added approach to diagnosis. Pediatr Radiol. 2018;48(5):735–744. doi:10.1007/s00247-018-4093-0.27 Distributed under the terms of the Creative Commons Attribution 4.0 International License (http://creativecommons.org/licenses/by/4.0/). No changes have been made to the images or the image description).

The treatment of TT is surgical detorsion. Manual detorsion should be attempted if surgery is not an immediate option; however, prompt referral should not delay this maneuver (Sharp, 2013). The maneuver comprising manually opening the testicle from medial to lateral can relieve pain and confirm the diagnosis. If history and physical examination suggest TT, immediate surgical exploration is indicated and should not be postponed in order to perform imaging studies. If in doubt, urgent urological consultation should be requested. Delayed intervention is associated with nonviability of the testicle, thus leading to untoward consequences. Rates of testicular salvage are better when surgery is performed within 7–12 hours of symptom onset (Laher, 2020).

URINARY STONE DISEASE/URETERAL COLIC (URC)/ PYELONEPHRITIS

Urinary Stone Disease

Up to the age of 70, 11% to 16% of males and 7% to 8% of females are affected by urinary stone disease (USD) in the population. It recurs in one of two patients with the diagnosis within 10 years. The incidence is thought to have doubled from 1994 to 2017, probably due to more sedentary lifestyle and liberal use of diagnostic modalities (Table **3**).

Table 3. Groups at risk for USD include the following.

Obesity
Low fluid intake (such as bakery workers, Alzheimer's disease)
Elderly,
Caucasians,
Low socioeconomic status,
Diabetes, pancreatitis
Gout
Hyperparathyroidism

The cause of ureteral colic (UrC) in a patient with USD is obstruction of the urinary flow with particles such as stones or clots. Stones are mostly composed of calcium oxalate or calcium phosphate. Often, when the stones formed in the kidney partially break off and fall into the ureter, they cause obstruction and therefore UrC.

As the stones move distally along the ureter, the lumen diameter narrows. There is a narrowing and high risk of obstruction of the urinary flow by the stone at three points: 1) the ureteropelvic junction (UPJ), 2) the area where the ureter intersects the iliac vessels, 3) the ureterovesical junction (UVJ) (Shoag, 2015).

Stones can sometimes pave the way for infection. UrC should not be clarified in the diagnosis of UC without distinguishing APN and pyonephrosis. **Aortic aneurysm rupture** should be excluded in the early period of UrC in middle-aged and older patients.

Examination and Evaluation

USD usually presents with UrC, severe flank pain, nausea/vomiting, and hematuria. Blunt and mild to moderate side/flank/groin pain may also turn into persistent severe colic pain. Referred pain in the vulvae or testicles may occur. Sweating may occur, vomiting is mostly triggered after prolonged UrC. Such findings may lead to misdiagnosis. There are many patients diagnosed with pancreatitis due to vomiting, epididymoorchitis, cystitis, PID or UTI due to referred pain.

Most patients with UrC are recognizable even on inspection. The typical appearance is young or middle-aged men who cannot find a comfortable position and writhe continuously or intermittently. Although most patients have a previous history of stone disease, it is not a rule.

Pill information: Think more than twice if you are diagnosing urolithiasis/renal colic for the first time in an elderly patient. Many life-threatening diagnoses such as aortic catastrophes may be missed.

Abdominal examination is normal except for a marked tenderness at the costovertebral angle on the involved kidney and there is no guarding.

As the renal and ureteral stimuli enter the spinal canal between T11 and L2, it will be a visceral pain. Therefore, a pain sensation coincides with many digestive system organs and genitals.

If there is fever, and/or shaking chills, you should seek for alternative diagnoses such as APN, urosepsis etc., because these are not expected in UrC.

Pulses on all four directions should be checked, the presence of murmur should be sought, and the aorta should be examined with USG to exclude **aortic pathologies**. It should be noted that a dissecting or ruptured aortic aneurysm is a good UrC mimic.

There may be **macroscopic hematuria** in UrC, but its absence does not exclude the diagnosis. Fever is unexpected, and if present, infection should be investigated and ruled out. Mostly, the stone falling into the bladder can halt the pain immediately, but in some patients, there may be obstruction at the vesicourethral entrance. Although it is accepted that stones smaller than 7-8 mm can pass without intervention with the help of ureteral peristalsis and urine flow, it is not 100% the rule.

Costovertebral angle tenderness is valuable when present, but is typically found in only 1 in 2 patients. (Ingimarsson 2016).

Work Up

- Blood urea nitrogen, creatinine, glucose can be measured.
- Erythrocytes in **urinalysis,** or hematuria positivity *via* midstream urine stix are found in 4 out of 5 patients with confirmed stones.
- A urine pH above 7.6 suggests infection with urealytic microorganisms.

Do not consider a diagnosis based on urinalysis. There are many cases of both false negative and false positive. For example, in aortic dissection or aneurysm, UrC + significant hematuria may be present, while there may be no findings in the urinalysis in a case with confirmed UrC.

Radiological Diagnosis

- Since 90% of the stones are radiopaque, **x-ray** may be ordered to see the culprit stones. However, the real-life witnesses that films are still only 50% sensitive and 70% specific for urinary stones. The culprit stone(s) is/are usually seen in the pelviureteric and ureterovesical junctions. It should be known that the ureters are adjacent to the transverse processes of the spines in imaging.
- The visualization of a stone in the ureter or kidney in a painful patient does not mean that the source of the problem is identified. You should still exclude more serious diagnoses.
- USG/POCUS is a very valuable bedside noninvasive imaging method to expedite ruling out many differential diagnoses in most patients (Fig. **4**). For example, USG can reveal a gallstone in a patient with right-side "renal colic".
- USG takes priority as a diagnostic tool in pregnant women.
- Non-contrast CT is a frequently used diagnostic tool since it is 95% sensitive and 95% specific. It is also advantageous to exclude other DD and to plan the interventions.
- IV urography is best in situations where CT is unavailable or not preferred. It is also very useful when planning endoscopic and surgical treatment. A delay of 5 minutes or more in the nephrogram phase is the typical finding of urinary obstruction.

Red flags: if you have any of the following, you are not dealing with an ordinary UrC patient. You had better keep the patient in the hospital.

- Age>50 and the first time with a diagnosis of kidney stone

- Fever
- Hemodynamic abnormality
- Solitary kidney
- Transplanted kidney

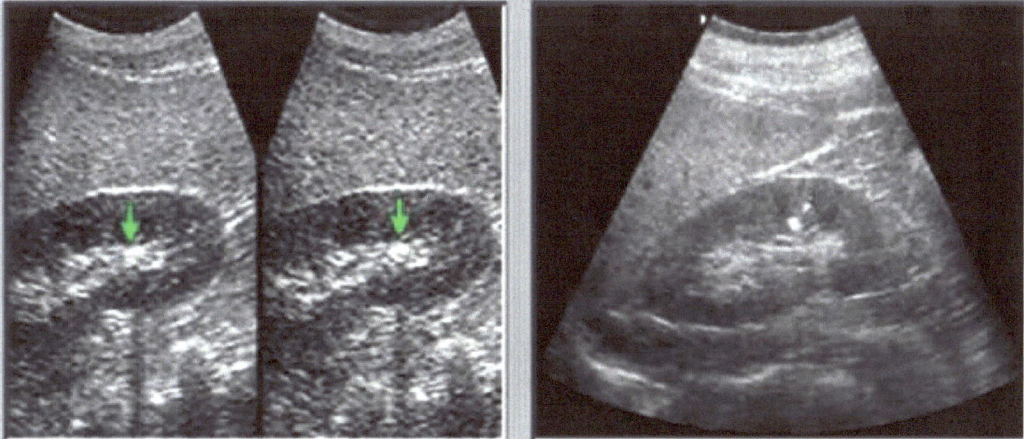

Fig. (4). Kidney stones are sometimes hard to visualize because they have low contrast. Small stones are difficult to image in those without hydronephrosis. However, the kidney stone is more hyperechoic than the renal hilum. Posterior acoustic shadow can be observed.

Urinary Tract Infection (UTI) including Acute Pyelonephritis (APN)

UTI is a major cause of AP and is encountered very commonly both in children and adults. The condition. The infections have a significant predilection to female sex in all age groups, except in early infancy and in elderly men with instrumentation or prostate diseases.

Special groups deserve attention, because of high morbidity and mortality in case of missed or delayed management in the acute setting. For example, UTI is the most common infection in kidney transplant recipients (Coussement, 2020). The clinical presentation varies from asymptomatic bacteriuria to APN affecting the kidney allograft.

Pediatric considerations *Escherichia coli* is prominent among causative agents. Accurate diagnosis is expedited *via* collection of a midstream or uncontaminated urine specimen. Urinary USG is indicated in all young children with first febrile attack of UTI and in older children with recurrent episodes (Mattoo, 2021). Anatomical abnormalities such as, vesicoureteral reflux associated with UTI warrant surgical intervention.

Advanced imaging: CT and MRI can help visualize conditions resistant to conventional treatments and supportive measures. These include APN, intrarenal and perinephric abscesses, pyonephrosis, chronic pyelonephritis, emphysematous UTIs, xanthogranulomatous pyelonephritis, tuberculosis, fungal infection, corynebacterium infection, ureteritis, complicated cystitis, various forms of urethritis and prostatic diseases (abscess and malignancies) (El-Ghar, 2021).

USD+pyelonephritis Case Presentation: (Figs. **5** and **6**).

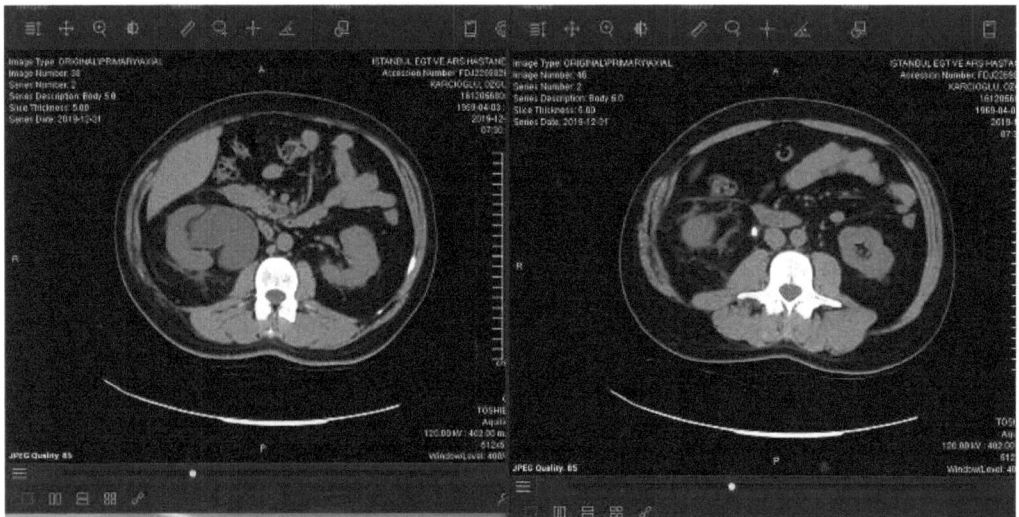

Fig. (5). A 53-year-old male physician (the writer of the chapter) with a stone at the ureteropelvic junction causing Grade II-III hydronephrosis. He was treated with nephrostomy+ESWL (lithotripsy).

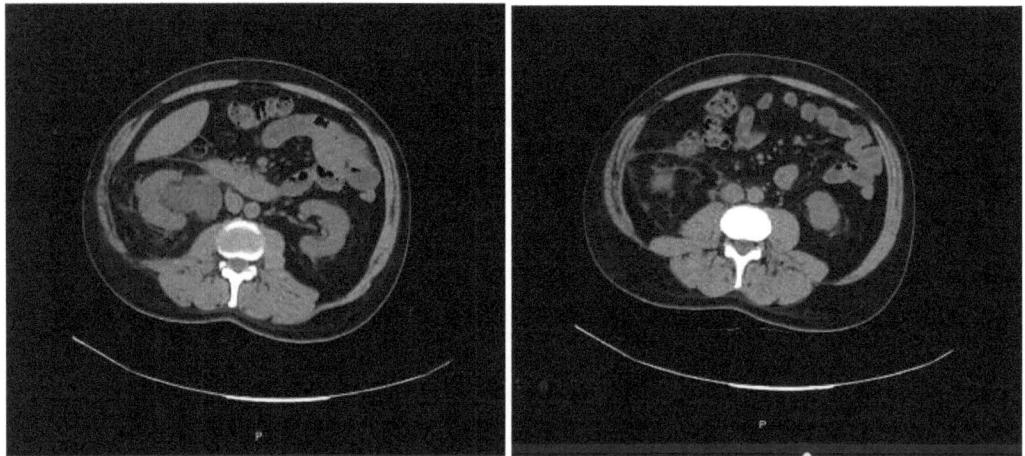

(Fig. 6) contd.....

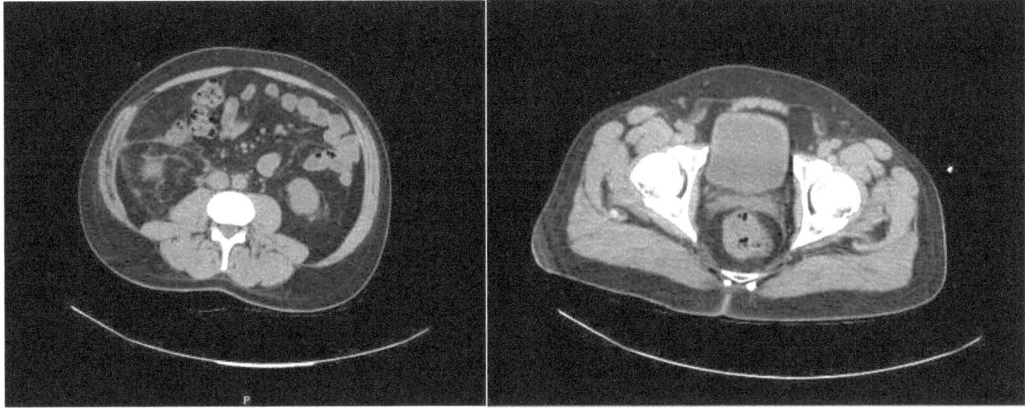

Fig. (6). 12 days later in the above patient. The right kidney collecting system is grade 3-4 wide. In the right kidney collecting system, a minimal density that may be significant in terms of hydronephrosis is observed. Right proximal ureter is widened. The dirty appearance around the ureter continues which is compatible with pyelonephritis.

MANAGEMENT

Pill information: Stone progression does not accelerate with overt hydration, but the patient should not remain dehydrated. A little plus-balance can be maintained. Nifedipine administration is also not helpful.

Pill information: Tamsulosin does not have any additive effect in small stones, but there is evidence that it accelerates passage and stone excretion in stones larger than 7 mm (Gottlieb, 2018). However, findings that it does not have a significant effect on the passage of stones up to 9 mm have also been published (Meltzer. 2018).

Pain management: Various agents including paracetamol or NSAIDs such as - oxicam or profen groups are the first line treatment. Opioids are reserved for treatment failure. The control of vegetative cortex can be accomplished with ondansetron as first choice (de la Encarnación Castellano, 2021). As salvage therapy, IV opioid or lidocaine can also be administered by titration according to the patient. In particular, there is information that IV paracetamol leads to a better or equivalent effect than morphine. Oral analgesia may also be tried if there is no excessive vomiting.

In accord with the findings of a meta-analytic study (50 studies including 5734 participants), NSAIDs are an effective treatment for renal colic when compared to placebo or antispasmodics (Afshar, 2015). NSAIDs were significantly more effective than hyoscine in pain reduction (5 comparisons, 196 participants: RR 2.44, 95% CI 1.61 to 3.70). The combination of NSAIDs and antispasmodics was not superior to NSAIDs only (9 comparisons, 906 participants: RR 1.00, 95% CI 0.89 to 1.13).

In brief, the addition of antispasmodics to NSAIDS does not result in better pain control. Considering systemic adverse effect potential, antispasmodics, anticholinergics have no place in the management of renal colic.

The **ondansetron/granisetron** group has priority against vomiting (Jokar, 2018).

Metoclopramide is not a reasonable option and may cause akathisia, especially in rapid infusions.

Antibiotic Therapy in UTI and APN

Oral antibiotic therapy for 7 to 10 days is prescribed for uncomplicated cases that respond well to the treatment (Mattoo, 2021).

Causative agents get more and more resistant to many antibiotics, and clinicians must be warned against indiscriminate use of antimicrobials in suspect patients with UTI.

Recently, the American College of Physicians issued a "Best Practice Advice" guide which recommended that *"in women with uncomplicated bacterial cystitis, clinicians should prescribe short-course antibiotics with either nitrofurantoin for 5 days, trimethoprim-sulfamethoxazole for 3 days, or fosfomycin as a single dose (Lee, 2021). In men and women with uncomplicated APN, clinicians should prescribe short-course therapy either with fluoroquinolones (5 to 7 days) or trimethoprim-sulfamethoxazole (14 days) based on antibiotic susceptibility."*

Tips for Disposition

- Patients without urinary obstruction and hydronephrosis and whose symptoms improve adequately can be discharged and scheduled for the outpatient follow-up.
- Patients whose pain does not relieve and whose obstruction continues are hospitalized. Patients with pyelonephritis, transplants or kidney failure should also be consulted and kept in hospital.
- Err on the patient's side, if you are hesitant to admit or discharge the patient, especially in situations urinary obstruction and hydronephrosis have not been ruled out.

Gynecological Pain: Ovarian Torsion, PID

"Gynecological pain" is a group of entities that is more difficult to evaluate compared to other causes of AP. The tendency to disclose the complaint socially in some cultural conditions and the deficiencies in taking an elaborate history by the healthcare personnel lead to an increased likelihood to misdiagnose these diseases or delayed management.

- **Ectopic pregnancy (EP):** AP in early (sometimes not yet known) pregnancy may be due to ectopic pregnancy (EP) or missed/incipient abortion.
- **Pain associated with the menstrual cycle:** First, any vaginal bleeding should be considered as associated with an EP or abortion. Dysmenorrhea is periodic pain that reaches its peak in the first days of menstruation. NSAIDs are primarily used in the management. Occasionally, opiates may be used if symptoms are very severe.
- **Endometriosis** is the living of endometrial tissue outside the uterus by forming cysts and adhesions. They most often present with dysmenorrhea between the ages of 8 and 30 years. Infertility and dyspareunia are also common complaints.
- **Corpus luteum cyst rupture (chocolate cyst)** develops in the premenstrual period, causing severe pain and bleeding.
- **Mittelschmerz** is the extrusion of the follicle cyst near the middle of the menstrual cycle, causing severe pain. It can masquerade AAp, PID etc. It usually does not prompt admission and can be followed on an outpatient basis.
- **Ovarian torsion (OT)** causes unilateral sharp and severe pain. There is tenderness on both abdominal palpation and vaginal/cervical exam.

The mechanism is understood with dual blood supply of the organ from the ovarian arteries and uterine arteries. Twisting of the ligaments can lead to venous congestion, edema, compression of arteries, and, if untreated, loss of blood supply to the ovary. The main risk factor for ovarian torsion is an ovarian mass that is 5 cm in diameter or larger (Guile, 2021). Pregnancy, as well as patients undergoing fertility treatments, are high risk due to enlarged follicles on the ovary (Mahonski, 2019).

Almost half (46%) of OT were found to accompany neoplasms, while the other half (48%) were associated with ovarian cysts. Of these masses, 89% were benign, and 80% of patients were under age 50. Therefore, reproductive-age females are at greatest risk of torsion (Varras, 2004).

It is the fifth most common emergency condition in gynecologic entities. However, the diagnosis is often missed because of the subtlety of the signs and symptoms, physical examination findings, and radiological characteristics. It has the potential to be confused with many acute abdomen-related diagnoses.

Evaluation and DD: Acute-onset pain with high severity to elicit nausea or vomiting should raise concern for OT, especially if an adnexal mass is palpated on examination. On the other hand, insidious and persistent AP suggests infection and/ or inflammation. Pain may be reflected in the legs, genitalia and back. Vaginal discharge, bleeding, delayed menstruation may provide important clues.

Nausea and vomiting occur in a majority (70%) of women with OT. The percentage is higher than the frequency with which these symptoms manifest with other gynecologic causes of pelvic pain (Dawood, 2021).

A complete blood count, metabolic panel, and a serum beta-hCG should be ordered. Anemia, if any, may indicate a torsion resulting in bleeding. Beta- hCG has great importance because of high risk of OT conveyed by pregnancy. These laboratory abnormalities are mostly non-specific, and the lab values can be normal in presence of OT (Guile, 2021).

Imaging: USG (especially color Doppler) and laparoscopic visualization are inappreciable in both diagnosis and management. The presence of color Doppler flow or contrast enhancement only suggests that an ovary is still viable and should not be used to exclude the diagnosis of torsion (Table **4**) (Strachowski, 2021). Clinicians are sometimes falsely reassured by normal vascularity, as arterial perfusion can be maintained until relatively late in the course of OT (Dawood, 2021).

Table 4. Imaging characteristics with high positive and negative predictive values in the diagnosis of ovarian torsion.

Favoring ovarian torsion	Excluding ovarian torsion
Asymmetric ovarian enlargement (edematous ovary migrated to the midline), Peripherally displaced follicles, Visualization of free fluid besides the ovaries, Multiple foci of stromal bleeding The whirlpool sign (twisted vascular pedicle), Abnormal ovarian location Uterus pulled towards the affected ovary Bleeding with absence of internal flow or enhancement (indicates infarction)	Symmetric nonenlarged ovaries in a normal location (with USG or CT)

Figs. (**7** and **8**) demonstrate examples of imaging studies (CT and MRI) in patients with ovarian diseases.

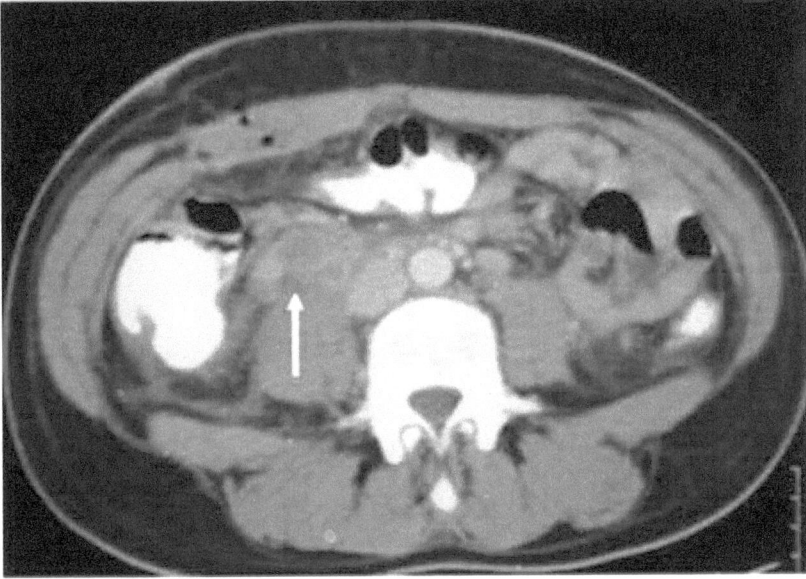

Fig. (7). Abdominal CT (arrow) showing thrombosis of the right ovarian vein.

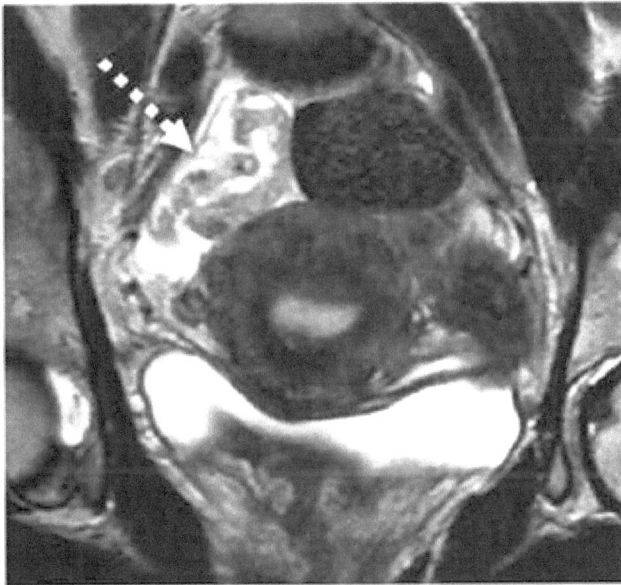

a)

(Fig. 6) contd.....

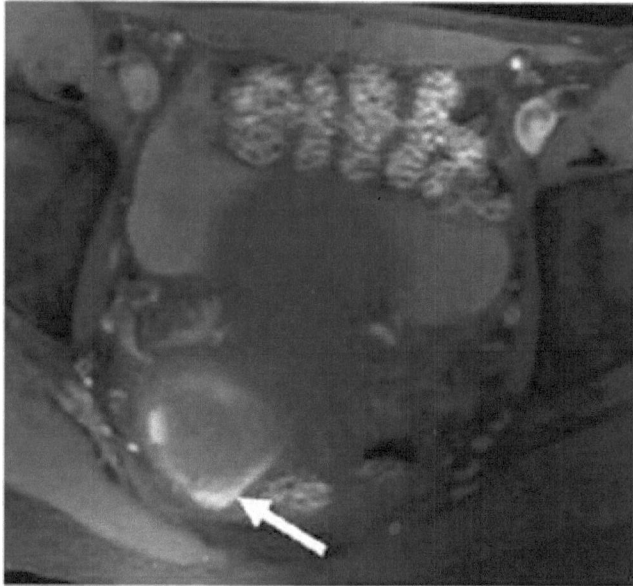

b)

Fig. (8). A woman in her thirties was admitted due to severe abdominal pain and vomiting. **(a)** T2-weighted magnetic resonance images demonstrate the right ovary with edema and a twisted edematous pedicle (arrow), consistent with adnexal torsion. **(b)** Axial T1-weighted image depicts high signal intensity (arrow) at the periphery of the right ovary, consistent with bleeding and indicative of ovarian infarction.

Treatment: The definitive management is surgical detorsion achieved as early as possible. Supportive treatment comprises hydration, antiemetics (ondansetron) and analgesia (mostly opiates). salvage of the ovary should be attempted especially in young women. The viability of the involved tissues can be judged by visualization. Laparoscopic surgery with direct visualization of a twisted ovary will generally be successful. A dark, enlarged ovary with hemorrhagic lesions may have compromised blood flow but is often salvageable (Bider, 1991).

Pelvic inflammatory disease (PID) is an infection of the upper genital tract in sexually active women.

The National Health and Nutrition Examination Survey 2013–2014 data (US) cite that 4.4% of young women (between the ages 18 and 44, 2.5 million women) had a history of PID (Kreisel, 2017).

If the infection has spread from the cervix to the uterus, it is called endometritis.

Mild to moderate PID has the prerequisites of exclusion of any tubo-ovarian abscess.

• **Severe disease** comprises severe clinical course and/or the identification of a tubo-ovarian abscess.

If the fallopian tubes are involved, it is mostly referred to as salpingitis whilst the term oophoritis is used should it inflict the ovaries. In the advanced cases it is called peritonitis, when there is peritoneal involvement. The severity can also vary from very mild to very severe, abscess formation. Involvement is often bilateral. 9/10 are sexually transmitted. All sexually active women of childbearing age are at high risk for all forms of PID.

Commonly isolated causative agents of PID *include Chlamydia trachomatis* and *Neisseria gonorrhoea. Chlamydia trachomatis* most commonly causes formation of isolated lesions and results in pelvic chlamydial infection. *Neisseria gonorrhea* causes pelvic gonococcal infection, and M. tuberculosis causes pelvic tuberculosis infection. *Mycoplasma hominis, Ureaplasma urealyticum* can also be detected. **Polymicrobial infection** is responsible in 35% of cases. Epithelial damage from infections such as *Chlamydia trachomatis* or *Neisseria gonorrhoeae* may pave the way to opportunistic infection from other bacteria.

Serious morbidity results from PID; about 20% of affected women become infertile, 40% develop chronic pelvic pain, and 1% of those who conceive have an ectopic pregnancy (Ross, 2014).

Radiology: Symptoms are more severe than radiological findings. There may be almost no signs in the early (in the stage cervicitis). In the late period, an adnexal mass with inflammatory changes around it can be visualized. In this advanced stage, tubes and ovaries may be indistinguishable from each other.

USG Findings	CT Findings
• Thick/dilated fallopian tubes • Incomplete septa in the tube(s) • Increased vascularity around the tube • Echogenic fluid in the tube (pyosalpinx) • cogwheel sign: cross-sectional view of thickened loops in tubes. • "beads on string" view	• Thickened fallopian tubes: >5 mm with contrast-enhanced wall • thickening of the uterosacral ligaments • Complex free fluid in the Douglas pouch • Pelvic fat streaks or heterogeneity • Ill-defined uterine border • Reactive lymphadenopathy (paraaortic and paracaval)

Figs. (**9** - **12**) give examples of imaging studies in patients with PID.

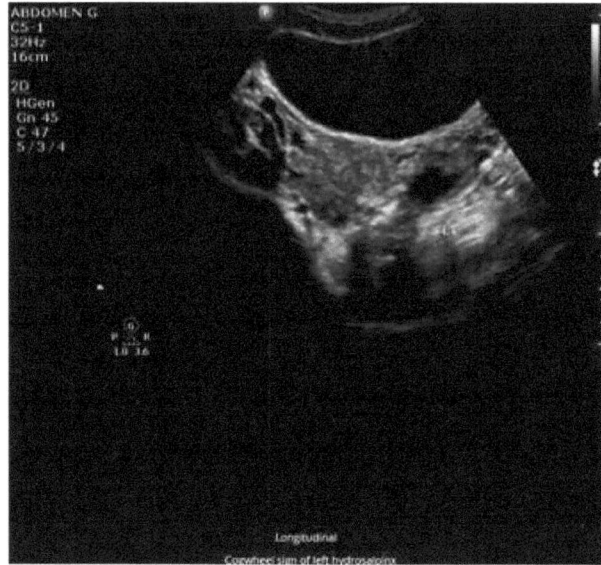

Fig. (9). Trans-abdominal USG shows dilated fluid-filled left salpinx. Thickened endosalpingeal walls are visualized in the transverse plane. There is no effusion in the Douglas pouch.

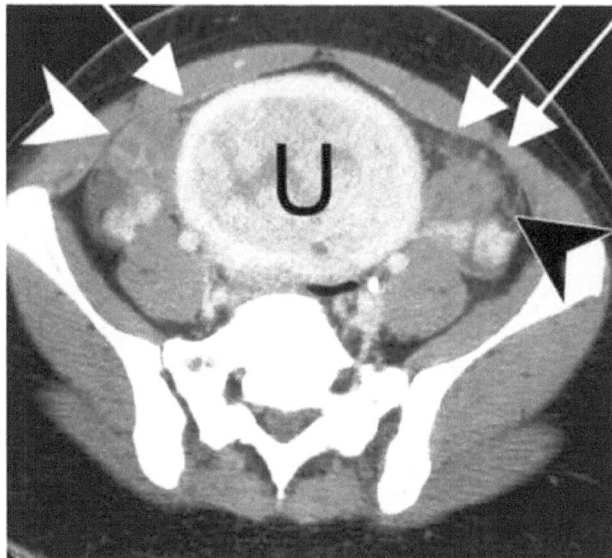

Fig. (10). Tomographic appearance of premature PID in a woman in her 33. In contrast-enhanced CT, abnormal enhancement of the ovaries (arrowheads) can be observed together with periovarian and peritoneal inflammation (arrows). Enlarged myomatous uterus (U) was detected incidentally.

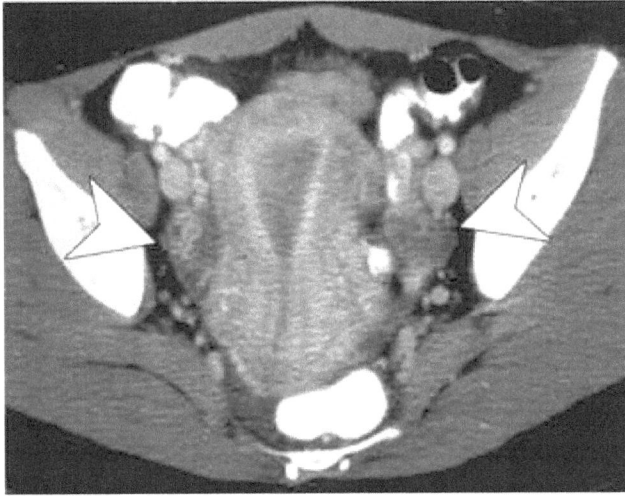

Fig. (11). Contrast-enhanced CT in a 25-year-old woman with PID. Abnormal enhancement of the endometrium and fluid accumulation due to endometritis are observed. It is also noted that the ovaries are enlarged (arrowheads).

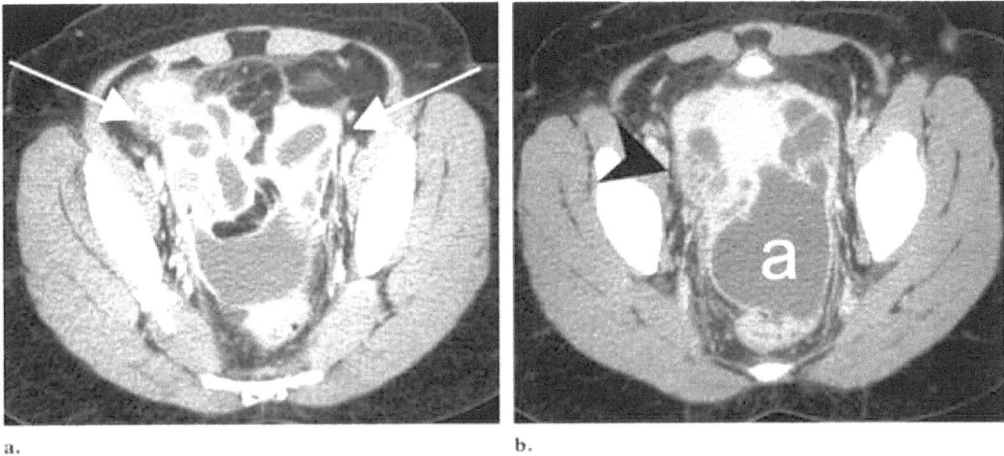

a.   b.

Fig. (12). Advanced PID in a woman in her 43. Contrast-enhanced CT scan sections show dilated fallopian tubes filled with complex fluid (a: arrows), inflammatory collections adjacent to the right ovary (b: arrowheads), and cul-de-sac abscess of 7 -8 cm in diameter (marked with "a"). Findings are consistent with pyosalpinx and tubo-ovarian abscess.

Clinical presentation of the disease can be acute, chronic, or subclinical. As far as those referred to the hospitals, many patients are underdiagnosed.

The typical patient with PID is a young woman with bilateral lower abdominal tenderness, vaginal discharge, fever (>38 C), abnormal vaginal bleeding, dyspareunia, cervical and adnexal tenderness on palpation.

PID should be presumed primarily on clinical suspicion, and empiric treatment should be initiated expediently in sexually active young women or those at risk for STD and/or PID with consistent clinical findings.

Management principles: Give IV fluids. Urine analysis and vaginal/cervical swab, blood count, and erythrocyte sedimentation rate can be ordered. **Sex partner treatment** is also suggested in most sources.

Who should be consulted and admitted to hospital? It would be wise to consult in case of suspicion of PID early as antibiotic treatment and follow-up will be pursued by the gynaecologist (Table **5**).

Table 5. Admission criteria in patients with PID.

• Pregnancy
• Severe disease,
• Need for parenteral antibiotics
• Disease progression instead of outpatient treatment
• Accompanying tubo-ovarian abscess,
• Failure to exclude surgical emergencies

Treatment is often with empirical antibiotics, without isolation of the causative agent. This approach is vital for minimizing the risk of important complications such as tubal obstruction and infertility.

According to the CDC, IM/oral therapy is an option in treating mild to moderate acute PID. In patients who do not respond to IM/oral therapy within 72 hours, a re-diagnostic evaluation should be made and a transition to IV therapy should be considered.

Recommended IM/oral Treatment Regimens

- **Ceftriaxone** 250 mg IM (single dose)+
- **Doxycycline** 100 mg oral 2x1; 14 days+/-
- **Metronidazole** 500 mg oral 2x1; 14 days

or

- **Cefoxitine** 2 g IM in a single dose and **Probenecid**, 1 g orally administered concurrently in a single dose+
- **Doxycycline** 100 mg oral 2x1; 14 days+/-
- **Metronidazole** 500 mg oral 2x1; 14 days

or

- Other parenteral 3rd generation **cephalosporine** (ceftizoxime or cefotaxim)+
- **Doxycycline** 100 mg oral 2x1; 14 days+/-
- **Metronidazole** 500 mg oral 2x1; 14 days

A two-week regimen of metronidazole is especially indicated in the setting of bacterial vaginosis, trichomoniasis, or recent uterine instrumentation (Curry, 2019). Otherwise, management principles are the same in patients with intrauterine devices or HIV positivity.

Failure in the treatment of PID can pave the way to untoward results such that intractable or chronic pelvic pain, infertility, ectopic pregnancy, and intraabdominal infections (Table **6**). Almost one in six women with salpingitis develops infertility.

Table 6. Complications of PID mostly result from delay or failure in management and comprise severe illnesses.

• Tubo-ovarian abscess
• Pyosalpinx
• Infertility
• Peritonitis
• Ovarian vein thrombosis
• Bowel obstruction as a result of adhesions (brid ileus)
• Fitz-Hugh-Curtis syndrome
• Increased risk of ectopic pregnancy
• Chronic pelvic pain (can be multifactorial)

Trends: Prevalence of diseases inflicted by organisms such as gonorrhea and chlamydia are rising, though studies pointed out an overall decline in PID incidences. This is especially worrisome with the rise of antibiotic-resistant *Neisseria gonorrhoeae*.

CONCLUSION

Urogenital tract diseases encompass a wide spectrum of disorders ranging from unimportant birth defects to life-threatening infections such as pyelonephritis and urosepsis. A patient with abdominal pain should be evaluated with proper history taking and physical examination including urogenital system in both sexes. Management of UTIs and GTDs is the key to ensure proper sexual development, function, and fertility as well as prevent serious morbidity and mortality. Medical emergencies such as testicular torsion, ruptured ovarian cysts, ovarian torsion and severe PID cause acute abdominal pain that prompts urgent intervention with admission to the hospital. All these conditions may warrant medical therapy and/or surgical intervention, in collaboration with medical and surgical specialists to ensure optimal outcomes.

REFERENCES

Afshar, K., Jafari, S., Marks, A.J., Eftekhari, A., MacNeily, A.E. (2015). Nonsteroidal anti-inflammatory drugs (NSAIDs) and non-opioids for acute renal colic. *Cochrane Database Syst. Rev.,* (6), CD006027.
[http://dx.doi.org/10.1002/14651858.CD006027.pub2] [PMID: 26120804]

Azmat, C.E., Vaitla, P. (2021). Orchitis. *StatPearls.* Treasure Island (FL): StatPearls Publishing.
[PMID: 31985958]

Bandarkar, A.N., Blask, A.R. (2018). Testicular torsion with preserved flow: key sonographic features and value-added approach to diagnosis. *Pediatr. Radiol.,* 48(5), 735-744.
[http://dx.doi.org/10.1007/s00247-018-4093-0] [PMID: 29468365]

Başekim, C.C., Kizilkaya, E., Pekkafali, Z., Baykal, K.V., Karsli, A.F. (2000). Mumps epididymo-orchitis: sonography and color Doppler sonographic findings. *Abdom. Imaging,* 25(3), 322-325.
[http://dx.doi.org/10.1007/s002610000039] [PMID: 10823460]

Bider, D., Mashiach, S., Dulitzky, M., Kokia, E., Lipitz, S., Ben-Rafael, Z. (1991). Clinical, surgical and pathologic findings of adnexal torsion in pregnant and nonpregnant women. *Surg. Gynecol. Obstet.,* 173(5), 363-366.
[PMID: 1948585]

CDC. (2015). *Sexually Transmitted Diseases Treatment Guidelines.* https://www.cdc.gov/std/tg2015/pid.htm

Center for Disease Control and Prevention. (2015). http://www.cdc.gov/std/ tg2015/epididymitis.htm

Coussement, J., Kaminski, H., Scemla, A., Manuel, O. (2020). Asymptomatic bacteriuria and urinary tract infections in kidney transplant recipients. *Curr. Opin. Infect. Dis.,* 33(6), 419-425.
[http://dx.doi.org/10.1097/QCO.0000000000000678] [PMID: 33148983]

Crawford, P., Crop, J.A. (2014). Evaluation of scrotal masses. *Am. Fam. Physician,* 89(9), 723-727.
[PMID: 24784335]

Curry, A., Williams, T., Penny, M.L. (2019). Pelvic Inflammatory Disease: Diagnosis, Management, and Prevention. *Am. Fam. Physician,* 100(6), 357-364.
[PMID: 31524362]

Dawood, M.T., Naik, M., Bharwani, N., Sudderuddin, S.A., Rockall, A.G., Stewart, V.R. (2021). Adnexal Torsion: Review of Radiologic Appearances. *Radiographics,* 41(2), 609-624.
[http://dx.doi.org/10.1148/rg.2021200118] [PMID: 33577417]

de la Encarnación Castellano, C., Canós Nebot, À., Caballero Romeu, J.P., Galán Llopis, J.A. (2021). Medical treatment for acute renal colic. *Arch. Esp. Urol.,* 74(1), 71-79.
[PMID: 33459623]

El-Ghar, M.A., Farg, H., Sharaf, D.E., El-Diasty, T. (2021). CT and MRI in Urinary Tract Infections: A Spectrum of Different Imaging Findings. *Medicina (Kaunas),* 57(1), 32.
[http://dx.doi.org/10.3390/medicina57010032] [PMID: 33401464]

Gottlieb, M., Long, B., Koyfman, A. (2018). The evaluation and management of urolithiasis in the ED: A review of the literature. *Am. J. Emerg. Med.,* 36(4), 699-706.
[http://dx.doi.org/10.1016/j.ajem.2018.01.003] [PMID: 29321112]

Guile, S.L., Mathai, J.K. (2020). Ovarian Torsion. *StatPearls.* StatPearls Publishing.Treasure Island (FL):

[PMID: 32809510]

Hata, J. Seeing the unseen, new techniques in vascular imaging: superb micro-vascular imaging; Published 2014.. (2014). https://eu.medical.canon/wp-content/uploads/sites/2/2015/01/Seeing- the-unseen-2014-- MI-on-Aplio-500.pdf. Accessed August 13.

Ingimarsson, J.P., Krambeck, A.E., Pais, V.M., Jr (2016). Diagnosis and Management of Nephrolithiasis. *Surg. Clin. North Am., 96*(3), 517-532.
[http://dx.doi.org/10.1016/j.suc.2016.02.008] [PMID: 27261792]

Jokar, A., Khademhosseini, P., Ahmadi, K., Sistani, A., Amiri, M., Sinaki, A.G. (2018). A Comparison of Metoclopramide and Ondansetron Efficacy for the Prevention of Nausea and Vomiting In Patients Suffered From Renal Colic. *Open Access Maced. J. Med. Sci., 6*(10), 1833-1838.
[http://dx.doi.org/10.3889/oamjms.2018.302] [PMID: 30455758]

Kanda, T., Mochida, J., Takada, S., Hori, Y., Yamaguchi, K., Takahashi, S. (2014). Case of mumps orchitis after vaccination. *Int. J. Urol., 21*(4), 426-428.
[http://dx.doi.org/10.1111/iju.12305] [PMID: 24164648]

Karaca, L., Oral, A., Kantarci, M., Sade, R., Ogul, H., Bayraktutan, U., Okur, A., Yüce, I. (2016). Comparison of the superb microvascular imaging technique and the color Doppler techniques for evaluating children's testicular blood flow. *Eur. Rev. Med. Pharmacol. Sci., 20*(10), 1947-1953.
[PMID: 27249591]

Kaver, I., Matzkin, H., Braf, Z.F. (1990). Epididymo-orchitis: a retrospective study of 121 patients. *J. Fam. Pract., 30*(5), 548-552.
[PMID: 2332745]

Kreisel, K., Torrone, E., Bernstein, K., Hong, J., Gorwitz, R. (2017). Prevalence of Pelvic Inflammatory Disease in Sexually Experienced Women of Reproductive Age - United States, 2013-2014. *MMWR Morb. Mortal. Wkly. Rep., 66*(3), 80-83.
[http://dx.doi.org/10.15585/mmwr.mm6603a3] [PMID: 28125569]

Laher, A., Ragavan, S., Mehta, P., Adam, A. (2020). Testicular Torsion in the Emergency Room: A Review of Detection and Management Strategies. *Open Access Emerg. Med., 12*, 237-246.
[http://dx.doi.org/10.2147/OAEM.S236767] [PMID: 33116959]

Lee, R.A., Centor, R.M., Humphrey, L.L., Jokela, J.A., Andrews, R., Qaseem, A., Akl, E.A., Bledsoe, T.A., Forciea, M.A., Haeme, R., Kansagara, D.L., Marcucci, M., Miller, M.C., Obley, A.J. (2021). Appropriate Use of Short-Course Antibiotics in Common Infections: Best Practice Advice From the American College of Physicians. *Ann. Intern. Med., 174*(6), 822-827.
[http://dx.doi.org/10.7326/M20-7355] [PMID: 33819054]

Mahonski, S., Hu, K.M. (2019). Female Nonobstetric Genitourinary Emergencies. *Emerg. Med. Clin. North Am., 37*(4), 771-784.
[http://dx.doi.org/10.1016/j.emc.2019.07.012] [PMID: 31563207]

Mattoo, T.K., Shaikh, N., Nelson, C.P. (2021). Contemporary Management of Urinary Tract Infection in Children. *Pediatrics, 147*(2), e2020012138.
[http://dx.doi.org/10.1542/peds.2020-012138] [PMID: 33479164]

McConaghy, J.R., Panchal, B. (2016). Epididymitis: An Overview. *Am. Fam. Physician, 94*(9), 723-726.
[PMID: 27929243]

Meltzer, A.C., Burrows, P.K., Wolfson, A.B., Hollander, J.E., Kurz, M., Kirkali, Z., Kusek, J.W., Mufarrij, P., Jackman, S.V., Brown, J. (2018). Effect of Tamsulosin on Passage of Symptomatic Ureteral Stones: A Randomized Clinical Trial. *JAMA Intern. Med., 178*(8), 1051-1057.
[http://dx.doi.org/10.1001/jamainternmed.2018.2259] [PMID: 29913020]

Mesquita, R.D., Rosas, J.L. (2017). Adult Acute Scrotal Edema - When Radiologists Can Help to Avoid Unnecessary Surgical Treatment. *J. Radiol. Case Rep., 11*(8), 24-30.
[http://dx.doi.org/10.3941/jrcr.v11i8.3165] [PMID: 29299103]

Ross, J. (2014). Pelvic inflammatory disease. *Clin Evid Handbook,* (June), 557-558.

Sharp, V.J., Kieran, K., Arlen, A.M. (2013). Testicular torsion: diagnosis, evaluation, and management. *Am. Fam. Physician, 88*(12), 835-840.
[PMID: 24364548]

Sheth, K.R., Keays, M., Grimsby, G.M., Granberg, C.F., Menon, V.S., DaJusta, D.G., Ostrov, L., Hill, M., Sanchez, E., Kuppermann, D., Harrison, C.B., Jacobs, M.A., Huang, R., Burgu, B., Hennes, H., Schlomer, B.J., Baker, L.A. (2016). Diagnosing Testicular Torsion before Urological Consultation and Imaging: Validation of the TWIST Score. *J. Urol., 195*(6), 1870-1876.
[http://dx.doi.org/10.1016/j.juro.2016.01.101] [PMID: 26835833]

Shoag, J., Tasian, G.E., Goldfarb, D.S., Eisner, B.H. (2015). The new epidemiology of nephrolithiasis. *Adv. Chronic Kidney Dis., 22*(4), 273-278.
[http://dx.doi.org/10.1053/j.ackd.2015.04.004] [PMID: 26088071]

Strachowski, L.M., Choi, H.H., Shum, D.J., Horrow, M.M. (2021). Pearls and Pitfalls in Imaging of Pelvic Adnexal Torsion: Seven Tips to Tell It's Twisted. *Radiographics, 41*(2), 625-640.
[http://dx.doi.org/10.1148/rg.2021200122] [PMID: 33646910]

Tracy, C.R., Steers, W.D., Costabile, R. (2008). Diagnosis and management of epididymitis. *Urol. Clin. North Am., 35*(1), 101-108, vii.
[http://dx.doi.org/10.1016/j.ucl.2007.09.013] [PMID: 18061028]

Trojian, T.H., Lishnak, T.S., Heiman, D. (2009). Epididymitis and orchitis: an overview. *Am. Fam. Physician, 79*(7), 583-587.
[PMID: 19378875]

Varras, M., Tsikini, A., Polyzos, D., Samara, Ch., Hadjopoulos, G., Akrivis, Ch. (2004). Uterine adnexal torsion: pathologic and gray-scale ultrasonographic findings. *Clin. Exp. Obstet. Gynecol., 31*(1), 34-38.
[PMID: 14998184]

Velasquez, J., Boniface, M.P., Mohseni, M. (2021). Acute Scrotum Pain.*StatPearls..* Treasure Island, FL: StatPearls Publishing. https://www.ncbi.nlm.nih.gov/books/NBK470335/ Updated 2021 Jul 18 Internet.

CHAPTER 8

"Chronic" Abdominal Pain in the Acute Setting: Functional Bowel Diseases, Irritable Bowel Syndrome (IBS) and Cancer-related Pain

Abstract: Chronic abdominal pain is a very common condition all over the world. Although not expected to present emergently, acute exacerbations of chronic pain or the slightest change that worsens the patient's condition (*e.g*, acute-onset diarrhea, vomiting, or loss of appetite) will trigger admissions to ED. Functional bowel diseases include irritable bowel syndrome (IBS, a.k.a. spastic colon), functional bloating, functional constipation, functional diarrhea, and unspecified functional bowel disorders. Epidemiologic, pathophysiologic and therapeutic studies of functional bowel diseases, employed the Rome Criteria with universal validity. Patients with malignancy can experience different types of cancer-related pain at any time during the disease process, perceived by the organs or systems involved.

Keywords: Abdominal pain, Cancer-related pain, Chronic abdominal pain, Functional bowel diseases, Irritable bowel syndrome, Spastic colon, Rome Criteria.

Evaluation and history should be focused towards differentiating benign functional disease from organic disease with serious outcomes. For example, significant recent weight loss, hypovolemia or cachectic appearance, signs of blood loss, and *de novo* anemia warrant further investigation to exclude organic etiology (Table **1**). In contrast, the laboratory values are expected to be normal in the case of "functional" abdominal pain (AP). **Irritable bowel syndrome (IBS)** may be considered in a patient with bowel habit changes accompanying AP.

Iron deficiency, if diagnosed, should suggest celiac disease, IBD (including ulcerative colitis/ Crohn's disease) or malignancy. As an accurate biomarker, detection of **fecal calprotectin** supports the presumptive diagnosis of IBD and helps to direct patients to colonoscopy. **Chronic pancreatitis** may be the cause of chronic AP, especially in patients with a history of previous pancreatitis attacks, alcoholism or gallstones. The flip side is that some patients without a previously

Ozgur KARCIOGLU, Selman YENİOCAK, Mandana HOSSEINZADEH & Seckin Bahar SEZGIN

diagnosed risk factors mentioned above can also present with recurrent AP which will some day be diagnosed with 'chronic AP' in the ED, as a challenge for the physicians.

Table 1. The following tests may be requested in the patient with chronic AP.

• CBC+ leukocyte formula
• Electrolyte, BUN, creatinine, glucose
• Calcium
• ALT/AST, alkaline phosphatase, bilirubin
• Lipase/amylase
• Serum iron, iron binding capacity, ferritin
• Transglutaminase

DD of IBS and other functional disorders should include a broad range of disorders causing AP at some point of the disease course (Table **2**).

Table 2. Uncommon causes of abdominal pain include the following entities.

• AAA- Abdominal aortic aneurysm
• Abdominal compartment syndrome
• Abdominal migraine
• Acute intermittent porphyria
• Angioedema (hereditary or due to ACE inhibitor)
• Celiac artery compression syndrome
• Chronic abdominal wall pain
• Colonic pseudoobstruction
• Eosinophilic gastroenteritis
• Epiploic appendagitis
• Familial Mediterranean Fever (FMF)
• Parasite-Helminth infections
• Herpes zoster
• Hypercalcemia
• Hypothyroidism
• Chronic lead poisoning
• Meckel's diverticulum
• Paroxysmal nocturnal hemoglobinuria (PNH)
• Pseudoappendicitis
• Causes of "pulmonary abdominal pain" (lower lobe pneumonia)
• Rectus sheath hematoma
• Renal infarction
• Lower rib-related pain
• Sclerosing mesenteritis
• Somatization

Irritable Bowel Syndrome (IBS); a.k.a. Spastic Colon

IBS is a functional disorder that causes occasional disturbances in the GIS and chronic AP associated with remarkable changes in bowel habits.

It is more common in the urban young population and women. Incidence figures of 5% to 20% have been reported in different geographic regions. The continent with the highest frequency is South America with 21%. It is rare over 50 years of age. The prevalence of IBS in Turkey has been found 5% in males, 7.4% in females and 6.3% overall, and there is a female predominance (around 2/3) (Celebi, 2004).

The mechanism that is most emphasized can be summarized as **"the nerves that carry messages from the gut to the brain are working too hard"** (Table **3**).

Table 3. The mechanisms focused on the etiology of IBS are as follows.

• Changes in intestinal motility,
• Visceral hypersensitivity,
• Intestinal barrier dysfunction,
• Intestinal bacterial overgrowth and
• Changes in intestinal flora,
• Intestinal mucosal inflammation,
• Genetic and epigenetic changes,
• Brain-intestinal system interaction
• Psychosocial problems.

Findings in the History and Examination

There is colic/cramp-like AP with exacerbations in the history. Symptoms are mostly intermittent and there may be asymptomatic periods for weeks in between. The most disturbing ones following AP are the feeling of urgency to defecate, bloating and increased number of defecations.

The severity of attacks changes over time. The location and definition of AP also varies from patient to patient. There may be patients who are relieved by defecation, as well as those with tenesmus and increased pain with defecation. **Bloating** is a prominent complaint.

Medication history should be taken carefully, as the side effects of some drugs can cause bloating and mimic IBS. Oral antidiabetic use should be questioned, especially in diabetic patients as diabetic gastroparesis should also be in the DD.

Recurrent and alternating episodes of diarrhea and constipation are typically seen. Diarrhea may occur in the morning and after meals, is usually small in volume and does not contain blood. When there is an attack of constipation, the stool becomes hard and shaped, sometimes associated with pain. AP is not accompanied by loss of appetite and weight loss and is usually not expected to progress or worsen.

Physical examination is usually normal. There may be mild tenderness in the abdomen. Rectal examination is important as in any abdominal examination, it can identify dyssynergic defecation supporting a diagnosis of IBS.

Diagnosis: No laboratory markers could be identified. Diagnosis is fortified by history and examination findings.

Lactose intolerance is one of the diseases that IBS is most confused with. These people cannot digest lactose, known as milk sugar. Drinking large amounts of milk or consuming dairy products can cause episodes of gas, bloating, cramps and diarrhea in these people. When the complaints are apparently associated with ingestion of milk, consumption of milk and dairy products should be limited or eliminated. In some cases, the administration of external enzyme preparations may lead to relief of symptoms. If symptoms improve significantly following cessation of dairy products for 2 weeks, we will be closer to the diagnosis.

The Rome IV criteria are used quite often and are helpful (Table 4)

Table 4. Rome IV criteria.

- Two or more of the following with at least one AP attack per week in the past three months.
● Defecation-related AP.
● Change in defecation frequency.
● Change in stool shape.

Subtypes in IBS are determined by stool consistency. The Bristol stool form scale is used to evaluate stool consistency.

Constipation-dominant IBS (IBS-C) hard stools are found in more than 25% of (types 1-2) and watery stools in less than 25% (types 6-7) of all defecation events. In diarrhea-dominant IBS (IBS-D), watery stools (types 6-7) are present in more than 25% of stools and hard stools constitute less than 25%. If both hard and watery stools are present in more than 25% of the stools, it is called mixed type IBS (IBS-M). If both types of defecation are present in less than 25% of defecations, they are called unclassified IBS (IBS-U) (Fig. **1**).

Definition of stool	points	Illustration
Discrete ball-like small hard parts	1	
Sausage-like confluent hard parts	2	
Sausage-like including fractures on the surface	3	
Sausage or snake-like, smooth or soft	4	
Well-bordered big parts	5	
Ill-bordered parts, like rice	6	
Watery, no hard parts	7	

Fig. (1). Bristol Stool Form Scale is used to classify IBS subtypes.

IBS subtypes are important in the management (Table 5). In their comprehensive systematic review, Gadour *et al.* reported that 50.4% of the patients diagnosed with IBS by the Rome II and III criteria had IBS-D, 13.8% had IBS-C, 30.3% had IBS-M, and 3.5% had IBS-U (Gadour, 2021). The IBS-D subtype was found to be associated with high alcohol intake.

Clinicians should be alerted about alarm symptoms (red flags) in patients considered to have FBD, together with exacerbating factors for the disease (Table **6** and **7**).

Table 5. IBS subtypes include the following.

Subtype definition	Prevalence reported in the systematic review by Gadour *et al.*, 2021.
1. IBS with predominance of constipation (C)	50.4%
2. Diarrhea-dominated IBS (D)	13.8%
3. IBS with mixed-type bowel habits: Intestinal motility in which diarrhea and constipation are reported concurrently. (M)	30.3%
4. Unclassified IBS: The group that is not consistent with any of three previous categories. (U)	3.5%

Table 6. Alarming symptoms (red flags) in a patient with suspected FBD.

1 Recent onset of symptoms and rapid deterioration
2 Onset of symptoms after age 45 to 50
3 Weight loss, fever, anemia, bloody stools (occult blood positivity)
4 Symptoms wake the patient up at night
5 Family history of GI cancer, IBD or celiac disease
6 Recent use of antibiotics
7 Having a history of travel to countries at risk of infection/infestation
8 Arthritis or skin manifestations, malabsorption, thyroid dysfunction

Table 7. Factors that exacerbate symptoms in IBS.

1. Overeating
2. Foods that increase gas production in the colon (fermentable oligo-, di-, monosaccharide, and polyol (FODMAPs)
3. Cereals (wheat, oats, rye, barley)
4. Chocolate, dairy products
5. Alcohol, tea, coffee, cola drink
6. Medicines
7. Surgical intervention
8. Psychological disorders
9. Seasonal changes
10. Menstrual cycle
11. Non-compliance with treatment

Imaging and Endoscopy Principles

Patients under 50 years of age, without alarm symptoms, and with typical IBS symptoms, do not require additional imaging. Although the advanced evaluation method varies from patient to the patient, endoscopy, colonoscopy, biopsy and abdominal CT can be used. Colonoscopy is indicated especially in cases over 50 years of age, where cancer cannot be excluded easily. When colonoscopy is performed in patients with IBS-D, random biopsies should be performed to rule out microscopic/lymphocytic colitis.

Recently, it has been demonstrated that CT-colonoscopy imaging is useful in distinguishing IBS subtypes (Ohgo, 2016). The descending colon diameter and transverse colon length were significantly smaller in the IBS-D group (Fig. **2**).

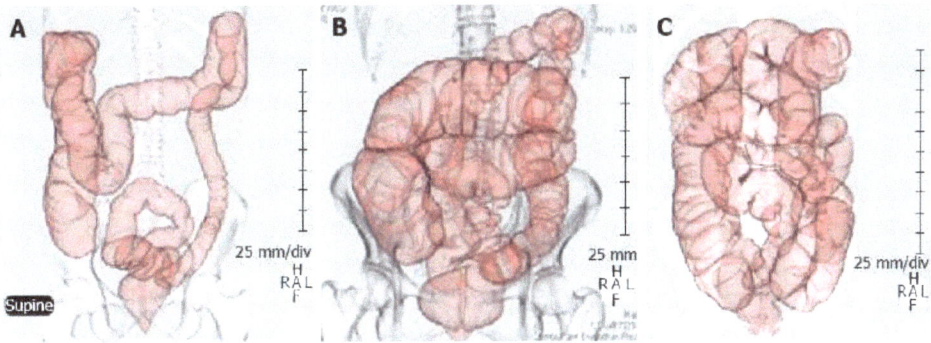

Fig. (2). IBS appearance on CT-colonography. A: Typical diarrhea-predominant IBS (IBS-D); B: Constipation-predominant IBS (IBS-C); C: Typical functional constipation.

WHICH TESTS ARE REQUESTED FOR GAS AND BLOATING?

Often a test is not required. The important factor is what happens in addition to the expected signs and complaints with the disease. For example, if there are symptoms such as weight loss, anemia, blood in the stool, fever, vomiting in addition to diarrhea, appropriate tests should be performed to rule out entities other than IBS (Table **8**).

Table 8. Diagnostic tests in irritable bowel syndrome.

Test	Explanations-notes
Basic blood tests (*i.e.*, CBC, CRP, ESR)	These are basic work up in the absence of red flag signs.
Celiac serology	Recommended in IBS-M and IBS-D subtypes to exclude Celiac disease

(Table 8) cont.....

Test	Explanations-notes
Basic blood tests + thyroid functions + Celiac serology + HIV work up	Recommended in the presence of red flag signs.
Stool examinations (Parasites, eggs, amoebic cysts, Clostridium difficile toxin, and others endemic in the region)	Recommended in the presence of red flag signs.
Abdomen imaging (USG, CT, Barium studies)	Recommended in the presence of red flag signs.
Colonoscopy	Recommended in the presence of red flag signs or above 50 years of age
Breath test to exclude lactose intolerance	Clinical suspicion persists after dietary restrictions

Management Strategy

Management workflow in IBS should reflect the light of evidence-based medicine (Fig. **3**).

Fecal Microbiota Transplantation (FMT): While there is currently no proven treatment for IBS, some authors have pointed out that FMT appears to be promising. El-Salhy *et al.* cited that the dose of the fecal transplant is also an important factor influencing the outcome of FMT for IBS (El-Salhy, 2021). Likewise, donor-dependent variations occur with regard to the efficacy of FMT in patients with IBS. Administration of the FMT to either the small or large intestine as well as single or repeated procedures also have an impact on the outcome, but the optimal route and repetition of administration remain to be determined. The procedure appears to be safe, as a 1-year follow-up of IBS patients who received FMT showed that adverse events of abdominal pain, diarrhea, and constipation were both mild and self-limiting.

Peckham *et al.* assessed the effectiveness and safety of clinical and individualized homeopathic treatment for IBS *via* high-quality studies in the literature (Peckham, 2021). At short-term follow-up of two weeks, global improvement in symptoms was experienced by 73% of asafoetida participants compared to 45% of placebo participants (RR 1.61, 95% CI 1.18 to 2.18; 2 studies, very low certainty evidence). The authors concluded that the results for the outcomes are uncertain. Thus, no firm conclusions regarding the effectiveness and safety of homeopathy for the treatment of IBS can be drawn.

Patient with suspected IBS (abdominal pain episodes, change in bowel habits and stool forms, relief with defecation)

Search for alarm features (red flags)

History
Age>50 years
Weight loss
Family history of GI malignancy
Severe / copious diarrhea
Febrile episodes, chills
Travel to endemic regions
Nocturnal symptoms
Hematochezia

Physical exam findings
Arthritis, rash/skin lesions, lymphadenopathy, abdominal mass

Red flag present

Red flag absent

Focused diagnostic work up

Diagnosis of IBS is established and therapy should be started based on predominant symptoms

No improvement

Reassess symptoms in 4-6 weeks

Improvement

Continue treatment

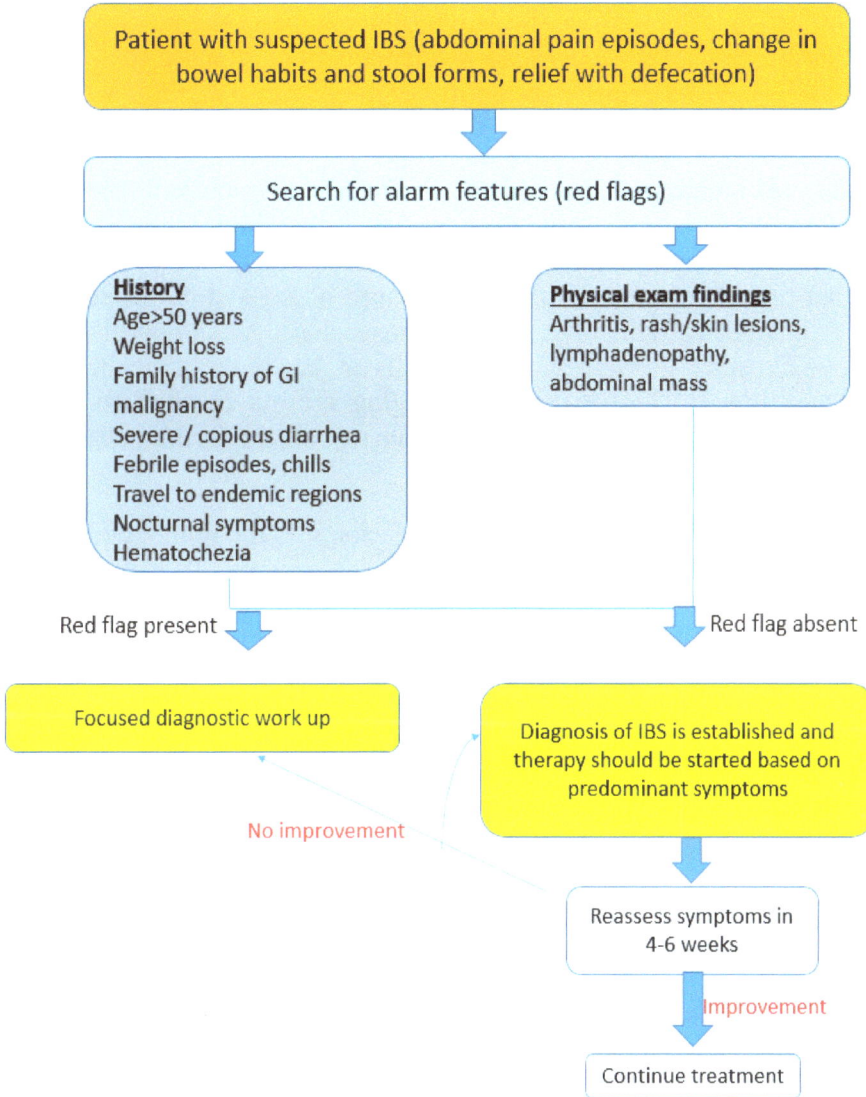

Fig. (3). The management algorithm of IBS. First of all, alarm findings /red flags are excluded and re-evaluated 4 to 6 weeks after treatment is started.

TREATMENT

A majority (70%) of patients have mild disease. Those who have psychological disorders or are under psychological stress, those with moderate to severe AP or diarrhea, those with fear of cancer, and women are more likely to consult a doctor. For this reason, it takes priority to instill confidence in patients, to explain that they do not turn into cancer (at least in the short term), and to comfort them.

Role of diet in the management of IBS: Diet plays an important role not only in the pathophysiology of IBS, but also as a tool that improves symptoms and quality of life. The density of gut endocrine cells is low in IBS patients, and it is believed that this abnormality is the direct cause of the symptoms seen in those with IBS. A low fermentable oligo-, di-, monosaccharide, and polyol (FODMAP) diet and FMT restore the gut endocrine cells to the level of healthy subjects. Changing to a low-FODMAP diet or changing the gut bacteria through FMT improves IBS symptoms and restores the density of endocrine cells (El-Salhy, 2019).

In patients with mild and intermittent IBS attacks, it is recommended to regulate diet and lifestyle instead of regular or lifelong treatment. **Pharmacological treatment** is recommended for patients with moderate symptoms and those with mild symptoms who do not respond to diet and lifestyle changes. The patient should stay away from the aggravating factors in Table **7**.

Many studies have emphasized the important role of microflora in the pathogenesis of IBS (Parkes *et al.* 2008). A meta-analysis of 20 randomized controlled trials involving 1404 patients found that global IBS symptoms improved in probiotic users (RR = 0.77, 95% CI 0.62–0.94) (McFarland and Dublin, 2008). In a double-blind study on patients with IBS, S. boulardii improved quality of life *versus* placebo (Choi *et al.* 2011). These findings are also in line with earlier well-designed studies in France (Bennani, 1990; Maupas *et al.* 1983). A retrospective analysis showed that S. boulardii and mebeverine treatment led to positive outcomes in IBS, and S. boulardii had beneficial effects on IBS symptoms and quality of life.

Additional Pharmacological Treatment

Antispasmodic (spasmolytic) agents are the mainstay of treatment for abdominal pain. They are the most commonly used drugs in the treatment of IBS, and they show their effects by reducing the contractility of intestinal smooth muscles. Antispasmodic + anxiolytic combinations may be beneficial in anxious patients. Another group of drugs is antidepressants. Tricyclic antidepressants and SSRIs are agents that act by modifying the perception of pain (Table **9**).

Table 9. Drug regimens used in IBS.

Drug Class	Chemical Compound and Dosage
Spasmolytics	Pinaverium bromide 150 mg/day, Otilonium bromide 30 mg/day, Hyoscine-N-butyl bromide 30-60 mg/day, Mebeverine 300 mg/day, Trimebutin maleate 300-600mg/day, Symetropium bromide 100 mg/day, Dicyclomine 20-80 mg/day, Peppermint oil 0.6-1.2 ml/day
Spasmolytics + Anxiolytic	Chlordiazepoxide + Clidinium bromide 30-60 mg/day, Medazepam + Hyoscine 60-80 mg/day, Diazepam + Oxyphencycline 14-21 mg/day,
SSRI	Citalopram 20 mg/day, Escitalopram 10 mg/day, Sertraline 25-100 mg/day Fluoxetine 10-40 mg/day Paroxetine 20-50 mg/day
Tricyclic antidepressants	Amitriptyline 10-150 mg/day, Imipramine 10-150 mg/day, Desipramine 10-150 mg/day, Nortriptyline 10-150 mg/day, Trimipramine 10-150 mg/day, Doxepine 10-150 mg/day,
Spasmolytics +Antiflatulant	Simethicone 320 mg/day, Alverin citrate + Simethicone 1080 mg/day,
Antibiotics	Rifaximin 1200 mg/day,
Probiotics	Saccharomyces boulardii 250-500 mg/day Bifidobacterium infantis 1 pack/day, Lactobacillus sp. 1-10x109 CFU/ day
Antidiarrheal agents	Loperamide 8-16 mg/day, Diphenoxylate/Atropine 15-20 mg/day,
5-HT3 antagonists	Alosetron 1-2 mg/ day,
Bulk-forming laxatives	Psyllium 2.5-30 gr/day, Methyl cellulose 1.5 gr/day, Calcium polycarbophil 2.5-5 gr/day,
Osmotic laxatives	Lactulose 10-20 gr/day, Polyethylene glycol 17 gr/day, Magnesium salts 30-60 ml/day, Sorbitol 70% 10-30 mg/day,
Contact laxatives	Sodium picosulfate 5-10 mg/day, Senoside A/B (anthraquinones) 15 mg/day, Bisacodyl 10-20 mg/day,

(Table 9) cont.....

Drug Class	Chemical Compound and Dosage
5-HT4 agonists	Tegaserod 12 mg/day, Prucalopride 2 mg/day,

What can be Done Apart From Diet And Medicine?

The usefulness of exercise can not be underestimated in these patients. Many patients benefit significantly from exercise in case of gas and bloating. For this, a significant exercise should be performed at least 3 to 4 times a week. The type of exercise to be pursued varies according to capabilities, time constraints and personal characteristics. But the most practical exercise is brisk walking until one gets tired.

Cancer as a Cause of AP

In patients over 50 years of age, the cause of unexplained AP may be cancer. On the other hand, AP constitutes 40% of the chief complaints among emergency admissions of cancer patients. In these patients, weight loss and the state of pain should be questioned and recorded with comparison to the past. Cancerous tissue itself can be the cause of AP, as well as the treatments and interventions pursued can lead to AP. In addition, all causes in the normal population can trigger acute AP in these patients. It was reported that 2.2% of the ED patients who had been discharged with a preliminary diagnosis of NSAP in 2011 were diagnosed with cancer within a year, and 1/5 of them died within a year. (Ferlander, 2018). Patients over 60 carry a substantially higher risk in this regard.

Due to the fact that the cancerous tissue is more fragile, bleeding may sometimes accompany AP. In most cases, anemia may be present as a result of chronic blood loss. Sometimes the pain may also indicate temporary or partial bowel obstruction. Perforation occurs more commonly in patients with cancer than in other patients. Findings can be masked in patients whose immune system is suppressed by certain treatments such as chemotherapy.

Further investigation is required in oncological patients with persistent vomiting and lack of oral intake and these patients should not be discharged from the hospital. Diagnosis can often be established after interpretation of contrast-enhanced tomography. Other patients, if stable, can be discharged and scheduled for outpatient follow-up (Ilgen, 2009) (Fig. **4**).

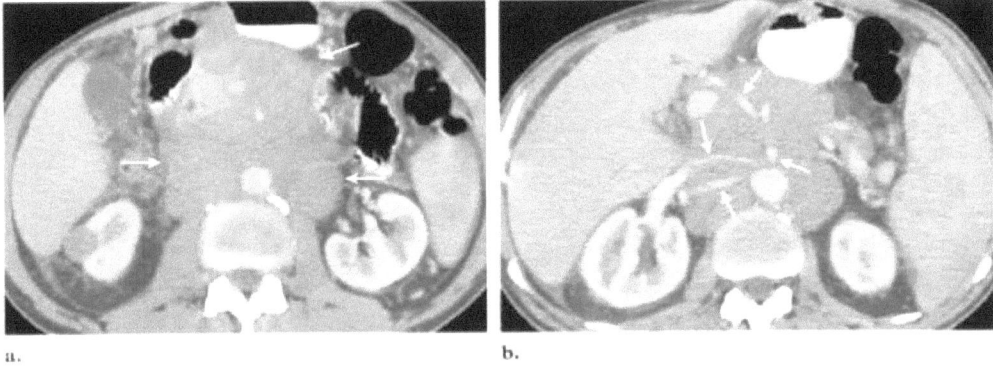

Fig. (4). CT images of a 42-year-old patient diagnosed with lymphoma demonstrate lymph nodes merged with each other. Section **(a)** shows a homogeneous conglomerated mass composed of mesenteric and retroperitoneal lymphadenopathy (arrows). **(b)** CT depicts that the mass surrounds but does not occlude the mesenteric vessels (arrows).

CONCLUSION

Functional bowel diseases comprise a group of conditions that are defined by signs and symptoms attributable to the gastrointestinal system, in the absence of organic causes identifiable by routine work up. IBS is associated with bowel habit changes accompanying AP. IBS subtypes include constipation or diarrhea-dominant entities and are based on stool form, which can be accomplished *via* the use of the Bristol Stool Form Scale. Physicians should be alert to screen patients with waxing and waning pain syndromes for malignant processes. On the other hand, patients with cancer-related pain should have proper management in terms of both pain relief and functional integrity.

REFERENCES

Akpinar, H, Kilic, B, Amanvermez, D (2000). Irritable bowel syndrome prevalance in Narlıdere district in Turkey. *8. United European Gastroenterology Weeks (UEGW)*. Belgium.

Bennani, A. (1990). Randomised trial of *Saccharomyces boulardii* in the treatment of functional colon disorders. *L'Objectif Medical, 73*, 56-61.

CAN G. (2015). *YILMAZ B. İrritabl Barsak Sendromunun Tanı ve Tedavisinde Yaklaşımlar. Güncel Gastroenteroloji 19/3.*. Eylül.

Celebi, S., Acik, Y., Deveci, S.E., Bahcecioglu, I.H., Ayar, A., Demir, A., Durukan, P. (2004). Epidemiological features of irritable bowel syndrome in a Turkish urban society. *J. Gastroenterol. Hepatol., 19*(7), 738-743.
[http://dx.doi.org/10.1111/j.1440-1746.2004.03367.x] [PMID: 15209618]

Choi, C.H., Jo, S.Y., Park, H.J., Chang, S.K., Byeon, J.S., Myung, S.J. (2011). A randomized, double-blind, placebo-controlled multicenter trial of *saccharomyces boulardii* in irritable bowel syndrome: effect on quality of life. *J. Clin. Gastroenterol., 45*(8), 679-683.
[http://dx.doi.org/10.1097/MCG.0b013e318204593e] [PMID: 21301358]

El-Salhy, M., Hatlebakk, J.G., Hausken, T. (2019). Diet in Irritable Bowel Syndrome (IBS): Interaction with Gut Microbiota and Gut Hormones. *Nutrients, 11*(8), 1824.

[http://dx.doi.org/10.3390/nu11081824] [PMID: 31394793]

El-Salhy, M., Hausken, T., Hatlebakk, J.G. (2021). Current status of fecal microbiota transplantation for irritable bowel syndrome. *Neurogastroenterol. Motil.,* *33*(11), e14157.
[http://dx.doi.org/10.1111/nmo.14157] [PMID: 34236740]

Ferlander, P., Elfström, C., Göransson, K., von Rosen, A., Djärv, T. (2018). Nonspecific abdominal pain in the Emergency Department: malignancy incidence in a nationwide Swedish cohort study. *Eur. J. Emerg. Med.,* *25*(2), 105-109.
[PMID: 27172392]

Gadour, E., Hassan, Z., Gadour, R. (2021). A Comprehensive Review of Transaminitis and Irritable Bowel Syndrome. *Cureus,* *13*(7), e16583.
[http://dx.doi.org/10.7759/cureus.16583] [PMID: 34322359]

Hasler, W.L., Owyang, C. (1817). Irritable bowel syndrome. *Textbook of Gastroenterology* Yamada, T., Owyang, C. (1817). JB Lippincott.(4th ed.). Philadelphia:

Ilgen, J.S., Marr, A.L. (2009). Cancer emergencies: the acute abdomen. *Emerg. Med. Clin. North Am.,* *27*(3), 381-399.
[http://dx.doi.org/10.1016/j.emc.2009.04.006] [PMID: 19646643]

Johannesson, E., Simrén, M., Strid, H., Bajor, A., Sadik, R. (2011). Physical activity improves symptoms in irritable bowel syndrome: a randomized controlled trial. *Am. J. Gastroenterol.,* *106*(5), 915-922.
[http://dx.doi.org/10.1038/ajg.2010.480] [PMID: 21206488]

Lovell, R.M., Ford, A.C. (2012). Global prevalence of and risk factors for irritable bowel syndrome: a meta-analysis. *Clin. Gastroenterol. Hepatol.,* *10*(7), 712-721.e4.
[http://dx.doi.org/10.1016/j.cgh.2012.02.029] [PMID: 22426087]

Maupas, J.L., Champemont, P., Delforge, M. (1983). Treatment of irritable bowel syndrome with *Saccharomyces boulardii*: a double-blind, placebo-controlled study. *Med. Chir. Dig.,* *12*, 77-79.

McFarland, L.V. (2010). Systematic review and meta-analysis of *Saccharomyces boulardii* in adult patients. *World J. Gastroenterol.,* *16*(18), 2202-2222.
[http://dx.doi.org/10.3748/wjg.v16.i18.2202] [PMID: 20458757]

McFarland, L.V., Dublin, S. (2008). Meta-analysis of probiotics for the treatment of irritable bowel syndrome. *World J. Gastroenterol.,* *14*(17), 2650-2661.
[http://dx.doi.org/10.3748/wjg.14.2650] [PMID: 18461650]

Ohgo, H., Imaeda, H., Yamaoka, M., Yoneno, K., Hosoe, N., Mizukami, T., Nakamoto, H. (2016). Irritable bowel syndrome evaluation using computed tomography colonography. *World J. Gastroenterol.,* *22*(42), 9394-9399.
[http://dx.doi.org/10.3748/wjg.v22.i42.9394] [PMID: 27895427]

Parkes, G.C., Brostoff, J., Whelan, K., Sanderson, J.D. (2008). Gastrointestinal microbiota in irritable bowel syndrome: their role in its pathogenesis and treatment. *Am. J. Gastroenterol.,* *103*(6), 1557-1567.
[http://dx.doi.org/10.1111/j.1572-0241.2008.01869.x] [PMID: 18513268]

Peckham, E.J., Cooper, K., Roberts, E.R., Agrawal, A., Brabyn, S., Tew, G. (2019). Homeopathy for treatment of irritable bowel syndrome. *Cochrane Database Syst. Rev.,* *9*(9), CD009710.
[http://dx.doi.org/10.1002/14651858.CD009710.pub3] [PMID: 31483486]

Soares, R.L. (2014). Irritable bowel syndrome: a clinical review. *World J. Gastroenterol.,* *20*(34), 12144-12160.
[http://dx.doi.org/10.3748/wjg.v20.i34.12144] [PMID: 25232249]

Wald, A. (2019). Clinical manifestations and diagnosis of irritable bowel syndrome in adults. *UpToDate.*

CHAPTER 9

Special Groups and Abdominal Pain

Abstract: Specific patient groups have inherent characteristics when they suffer from diseases, including those of the digestive system and other causes of abdominal pain. Both diagnostic features and treatment measures differ regarding the patient's age, sex, previous medical / surgical history, and comorbid diseases. Pregnancy has its unique features in both anatomy and physiology of the woman which result in substantial variation in physical examination finding, radiological and laboratory adjuncts (*e.g.*, the location of the appendix is shifted away from its usual site and computed tomography is hardly ever used to diagnose etiologies of abdominal pain in pregnant women). Likewise, children have many differences in presentation, examination findings, work up and treatment principles, complicating the management process.

In addition, the pandemic disease has caused a paradigm shift in the evaluation of almost all diseases, including those with abdominal pain. Many data suggest a close relationship between COVID-19 and the digestive system. Patients with COVID-19 carry a high risk of digestive symptomatology including abdominal pain, nausea and vomiting, diarrhea and others. HIV (+) patients exhibit various GI symptoms such as diarrhea, abdominal pain and proctitis.

Healthcare providers should have robust knowledge of various forms of presentations and characteristics of special subgroups with abdominal pain in this regard, to prevent misdiagnoses and treatment errors in those patients.

Keywords: Acute abdominal pain, Acute appendicitis, Acute cholecystitis, COVID-19, Diverticulitis, Ectopic pregnancy, Elderly, Human Immunodeficiency Virus (HIV), Invagination, Mesenteric ischemia, Mesenteric lymphadenitis, Intussusception, Pregnancy.

PREGNANCY-RELATED ACUTE AP

Although the etiologies of AP in pregnancy are essentially similar to other patients, it is necessary to pay attention to some key issues.

Ectopic pregnancy (EP) is the development of the gestational sac implanted outside the uterus. It is estimated that 5 to 10 out of 100 pregnancies can be

Ozgur KARCIOGLU, Selman YENİOCAK, Mandana HOSSEINZADEH & Seckin Bahar SEZGIN

located ectopically. 96% of EPs are found in the ampulla or isthmus of the Fallopian tubes, 2% in the interstitial tissue of the uterus, and the remainder in the other intraabdominal sites.

EP is diagnosed most commonly in women who have had their first pregnancies or in multiparous women who have become pregnant for the first time after a long time.

EP is the most common cause of pregnancy deaths in the first trimester, resulting mostly from delayed diagnosis. Therefore, in every woman of childbearing age presenting with AP and/or vaginal bleeding, the diagnosis of EP should be presumed until it is ruled out. If the triad of pain+bleeding+syncope can be identified in a woman of child bearing age, the diagnosis is far more likely.

Among the risk factors are pathologies that slow down or stop the migration of the fertilized ovum to the uterus: PID, pelvic adhesions, endometriosis, *in vitro* fertilization, intrauterine device, use of progesterone-containing birth control pills, congenital anatomical variants, malignancies or other tumoral masses.

PATHOLOGY

EP Implanted In The Fallopian Tube can have 3 Potential Consequences

- Rupture towards the peritoneal cavity (tubal abortion)
- Spontaneous abortion (with varying degrees of pain and bleeding).
- Rupture into the tube (with varying degrees of pain and bleeding).

EP implanted in one of the uterine horns can be viable till the 10th to 14th weeks. Very rarely, there are intraperitoneal pregnancies reaching the term.

Clinical Presentation

The most common form of presentation is sudden onset lower abdominal pain and bleeding, associated with syncope or presyncope. Although not a rule, delayed menstruation can be noted. Nausea and vomiting are common. There may also be a history of irregular bleeding in different colors from time to time. Admissions can also be seen after one to four weeks of waxing and waning pain episodes.

EP risk factors, delayed menstruation, and pregnancy symptoms should be questioned, but none of them is a *sine qua non* for the diagnosis of EP. Findings compatible with hemorrhagic shock may be encountered. Fluid resuscitation is to be initiated even before the diagnosis is confirmed.

Abdominal findings can range from very mild pain to peritoneal irritation. Tenderness and sometimes a mass may be identified in bimanual vaginal examination if performed in the emergency setting.

The patients should be consulted with OB/GYN without waiting for verification of the diagnosis of EP.

Emergency Treatments and Consultations Should not be Delayed for the Results of the Laboratory Work Up

B-HCG levels are typically much lower than the expected gestational week, but the pregnancy test is positive.

Some recent studies investigated new markers such as serum protein calponin 2 (CNN2) as a biomarker for tubal EP (Zhang, 2021). Serum CNN2 concentration was found to be increased in those with EP than in women with viable intrauterine pregnancy (vIUP) and miscarriage. The serum CNN2 predicted EP from vIUP and miscarriage with areas under the curve (AUCs) of 0.931 (95% confidence interval: 0.889-0.975). Their data highlight the usability of serum CNN2 as a single marker for the diagnosis of EP.

Although transvaginal USG gives better results, it can also be started with transabdominal USG and findings such as significant Intraabdominal free fluid (pelvic hematocele) accelerate the diagnosis and management (Table **1**). On the contrary, visualization of an intrauterine pregnancy help ruling out EP and mandate a search for other DD which can explain the patient's findings such as a missed abortion, placenta previa, *etc*. (Fig. **1**).

Table 1. Findings that increase the likelihood of a diagnosis of EP with a compatible clinical scenario.

1 Extrauterine gestational sac, containing yolk sac or embryo
2 Adnexal ring sign
3 Adnexal mass
4 Significant free fluid in the abdomen, including Morison's pouch (hepatorenal space)
5 Complex free fluid (suggesting hemoperitoneum)
6 Pseudogestational sac
7 Weak decidual reaction
8 Blood in the endometrium

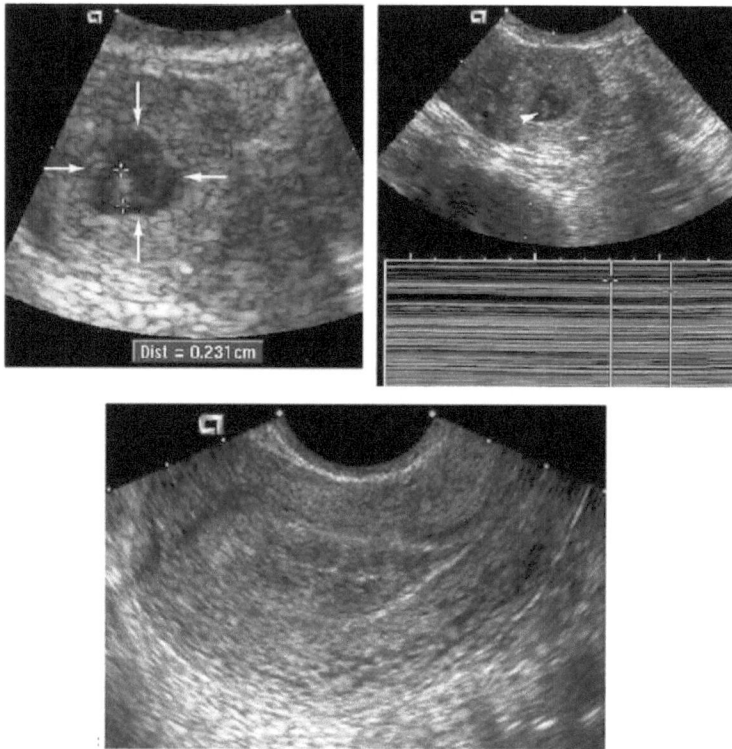

Fig. (1). Top left: Transvaginal view of the right adnexa showing a viable embryo in the extrauterine gestational sac. Top right: Cardiac activity of the embryo is observed in M-mode. Bottom: Sagittal transvaginal view shows no gestational sac within the thickened endometrium.

Initial management: Supplemental O_2 should be given, and fluid resuscitation should be performed *via* a wide-bore vascular access from two different sites. Transfusion of whole blood or blood products (*e.g.* packed RBC) should be adjusted in accord with the severity of shock states.

Kleihauer-Betke test is performed to search for fetomaternal bleeding. Administration of anti-D immunoglobulin may be required in eligible patients. If there is severe intra-abdominal bleeding, emergency operation is required together with resuscitative approaches.

In the emergency management, embolization of the bleeding uterine artery combined with methotrexate for broad ligament EP was also reported in a 30-year old primigravida (Bhinder KK, 2021) (Fig. **2**).

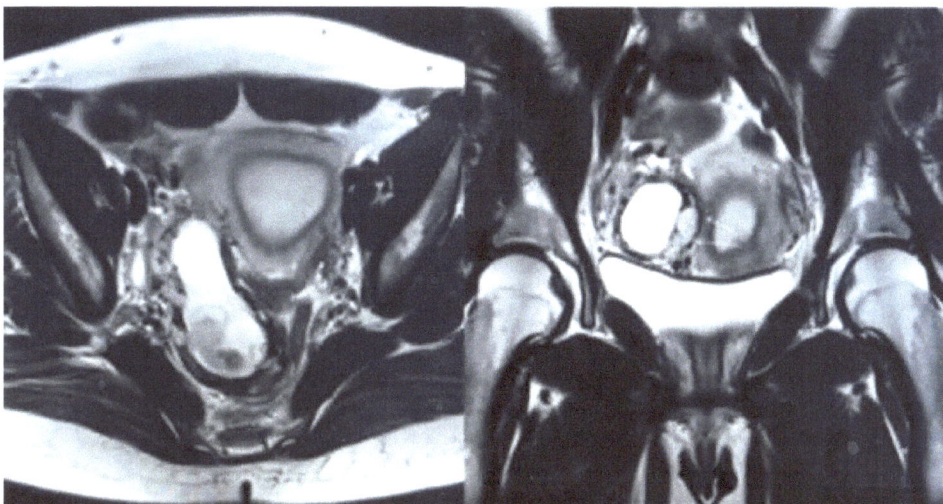

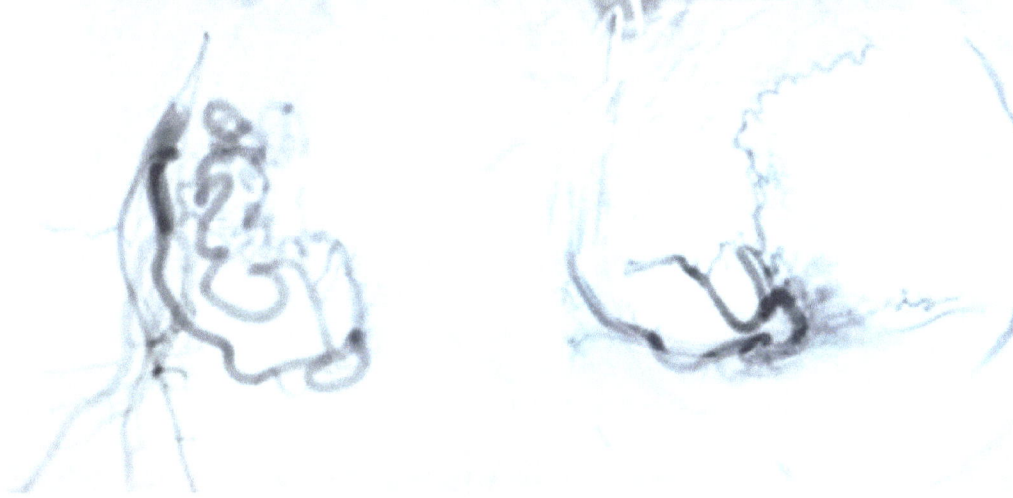

Fig. (2). A. Pelvic MRI depicted a single right-sided broad ligament-extra uterine pelvic ectopic pregnancy with extrinsic mass effect on the right lower uterine segment without frank myometrial invasion. B. Embolization of the right uterine artery stopped the contrast extravasation (Left: Pre-procedural, Right: Post-procedural angiogram.

Appendicitis in Pregnancy

AAp is the most common surgical nonobstetric emergency and cause of acute AP in pregnancy with a rate of 25%. AAp has been documented to have an incidence of 1/200 to 1/8000 in pregnancies (most frequently in Taiwan, least frequently in Mexico). Incessant acute-onset AP in the right lower quadrant is the most common complaint which is also the most reliable symptom leading to an accurate diagnosis. Table **2** shows the entities in the list of differential diagnosis of AAp in pregnancy and puerperial cases.

Table 2. Differential diagnosis of AAp in pregnancy and puerperial cases.

Non-OB/GYN Diagnoses	OB/GYN Diagnoses
Gastroenteritis	Rupture/hemorrhagic ovarian cyst
UTI/ Pyelonephritis	Adnexal torsion
Urinary stone disease	Salpingitis/ PID
Acute cholecystitis	Tubo-ovarian abscess
Acute pancreatitis	Abruptio placenta
Incarcerated hernia	Threatened abortion
Bowel obstruction	Degenerative fibroid
Tumor in the cecum	Chorioamnionitis
Mesenteric adenitis	Preeclampsia
Spontaneous rectus sheath hematoma (abdominal wall)	Ectopic pregnancy
Pulmonary Embolism	Premature labor
Right lower lobe pneumonia	Lig. Rotundum (round ligament) syndrome
Meckel's diverticulitis	Pelvic endometriosis
Sickle cell anemia (crisis)	
Stump app	
Inflammatory bowel disease	

On the other hand, fever and tachycardia are not sensitive findings. Since leukocytosis is usually found in pregnancy (especially in labor), it cannot be used in the diagnosis of AAp. Neutrophil granulocytosis can be diagnostic because it is a marker of bacterial infection, especially if there is no other source of infection.

USG is the preferred imaging modality, but its accuracy decreases in the last trimester. MRI is diagnostic when USG is not helpful.

Is there any difference in the Alvarado score?

Yes. The presence of right lower quadrant pain takes 1 and leukocytosis takes 2 points in the Alvarado score used in nonpregnant patients, but this situation is reversed in pregnant women. The left shift in the leukocyte formula is not scored in pregnant women. Thus, the calculation is made over 9 points.

Diagnostic Difficulties

1- Masking the findings: abdominal distension, displacement of organs in the abdomen, suppression of the inflammatory response

2- Changing appendiceal location with advanced pregnancy

3- Mistaken presumption that nausea, vomiting and AP are absolutely normal during pregnancy.

4- Expansion of the differential diagnosis list with pregnancy

5- Confusion of obstetric complications with the first signs of nonobstetric problems

Can I have a CT scan in case of suspected AAp during pregnancy?

Yes. If USG and laboratory data are not diagnostic, CT is performed in cases of suspected AAp in cases where there is no access to MRI or no experience in interpreting the MRI findings, following consultation with the OB/GYN (Fig. **3**). The decision to CT scan the patient in advanced pregnancy will certainly be easier than it is in early pregnancy. Due consent should be obtained from the patient and relatives.

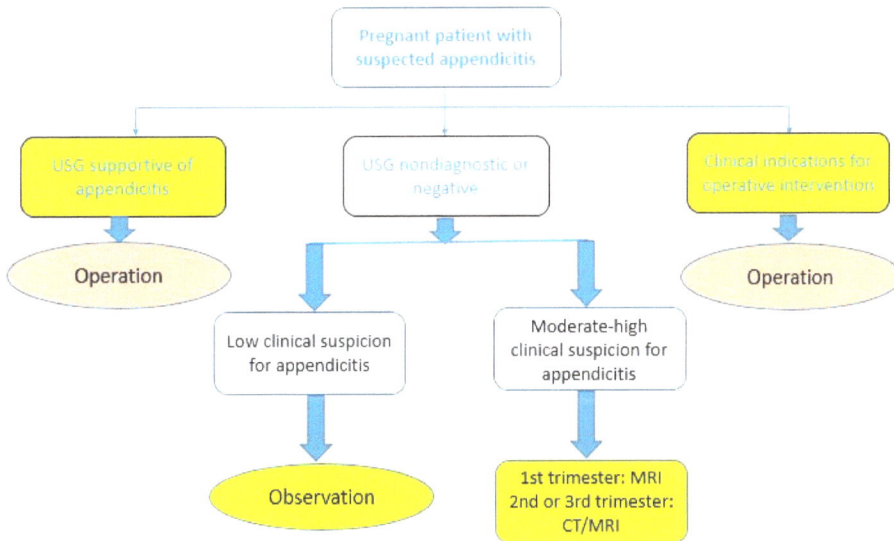

Fig. (3). Diagnosis and evaluation algorithm in case of suspected AAp in pregnancy. USG plays a pivotal role in the management, while CT can be obtained in the advanced pregnancy in the presence of moderate or high clinical suspicion. OR: Operation room.

What are the AAp findings on CT (Figs. **4 - 6**)?

- **Increased diameter of the appendix (>6 mm)**
- **Periappendiceal inflammation findings:**
  - **Fatty streaks,**
  - **phlegmon,**
  - **fluid collection,**
  - **intraluminal gas image**

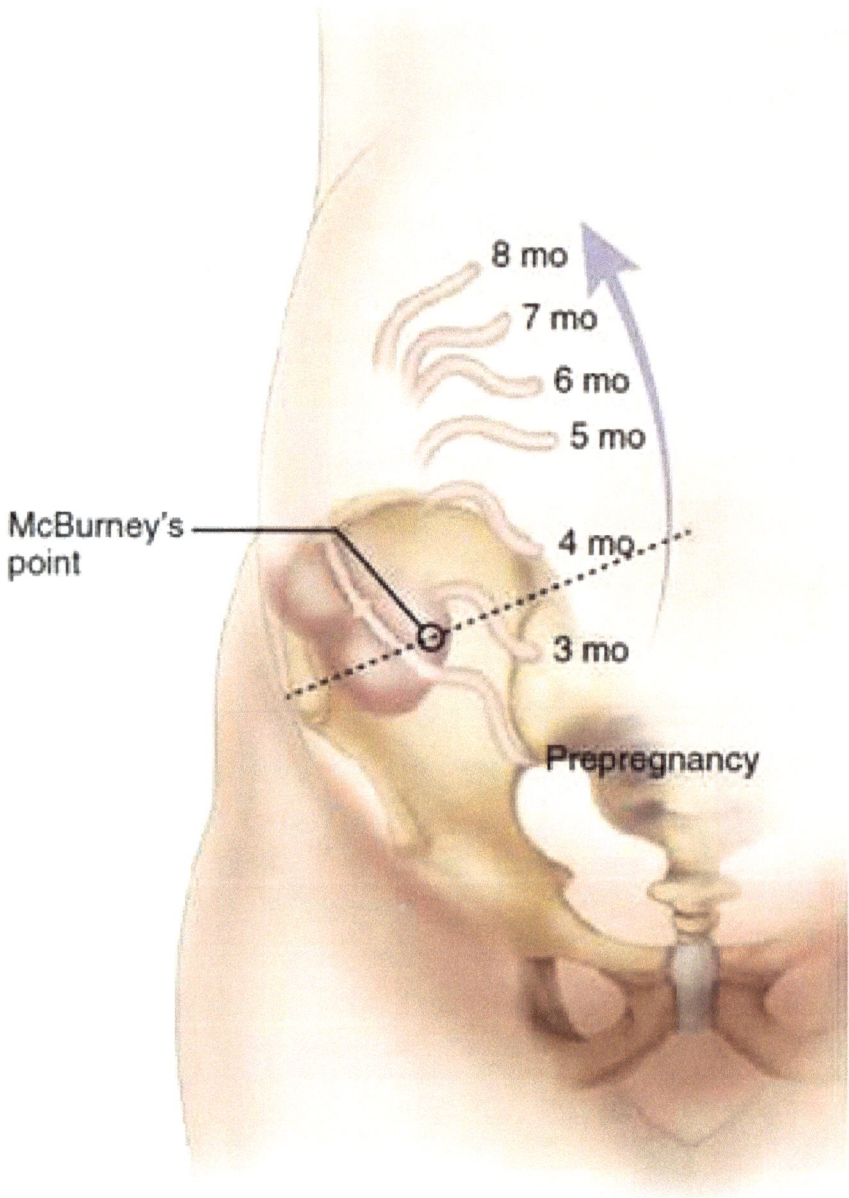

Fig. (4). The situation of the appendix changes in accord with the weeks of pregnancy.

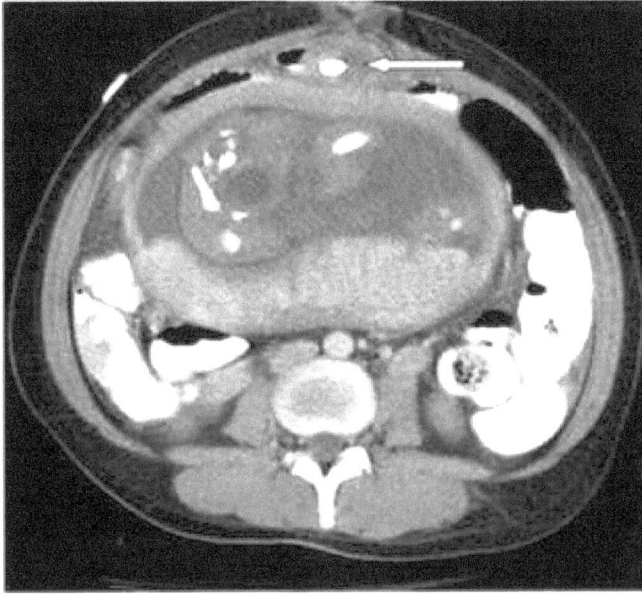

Fig. (5). In the tomographic view of a pregnant woman in her 29th week, fluid collection containing an enterolith below the umbilicus (arrow) and intrauterine pregnancy are observed at the same time.

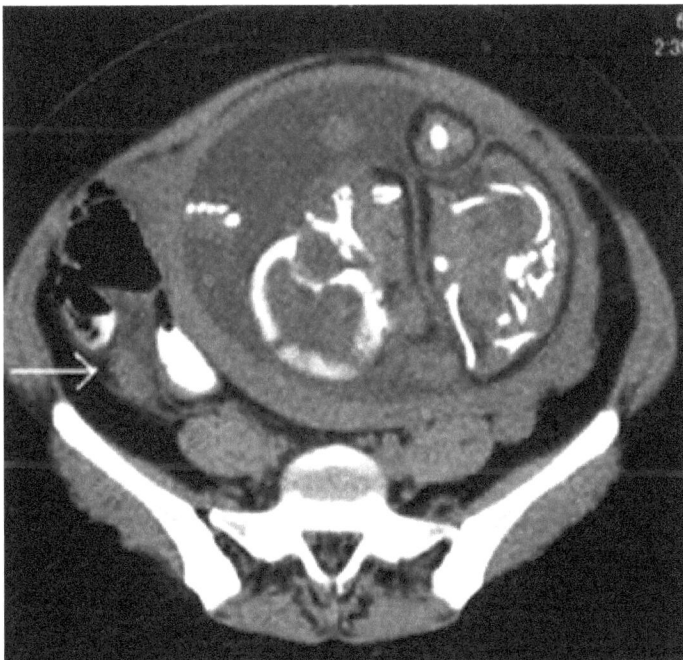

Fig. (6). Appendiceal thickening and periappendiceal fat streaks (arrow) on transverse section of CT with oral + IV contrast in a 27-week pregnant woman.

Management is Open or Laparoscopic Surgery

During pregnancy, AAp is most commonly detected in the second trimester (35% to 50%). It is more common in the multiparous, non-obese, constipated pregnant women and those with high socioeconomic status.

Maternal mortality increases when diagnosis is delayed for more than 24 hours. This delay is most commonly seen in the last trimester due to the vagueness of the findings and confusion with other findings. Although fetal mortality is quite low, it increases in cases of perforation and diffuse peritonitis leading to sepsis (Fig. 7).

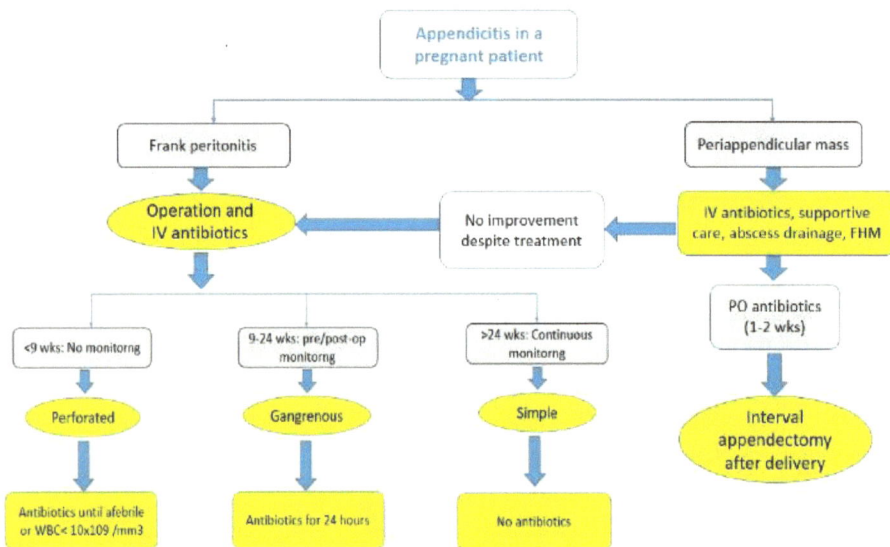

Fig. (7). Treatment algorithm in case of AAp in pregnancy. FHM: Fetal Heart Monitoring.

Acute Cholecystitis (AC) in Pregnancy

Pregnancy represents an essential risk for almost all biliary diseases, including acute cholecystitis, sludge formation in the gallbladder, and cholelithiasis (Table 3). In fact, the entities constitute a more significant health issue when ensuing in the early pregnancy, for the challenges during diagnostic and therapeutic procedures (*e.g.*, the hazards of radiation given with CT, general anesthesia in the operative treatment, *etc.*). On the other hand, when it emerges in the third trimester, the most common approach is to delay surgical procedures until after delivery to protect the fetus from these hazardous effects (Fong, 2019). Up-to-date guidelines underline that third-trimester cholecystectomy is safe for both maternal and fetal point of view.

Table 3. Differential diagnosis of the patient presenting with right upper quadrant pain in pregnancy. Patients are mainly divided into two groups in regard to the presence of jaundice.

With jaundice	Without jaundice
Stones in ductus communis	Inferior AMI
Hepatitis	AAp
Intrahepatic cholestasis	Pancreatitis
Preeclampsia-eclampsia	Symptomatic/perforated peptic ulcer
HELLP syndrome	Pyelonephritis/ urinary stone disease
Acute fatty liver of pregnancy	Radiculopathy
Hepatic malignancy	Herpes zoster (shingles)
Cholangitis	Perihepatitis (Fitz-Hugh- Curtis syndrome)
Hepatic vascular engorgement	Rib fracture/Rib margin pain
Hepatic hematoma	Pleural effusion
Pneumonia	Colon cancer (hepatic flexure)

Around 24.000 pregnant women with AC have recently been analysed in terms of changing surgical strategies between 2003 and 2015 (Cheng, 2020). The median age was 26 years. More than one-third (36%) were subject to non-operative management while almost 60% underwent laparoscopic cholecystectomy while open cholecystectomy was employed only in a minority (4%). Of note, laparoscopic cholecystectomy was more common after 2007 (odds ratio [OR] 1.333, $p<0.001$)

The common causes of acute abdomen, AAp and AC, can mostly be diagnosed with USG. In most cases with suspect USG findings or undiagnosed severe symptoms (Table **4**), CT is prompted as soon as possible (Reimer, 2021). On the other hand, MRI is safely recommended in pregnant women and infants with unclear ultrasound findings (Figs. **8 - 10**).

Table 4. A. Expected findings on USG that establishes the diagnosis of AC.

• AP lasting longer than 4 days
• Peritoneal findings
• C-reactive protein >75 mg/L
• Leukocytes >10,500 µL
• >500 mL free fluid
• Diminished mural contrast-enhancing

Table 4. B. Findings suggestive of common bile duct (CBD)/ductus communis obstruction in USG.

• Gallbladder stones are smaller than canal diameter
• Common bile duct (CBD)/Ductus communis diameter >7 mm
• Enlargement of the intra- and extrahepatic ducts

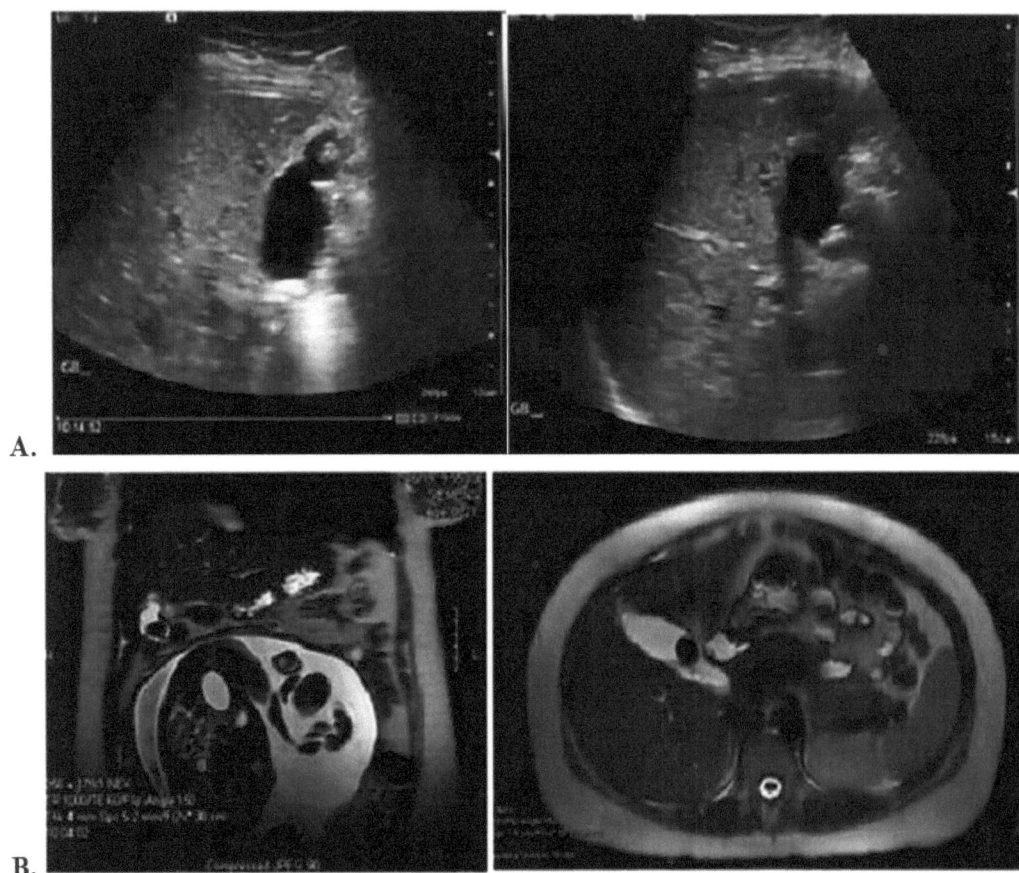

A.

B.

Fig. (8). A. Ultrasonographic findings of a nonmobile stone (~14 mm) in gallbladder neck and gallbladder wall with a thickness of 4 mm in a 22-year-old pregnant patient in 32nd week. **B.** MRCP transverse and sagittal views with 10 mm dilated CBD, stones, and visible fetus noted. She underwent a laparoscopic cholecystectomy with intraoperative cholangiogram (Ward, 2021).

Thin-section MRCP reconstruction shows that the fundus of distended gallbladder compresses the proximal CBD (arrow), causes intrahepatic biliary dilatation, and a normal diameter ductus communis is found distally (arrowheads). Finally, the image is consistent with Mirizzi syndrome.

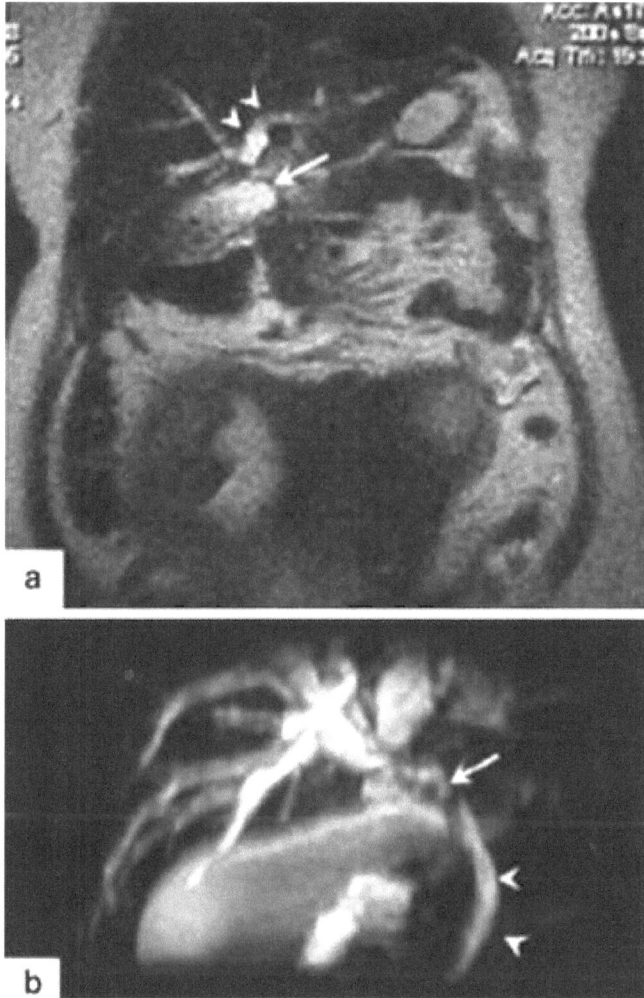

Fig. (9). Obstructive jaundice causing right upper quadrant pain in a 36-week pregnant woman in her 27. **(a)** Coronal T2-weighted single-shot fast spin-echo image of distal gallbladder and a gallstone (arrow) and intrahepatic biliary dilatation (arrowheads). **(b)** Thin-section MR cholangiopancreatography (MRCP) images show normal diameter distal to the CBD, and the ductus communis hepaticus compressed by distended gallbladder.

Other Causes of AP During Pregnancy

Nausea and vomiting (N/V) of Pregnancy: This constitutes the most common medical complaint recorded in pregnancy, which is encountered up to four in every five pregnancies, and hyperemesis gravidarum comprises less than 1% of pregnant women (Chen, 2012). These complaints can be associated with AP and a broad range of acute conditions to be considered in the DD. In addition to *de novo* conditions, there are some pregnant women with chronic conditions which trigger AP such as IBS, hypoperistaltic states (*e.g.*, hypothyroidism).

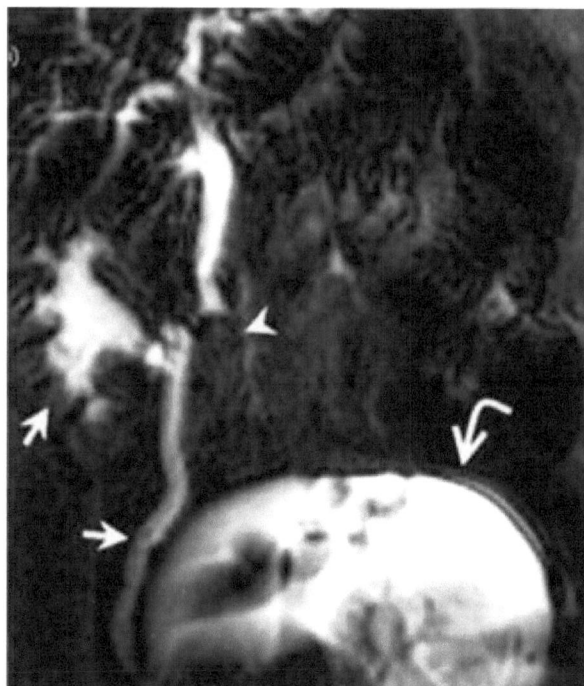

Fig. (10). Occlusion of CBD (arrowhead) and gravid uterus (curved arrow) in second trimester pregnancy in MR cholangiopancreatography (MRCP).

Pancreatitis: In fact, clinical laboratory criteria in the diagnosis of pancreatitis are not different from those of non-pregnant women. Physical examination of the patient with suspected pancreatitis rarely yields diagnostic information, as the organ lies in the retroperitoneal space. Grey-Turner's sign (ecchymosis or discoloration of the flanks) and Cullen's sign (periumbilical ecchymosis) are uncommon subcutaneous signs of severe acute necrotizing pancreatitis (Guldner, 2021) (Fig. **11**). These may be encountered in many other conditions with retroperitoneal haemorrhage therefore convey low sensitivity and specificity.

In case of suspicion of acute pancreatitis, gallstones and structures that can be visualized ultrasonographically should be distinguished by USG as soon as possible. The sensitivity of USG does not exceed 38% in discerning duct stones. Obesity and intestinal gases complicate the process. 54% of pancreatic pseudocysts can be recognized by USG.

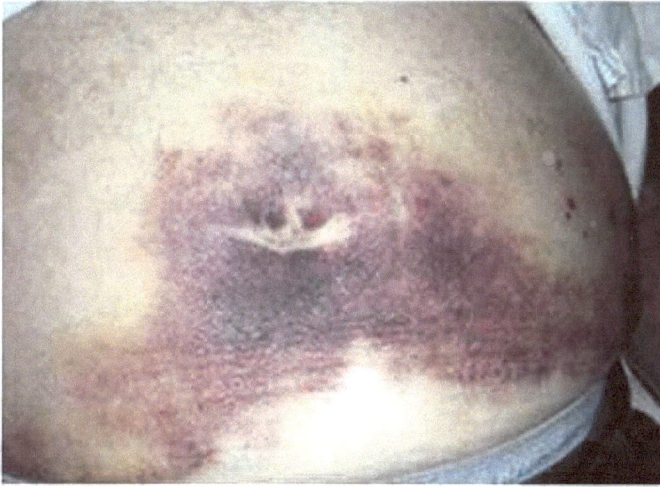

Fig. (11). Cullen's sign in a pregnant woman. It is rare, although it will be strongly suggestive of hemorrhagic pancreatitis when detected.

Acute pancreatitis in pregnancy is a rare occurrence and conveys an incidence rate below 0.1% in all pregnancies. There have been some case series reported very poor outcomes, with maternal mortality rates of 20%, while almost half of the feti are lost (Hughes, 2021).

Pancreatic disease ensues in the third trimester or the early postpartum period. The three commonest precipitating factors for pancreatitis are gallstones (65 to 100%), alcohol consumption and hypertriglyceridemia (Ducarme, 2014). Hypertriglyceridemia is exacerbated in pregnancy, due to elevated estrogen and insulin resistance. Ranson and Balthazar criteria can be used to evaluate the severity and treat the disease during pregnancy, although the validity of the Ranson criteria in pregnancy has not been studied.

Management principles consist of conservative treatment in early pregnancy and laparoscopic cholecystectomy in second trimester. In late pregnancy, however, conservative treatment or ERCP with endoscopic sphincterotomy, take priority (Ducarme, 2014). Laparoscopic cholecystectomy is the first choice in early postpartum period.

Tan *et al.* reported a case of gestational hypertriglyceridemia-induced pancreatitis in a primigravida at 31-weeks' gestation (Tan, 2021). The disease was complicated by impending preterm labor and metabolic acidosis requiring hemodialysis. In the management, therapeutic plasma exchange, followed by treatment with IV insulin, low-fat diet, and omega-3 proved successful. Triglyceride levels were stabilized after plasma exchange and the patient delivered the baby in term. The authors pointed out that management is challenging as risks and benefits of alternatives are to be weighed against fetal outcomes. Of note, a multidisciplinary approach is the key to achieve relief with respect to maternal and fetal welfare. In addition, a low-fat diet while ensuring adequate nutrition in pregnancy is important.

Operative conditions in pregnancy include empyema, spontaneous pneumothorax, and diaphragmatic hernia (Fig. **12**) (Whang, 2018).

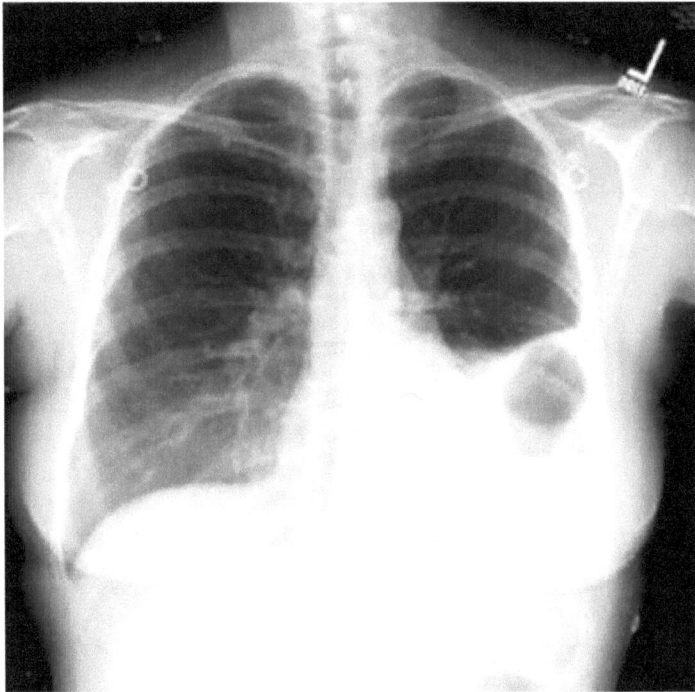

Fig. (12). Diaphragmatic hernia: colonic air-fluid levels in the left hemithorax.

Bochdalek hernia (BH) is a rare form of diaphragmatic hernia, which mostly presents with nonspecific manifestations and thus are frequently delayed to be recognized in the emergent situations. In a large series of BH, mean age of these patients was recorded to be 51 years with a male predominance (Machado, 2016). Precipitating factors were revealed in around one-fourth, with 5.3% of them being pregnant. The authors stressed on that BH should be viewed in the DD in patients who are admitted with abdominal and chest complaints concurrently.

ACUTE AP IN CHILDREN

Note: In this section, diagnoses such as AAp, biliary tract diseases and Meckel's diverticulum, which can be seen in adults and children, will not be focused on, but the diseases seen mostly/ exclusively in children will be emphasized.

Invagination/intussusception (I/I): I/I is most commonly diagnosed in toddlers and infants (6 months-1 years). A majority of the patients are idiopathic and around 1/10 will disclose a pathological lead point (Vandertuin, 2011). It is more common during seasonal changes, in spring and autumn. I/I occurs when the last part of the small intestine (ileum) enters the first part of the colon (cecum) (ileo-cecal invagination). Hyperperistaltic diseases such as diarrhea, (*e.g.* rotavirus outbreaks) may lead to I/I.

The last part of the small intestine, which is rich in lymphatic tissue, may become edematous with general systemic infections such as upper respiratory tract infections. This tissue prevents the retraction of the intestine, which has become invaginated for any reason, thus facilitating the development of I/I.

In brief, I/I should be taken into consideration in all pediatric cases, below the age of 3 years, with acute colic-like AP.

The child with I/I throws out at first whatever he/she ate, producing yellow-green vomitus stained with bile. As a rule, the child has no appetite. In the last stage, defecation begins in the form of "strawberry jelly", which is reflective of the ischemic tissue.

I/I can usually be diagnosed with X-ray and USG (Fig. **13**).

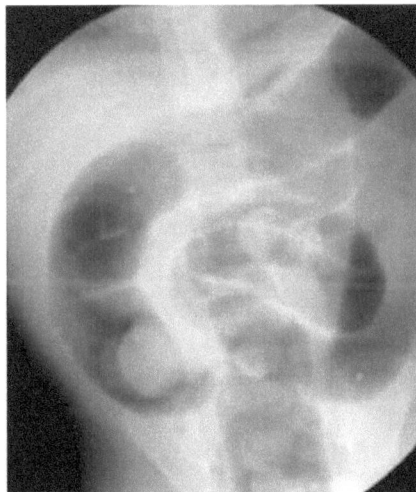

Fig. (13). In the pediatric patient with 4.5 cm invagination in the middle segment of the abdomen, reduction was performed with saline infusion under the guidance of USG.

In the initial management, vascular access should be opened, crystalloid fluid should be given, and pain should be relieved. Broad-spectrum antibiotics are administered.

The treatment strategy is almost entirely surgical in adults. In children, noninvasive approaches are the most successful strategy as opposed to others.

In the absence of evident perforation, nonoperative reduction can be undertaken using hydrostatic or pneumatic pressure with an enema.

Hydrostatic reduction with fluids: Barium or isotonic fluid is administered per rectum to intestines from a height of 1.5 meters under 150 mmHg pressure, guided and accompanied by USG. In this way, it is tried to restore the passage in the invaginated intestines. It can be repeated two or three times. Between 52% to 91% of success is recorded. In case of failure, open surgery is performed.

Pneumatic therapy: It is attempted to open the invaginated bowels by giving per rectal air to the intestines. The upper safe limit is 80 mmHg in infants and 110-120 mmHg in older children. The technique is successful in 70% to 88% of the cases.

Celiac disease is an immune-mediated disease that interacts with almost all body systems, mostly manifested with AP, fatigue and diarrhea. A great majority of the patients remain undiagnosed in the population. Consumption of gluten-containing food almost invariably precipitates the signs and symptoms in susceptible children. Damage in small intestinal mucosa, detection of celiac specific antibodies, human leukocyte antigen (HLA)-DQ2 or HLA-DQ8, and consistent clinical manifestations triggered by gluten intake are characteristics of the disease (Sahin, 2021). Gluten is abundant in cereal grains, namely, wheat, barley, rye, and oats.

Findings: Chronic or intermittent diarrhea without apparent cause, failure to thrive, weight loss, delayed puberty, amenorrhea, iron deficiency, attacks of nausea/ vomiting, attacks of AP and distension, constipation, recurrent aphthous stomatitis, and abnormal liver enzyme elevation, should warrant serologic tests for the disease. Table **1** indicates the changes assumed by the crypts and villi with respect to the type of the disease.

Table 1. The modified Marsh classification is used to classify changes in the crypts and villi in patients with Celiac disease.

-	IEL (Intraepithelial lymphocyte count/ 100 epithelial cells	Crypts	Villi
Type 0	< 40	Normal	Normal
Type 1	> 40	Normal	Normal
Type 2	> 40	Hypertrophic	Normal
Type 3a	> 40	Hypertrophic	Mild atrophy
Type 3b	> 40	Hypertrophic	Marked atrophy
Type 3c	> 40	Hypertrophic	Absent

Complications of the disease are seen in those noncompliant with diet. Hyposplenism, intestinal lymphoma, small bowel adenocarcinoma, and ulcerative jejunoileitis (Al-Toma, 2006).

Management: The only method proven to be effective is lifelong consumption of gluten-free diet. Significant improvements in symptoms, normalization of biochemical tests, and improvement in quality of life with the strict maintenance of the diet are reported in the literature (Husby, 2019).

MESENTERIC LYMPHADENITIS (ML)

ML is the painful state of lymph nodes in the mesentery due to inflammation and swelling. It is a common cause of AP in children and adolescents. Since AAp is confused with other childhood causes of acute AP such as Meckel's diverticulum, it may cause unnecessary radiological examinations, hospitalization, and even rarely operations. Viruses, bacteria, and parasites can trigger ML. Other than infections, lymphoma and some types of cancer can also cause ML.

Diarrhea triggered by Yersinia enterocolitica is particularly severe and is an excellent mimic of AAp. ML can also be seen in the course of HIV, tuberculosis infections, and Crohn's disease.

Findings: It causes AP mostly in the midline and right lower quadrant. Loss of appetite, increased leukocytes, nausea-vomiting and weakness may also be added, although none is specific.

Mostly, ML will heal once the infection that triggered the ML has been relieved and does not require additional treatment. However, NSAIDs and antibiotics may be necessary in some severe cases.

Diagnosis: Although the diagnosis can usually be made by USG, CT may be required in older patients to rule out serious diagnoses (Figs. **14** and **15**).

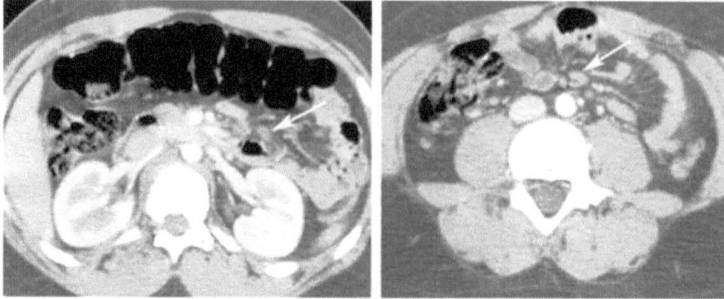

Fig. (14). A 17-year-old young man with the appearance of normal lymph nodes in CT which was obtained due to blunt abdominal trauma.

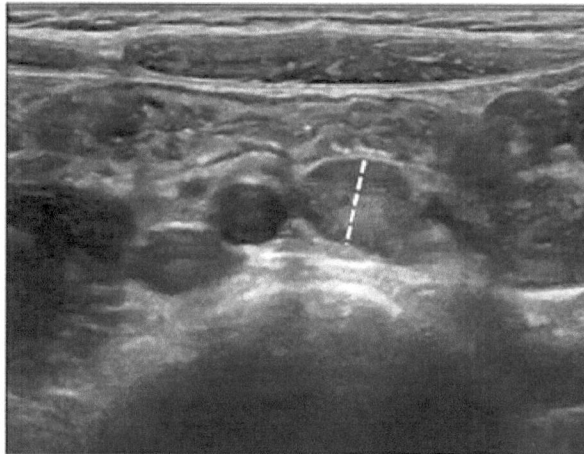

Fig. (15). Abdominal USG image of a six-year-old girl shows enlarged hypoechoic mesenteric lymph nodes. The largest node is 9 mm in diameter. The patient was diagnosed with acute nonspecific mesenteric lymphadenitis.

At least 3 lymph nodes with a short diameter of larger than 5 mm are noted in the right lower quadrant. Nodes are most commonly seen anterior to the right psoas muscle, sometimes in the mesentery. Ileal or ileocecal wall thickening (>3 mm) may be visualized. The appendix should also be interpreted as normal.

An interesting note: Children with ML or AAp are less likely to be diagnosed with ulcerative colitis in the future.

Work up in children: USG appears to be the most useful in children because they have thinner muscles and less abdominal fat. It has a sensitivity of 78 to 88% and a specificity of 83 to 94% for diagnosing AAp (Jones 2021). The main drawback is its operator dependence which is translated into being unable to rule out AAp *via* an equivocal or negative study.

COVID-19 and Children in Relation to AP

Many studies have pointed out a close relationship between COVID-19 infection and the digestive system. Multisystem Inflammatory Syndrome in Children (MIS-C) is an ominous manifestation of COVID-19 in children, which is associated with higher severity of clinical course (*i.e.*, >2/3 of cases in need of critical care). A systematic review disclosed that GI symptoms (>70%) comprised AP (34%) and diarrhea (27%), while rates of cough and dyspnea were recorded much lower (4.5% and 9.6%, respectively) (Radia, 2021). Authors emphasized that a higher incidence of GI symptoms were noted in MIS-C, when compared to the other children with COVID-19. In a small case series of children with MIS-C, Blumfield *et al.* reported that imaging modalities (ultrasound, CT, and radiography) disclosed ascites (38%), hepatomegaly (38%), bowel wall thickening (19%), gallbladder wall thickening (19%), mesenteric lymphadenopathy (13%), splenomegaly (6%), and bladder wall thickening (6%) (Blumfield, 2021).

SARS-COV-2 may enter cells directly *via* the ACE2 receptor, and interacts with the usual operation of the GI tract and liver. Disorders of the digestive system and COVID-19 are frequently linked, can worsen patient prognosis, and increase the death rates (Lei, 2021).

In another case series, fecal detection of viral RNA was noted in a minority of patients without GI symptoms (4%) (Park, 2021). Mean cycle threshold values from the time of quarantine to the time of fecal collection tended to be lower in patients with virus detected in fecal samples than in patients without virus in fecal samples. Shedding of virus into feces persisted until day 50 after diagnosis; fecal samples began to test negative before or at approximately the time that respiratory specimens also began to test negative.

Acute AP in the Elderly

Elderly individuals present somewhat differently to healthcare institutions. It is an important reason that diseases that cause autonomic neuropathy such as debility, diabetes and kidney diseases are frequently found in the elderly. Inability of the sympathetic nervous system to respond sharply as expected in young people, slowing of perception, electrolyte disorders, malignancy, decreased immunity, cognitive disorders such as Alzheimer's are other contributing factors. As a result, there is a decrease in diagnostic accuracy in proportion to age.

To be more specific, seniors present more frequently with vague, suspect, and nonspecific complaints and findings. Even in the case of peritonitis, findings such as generalized rigidity are less common than expected in these seniors. Fever, leukocytosis and elevated CRP are also less common. They also express their pain equivocally and less precisely.

Half to 60% of the elderly presenting to the ED with acute AP have an indication for admission to the hospital. A significant portion of inpatients are eventually operated on. Another important point is that in these patients there is a significant rate of missed diagnoses and delays. Since these patients have been screened with advanced laboratory and imaging modalities in recent decades, the accuracy in diagnosis has also increased. Within 2 weeks, 1/5 of all elderly cases with AP undergo operation and 5% die.

Due to these uncertain and vague presentations, the elderly with severe acute abdominal syndrome may be discharged incorrectly with diagnoses such as AGE, UTI, urinary stone disease or NSAP.

As a rule, consideration of benign diagnoses such as AGE and NSAP in the elderly after all other specific diagnoses have been excluded will prevent diagnostic delays and misses.

Approximately half of the elderly have gallbladder diseases, the same rate of diverticular diseases, and approximately 10% harbor AAA secondary to hypertension.

Biliary tract diseases are the most common diagnosis in the elderly presenting with acute AP. It is translated into 10% mortality in this group following the diagnosis of cholecystitis. Of note, cholecystitis is acalculous in 10% of patients which means that USG may not be helpful as expected in the younger counterparts. Another interesting point is that **fever, leukocytosis and jaundice, known as the "Charcot triad"** which is classically found in these patients, are not recorded in more than half of these patients.

DIVERTICULITIS

It is seen with an incidence of around 65% in developed countries over the age of 65. A great majority (85%) involves the left colon. Half of the elderly patients do not even have leukocytosis, and most are fever-free. Since only ¼ of them are positive for occult blood in the stool, this examination should not be relied upon as a diagnostic tool. The characteristics of the entity is explained in the relevant chapter.

Acute Appendicitis (AAp) The characteristics of the entity are explained in the relevant chapter.

Pill info: Although only 10% of the cases with AAp are over 60 years of age, half of the deaths are in this group. Half of elderly patients with AAp are already perforated at the time of diagnosis.

AAp is the most common surgical emergency in the general population, only secondary to abscess drainage. Advancing age is among the influential factors on preoperative diagnostic processes and the stage of the disease. Elderly patients constitute around 5% of the total pool of appendectomy cases. Gurleyik *et al.* reported that the perforation rate in the elderly was significantly higher than in others (P<0.001) (Gurleyik, 2003). The elderly comprised more than one-eighth of the perforated cases while only around 3% of non-perforated cases (P<0.001).

Fever and leukocytosis can be found in around half of the elderly cases. It is also interesting that one third of the cases do not localize the pain in the right lower quadrant. Because of all these, wrong diagnoses are recorded in approximately half of the cases.

Postoperative morbidity boosts with age, which was noted in more than one-third of the aged, in 73.8% of perforated, and in 11.9% of non-perforated cases (P<0.001). The mortality rate was 5.5% in the elderly group, 11.9% in patients with perforated, and 1.5% in patients with non-perforated AAp, while nobody died in patients younger than 50 years. Postoperative morbidity and mortality are considerably high in the elderly. The progression of the disease and the clinical courses of patients are worse in the elderly when compared to the younger groups. Perforation, sepsis and septic shock are the main causes of untoward consequences (Fig. **16**).

MRI FOR AAP?

The MRI criteria for appendicitis include the visualization of the enlarged appendix (over 7 mm diameter), wall thickening over 2 mm, peri-appendiceal fat stranding, fluid-filled appendix, or free fluid. These are consistent imaging criteria throughout the different modalities.

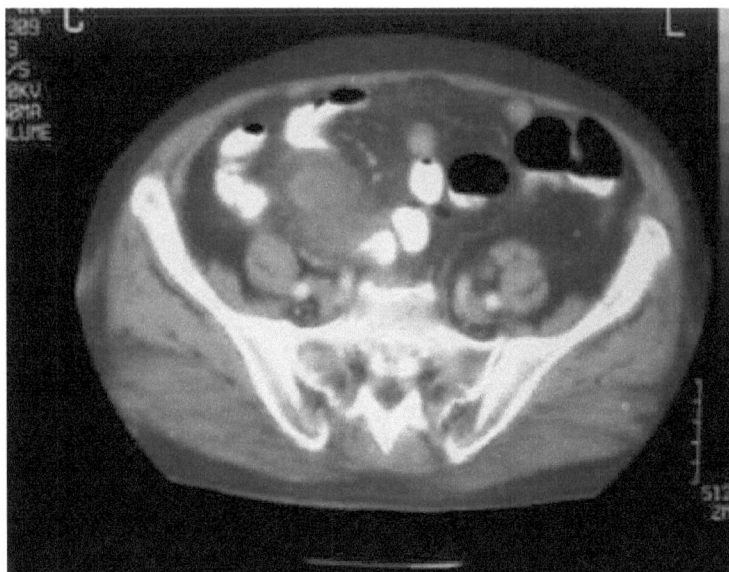

Fig. (16). An elderly woman in her 86, is admitted due to mild abdominal pain and an inflammatory mass is palpated in the right side of the abdomen. Ruptured AAp could only be disclosed during surgery.

MRI is also used to stage appendiceal neoplasms with its high accuracy in comparison to CT. The accuracy has risen to 90% by employment of diffusion-weighted imaging (DWI) (Jones, 2021). Solid tumors exhibit restricted diffusion in the involved tissue. Delayed gadolinium-enhanced imaging is performed *via* administration of PO and PR contrast which is associated with a sensitivity of 95% and specificity of 70% (Kim, 2018).

Mesenteric Artery Ischemia

There is a severe AP disproportionate to the degree of the symptoms. It has a mortality rate of around 80% once the diagnosis is established. It may be accompanied by vomiting and diarrhea, sometimes misleading the physician. Heart failure, previous AMI, and AF are risk factors. Non-occlusive mesenteric ischemia (NOMI) is also quite common. Contrast-enhanced abdominal CT is appropriate in cases where Doppler USG is not sufficient for diagnosis in a majority of cases (Fig. **17**).

Bowel-related Emergencies

Intestinal obstruction is present in 1 in 8 elderly people with AP. Among these, sigmoid volvulus is quite common and can be recognized by x-ray (Fig. **18**). Cancer-related occlusions are also quite common, and sometimes such an obstruction may be the first sign of malignancy.

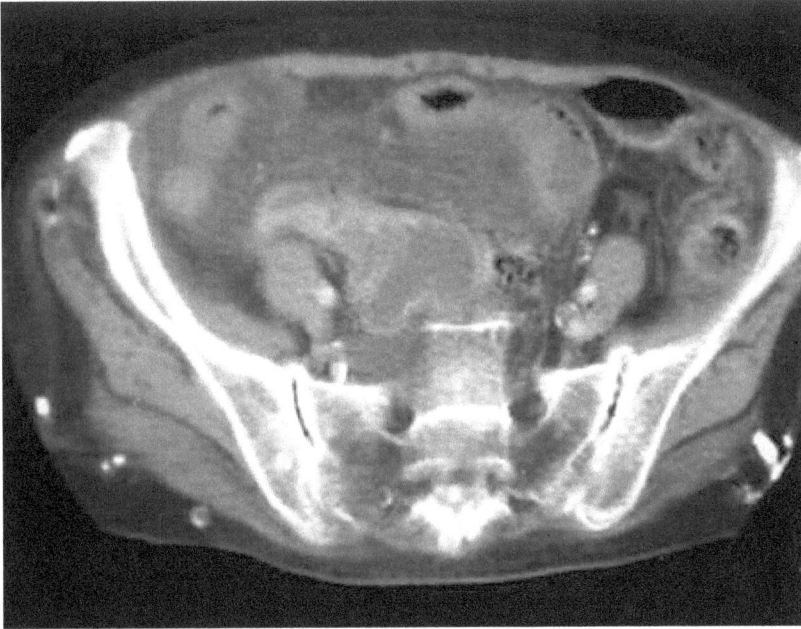

Fig. (17). 76-year-old woman presented with severe abdominal pain for 3 hours. Ischemic bowel was surgically resected. Annular intestinal wall edema is noted posteriorly.

The enlargement of the colon more than 9 cm is a harbinger of impending perforation. Sedentery life, immobility, constipation and use of laxatives are risk factors for volvulus.

Small Bowel Obstruction

Most commonly, adhesions from previous operations lead to obstruction (brid ileus). In the elderly, incarcerated hernia is seen more frequently than in young people with 30% and gallstone ileus with 20% (Fig. **19**).

AAA is mostly the disease of the elderly due to chronic hypertension. In the elderly, the male/female ratio increases to 7/1. While the mortality rate is 25% when it is diagnosed incidentally (in the hemodynamically stable patient), it increases to 80% when diagnosed emergently with rupture. In these cases, such as back pain, AP and shock findings such as tachycardia are seen less frequently or not recorded at all, compared to young people. Therefore, delay in diagnosis is common. 30% of the elderly with ruptured AAA receive misdiagnoses including renal colic or other benign diseases. The fact that it causes kidney damage and sometimes hematuria due to fistulization also contributes to this high rate of erratic practices. As a rule, aortic emergencies should be excluded before diagnosing renal colic in an elderly person.

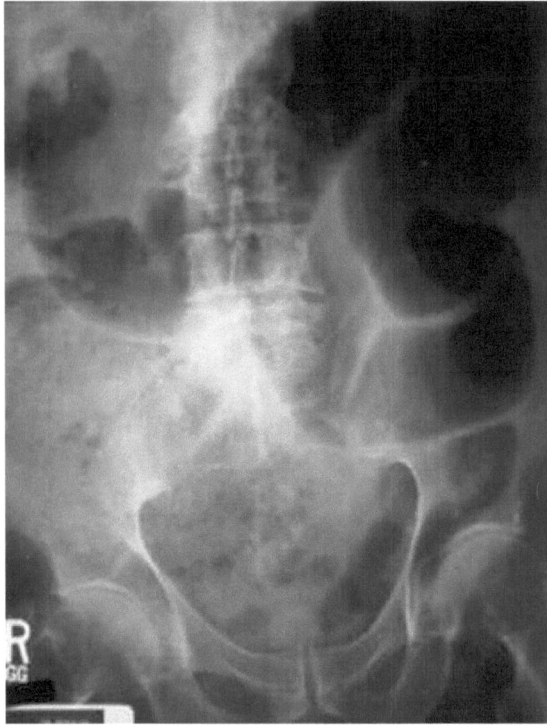

Fig. (18). An enlargement of the large bowels is observed on X-ray in a 90-year-old male patient who presented with abdominal pain for 4 days. A diagnosis of sigmoid volvulus and ischemic colon was made during the operation.

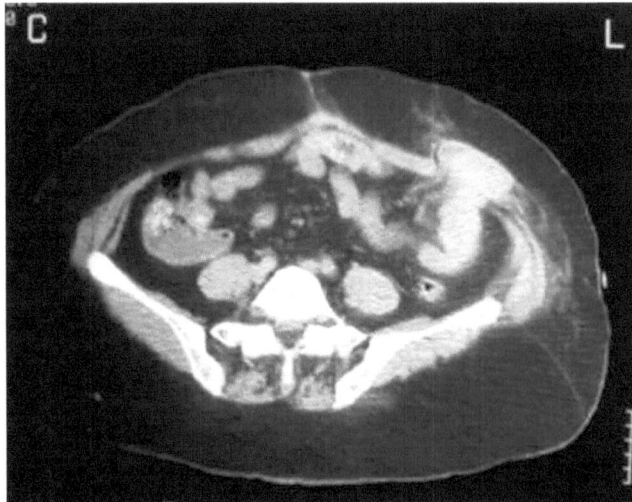

Fig. (19). CT section of a 64-year-old woman presenting with vague and moderate abdominal pain for two days. On examination, a tender mass is palpable in the left lower quadrant. Incarcerated ventral hernia image is observed in the same region.

Malignancies: 10% of the elderly who are discharged from the ED with the diagnosis of NSAP are eventually diagnosed with cancer. Cancer-related obstructions are seen in a very high proportion of ileus cases and perforations in the elderly compared to young people.

Lab Work Up

Increased anion gap may indicate severe intra-abdominal process, *e.g.* mesenteric infarction, ischemic colitis, and necrotizing pancreatitis. Normal liver function tests should not be relied upon because the expected elevation may not be seen in the elderly with acute cholecystitis. Lipase is a more reliable test for pancreatitis than amylase.

When considering UTI or pyelonephritis in women, sampling with a catheter gives more accurate results.

Taking blood cultures will be appropriate in acute AP cases presenting with fever or hypothermia, especially if sepsis is suspected.

Prothrombin time (PT) and activated partial thromboplastin time (aPTT) should be requested in patients with suspected liver failure, GI bleeding, moribund condition and sepsis.

Arterial blood gases (ABG) should be analyzed in patients with suspected ischemic bowel, DKA, sepsis, GIB and ruptured AAA. The most expedient way to see the hematocrit value in the last two entities is to request an ABG, although more developed and rapid technologies emerge nowadays. In the same group of cases, the lactate level should also be taken as soon as possible. Analysis of blood lactate levels in the first 20 minutes in sepsis affects even the prognosis favorably.

Blood group and cross-match should be ordered in those with suspected GIB and/or AAA and all patients with unstable clinical conditions such as sepsis/septic shock.

Bedside USG (POCUS) should be preferred for many reasons such as ease of performance and repetition, no radiation, noninvasiveness, and lack of side effects. POCUS should be performed immediately, especially in AAA/DAA and biliary system diseases.

USG is very useful in distinguishing between complicated AAp and noncomplicated ones, in this way, it can help decide whether to give antibiotics only and follow up or appendectomy is the priority.

CT should be preferred in suspected AAp cases and diverticular disease to establish diagnosis and to visualize the extent of the disease. It is 93% sensitive in diagnosing diverticulitis. However, waiting for the luminal cavity of the diverticulum for being filled with contrast in 2-3 hours is its drawback. In one study, when water-soluble contrast agent was given as an enema, the diagnostic sensitivity was 99% without oral or IV contrast. Barium enema should be avoided.

Shall we do a CT scan? In a prospective study (Millet et al, 2017), 'routine' non-contrast CT scan was associated with an increased rate of diagnosis in the ED from 76.8% to 85% and treatment decisions from 88.5% to 95.8% in 401 elderly patients ($\geq$75 years) presenting with nontraumatic AP. In addition, with this approach, unsuspected abdominal pathologies were detected at a rate of 30% (Fig. (**20**)).

With **non-contrast helical CT, ureteral and renal stones** are visualized with 95 to 100% sensitivity. Pelvic vascular calcifications, which are seen in a significant portion of the elderly, may complicate the diagnosis.

CT-angiography is especially preferred in mesenteric ischemia. MDCT has a sensitivity of 94% to 96%. At the same time, alternative diagnoses can mostly be identified with this method.

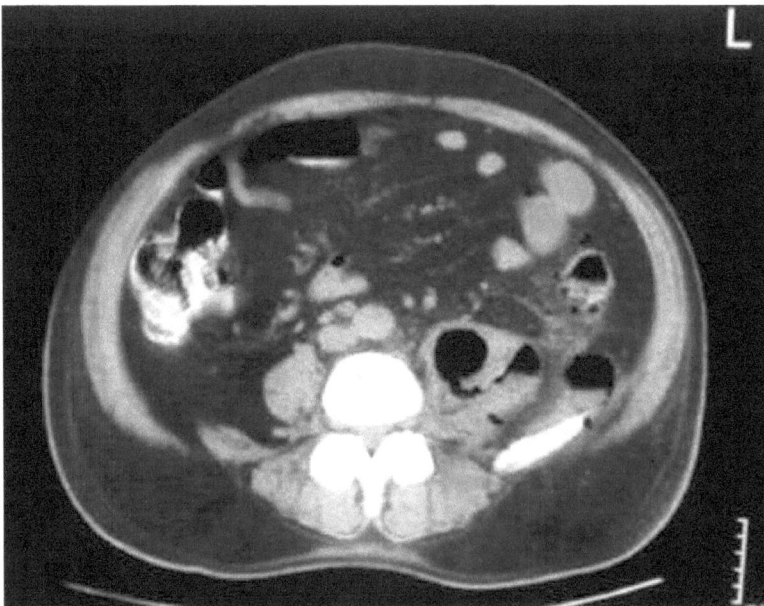

Fig. (20). Multiple diverticula in the descending colon (left) and increase in fat streaking (stranding) in a 62-year-old man presenting with left lower quadrant pain lasting for two weeks.

Specific Treatment/discharge Recommendations for the Elderly

Early cholecystectomy should be preferred in the elderly with acute cholecystitis. Operations started laparoscopically turn into open in ¼ of the elderly patients.

Hypotensive, tachycardic elderly patients with altered levels of consciousness should be admitted to the intensive care unit.

Pill information: The discharge decision of elderly patients with acute AP should be taken very cautiously, after thinking more than twice. Patients with suspected mesenteric ischemia, AAA/DAA, associated with abnormal vital signs cannot be discharged without consultation. "In-between" patients should also be consulted before being sent home.

IN CASES WHERE GIB IS CONSIDERED, GASTROENTEROLOGISTS SHOULD BE CONSULTED

Abdominal Pain in HIV (+) Patients (H+P)

H+P are referred to EDs with AP for a myriad of reasons similar with other patients. While some of these cases are followed up regularly by some specific centers, some others are not, which leads to higher rates of referral to EDs.

The diagnostic evaluation is not fundamentally different from other patients. However, important differences may also arise occasionally. The DD list is basically similar. CD4 cell counts should be checked for immune functions. Cytomegalovirus (CMV), Mycobacterium avium complex [MAC], cryptosporidium are among possible opportunistic infections and should be investigated. Neoplasms such as Kaposi's sarcoma and lymphoma are also quite common.

If there are signs of immune deficiency (CD4 <100 cells/microL) when H+P presents with AP, the clinician should be more liberal to proceed with further examination, including laboratory and radiological imaging. Cultures of stool and other suspected tissues would also be appropriate at this point.

Since odynophagia, stomatitis, dysphagia and diarrhea are also common in H+P cases, their treatment should also be commenced as necessary. In case of anorectal involvement and proctitis, tenesmus, pain during defecation, and incontinence are expected.

Lower GI bleeding is common in those with Kaposi's sarcoma and Bartonella infections. AP may or may not accompany these patients with GIB, therefore clinicians should be extremely alert to search for these findings, *e.g.*, digital rectal examination should be pursued routinely.

All these problems are more common in those who do not use antiretroviral therapy (ART). For example, it has been reported that one out of 6 cases (H+P) was diagnosed with chronic diarrhea. Drug-induced diarrhea should also be considered if diarrhea is the only symptom in those receiving ART.

Since it is a group to be managed in a multidisciplinary fashion that may have a poor prognosis, the threshold for consultation should be kept low when H+P presents with AP.

COVID-19 and GI Manifestations Including Abdominal Pain

In vitro studies showed that SARS-CoV-2 could enter into the GI epithelial cells by the ACE-2 receptors. These findings and fecal identification of viral RNA suggest the direct involvement of the GI tract in the course of pandemic disease (Deidda, 2021). Fecal–oral transmission route is a potential risk for transmission. The presence of the virus in the GI tract also represents a diagnostic opportunity. There are some patients with ongoing viral shedding through GI secretions when the oral swab test is negative and pose a threat to the public.

Although not very practical, it can be postulated that patients with high clinical suspicion of COVID-19 could undergo anal swab or stool viral test despite a negative throat swab for SARS-CoV-2.

A recent meta-analysis disclosed that GI complaints (nausea, vomiting, AP) and respiratory symptoms (shortness of breath, chest pain) were associated with severe COVID-19 (Li, 2021), Interestingly, this report ranked AP as an important poor prognostic factor in COVID-19 course, second only to immunosuppression (coefficient 24.7 and 53.9, respectively). GI symptoms were reported to be common in patients with COVID-19, the proportion of individuals with diarrhea was 9.5%, while AP and vomiting were less common (4.5%, and 4.7%, respectively). AP was significantly more common among those with severe disease in comparison to mild and moderate cases (p=0.01).

The frequencies of GI symptoms encountered in patients with COVID-19 comprised a wide array (3% to 41%) as underlined in a systematic review including 22 studies (Ye, 2021). GI complaints included AP, nausea, vomiting, diarrhea (most common), loss of appetite, belching, distension, and GIB. The severity of liver dysfunction was significantly associated with the severity of COVID-19. Of note, digestive system manifestations are crucial for early recognition and treatment. Atypical patients with the pandemic disease constituted a special group who will benefit from this opportunity.

The relationship between GI symptoms and severity of COVID-19 in adults Gayam *et al.* reported that cough, dyspnea, fever, GI symptoms, and myalgia were the predominant presentation among African-American patients admitted to hospital with COVID-19 (Gayam, 2021). The most common presenting symptoms were cough, myalgia, fever/chills, shortness of breath, and GI symptoms (nausea, vomiting, diarrhea, and AP), with a prevalence of 62.50%, 43.87%, 53.68%, and 27.21%, respectively. Nonetheless, GI symptoms were not among predictors of mortality.

How were the trends of non-urgent conditions and related admissions in the pandemic era? In general, outpatient visits for many urgent conditions remained relatively stable during the pandemic, however, non-urgent presentations decreased in 2020 and 2021, for fear of contracting the pandemic disease, concerns about the overcrowdedness of hospitals and EDs, and others. Giannouchos *et al.* disclosed that overall outpatient ED visits declined from mid-March to August 2020, particularly for non-medically urgent conditions which can be treated in other more appropriate care settings (Giannouchos, 2021). Fig. (**21**) shows that non-emergent conditions (nausea/vomiting and AP) related to GIS have gone relatively stable, in spite of certain waves throughout the pandemic period.

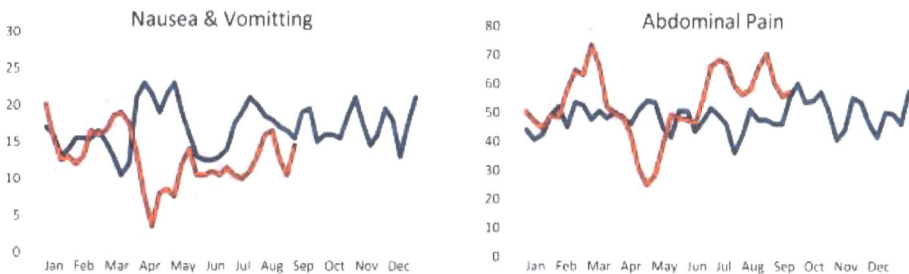

Fig. (21). Trends in weekly outpatient ED visits by less medically urgent conditions from January 1, 2019 to August 31, 2020 (Adapted from Giannouchos, 2021).

Chronic diarrhea (CD) in the acute setting or ED: CD is defined as experiencing more than 3 major bowel movements per day, loose stools, or stool weight >200 g/day for at least 4 weeks.

CD may not reflect an infectious source and may be the hallmark of a myriad GI and systemic illnesses or adverse effects of the medicines used (Hammer, 2021).

Patients with persistent and/or intractable diarrhea should undergo a thorough and detailed evaluation.

The essential goal in the management is establishing a robust diagnosis, directing a specific treatment to the specific causes and prevention of water and electrolyte imbalances, if any.

CONCLUSION

Although acute abdominal pain is a life-threatening medical emergency for all ages and sexes, specific subgroups have important features to be considered in both diagnostic and therapeutic processes. Ectopic pregnancy is the most common cause of shock and pregnancy deaths in the first trimester, resulting mostly from delayed diagnosis. Therefore, in every woman of childbearing age presenting with AP and/or vaginal bleeding, the diagnosis of EP should be sought for and definitely ruled out. Amid the pandemic waves, many studies have suggested a close relationship between COVID-19 and the digestive system. Patients with COVID-19 carry a high risk of digestive symptomatology including abdominal pain, nausea and vomiting, diarrhea and others. HIV (+) patients exhibit various GI symptoms such as diarrhea, abdominal pain and proctitis.

In brief, emergency treatments and consultations should not be delayed for the results of the laboratory work in conditions with acute abdominal pain.

REFERENCES

Al-Toma, A., Goerres, M.S., Meijer, J.W., Peña, A.S., Crusius, J.B., Mulder, C.J. (2006). Human leukocyte antigen-DQ2 homozygosity and the development of refractory celiac disease and enteropathy-associated T-cell lymphoma. *Clin. Gastroenterol. Hepatol., 4*(3), 315-319.
[http://dx.doi.org/10.1016/j.cgh.2005.12.011] [PMID: 16527694]

Bhinder, K.K., Sarfraz, A., Sarfraz, Z., Riaz, S., Aslam, S., Ameena, Z. (2021). Uterine artery embolization combined with methotrexate for broad ligament ectopic pregnancy in a 30-year old primigravida. *Radiol. Case Rep., 16*(8), 2248-2251.
[http://dx.doi.org/10.1016/j.radcr.2021.05.032] [PMID: 34188737]

Blumfield, E., Levin, T.L., Kurian, J., Lee, E.Y., Liszewski, M.C. (2021). Imaging Findings in Multisystem Inflammatory Syndrome in Children (MIS-C) Associated With Coronavirus Disease (COVID-19). *AJR Am. J. Roentgenol., 216*(2), 507-517.
[http://dx.doi.org/10.2214/AJR.20.24032] [PMID: 32755212]

Chen, X., Yang, X., Cheng, W. (2012). Diaphragmatic tear in pregnancy induced by intractable vomiting: a case report and review of the literature. *J. Matern. Fetal Neonatal Med., 25*(9), 1822-1824.
[http://dx.doi.org/10.3109/14767058.2011.640371] [PMID: 22098059]

Cheng, V., Matsushima, K., Sandhu, K., Ashbrook, M., Matsuo, K., Inaba, K., Demetriades, D. (2020). Surgical trends in the management of acute cholecystitis during pregnancy. *Surg. Endosc., 35*, 5752-5759.
[http://dx.doi.org/10.1007/s00464-020-08054-w] [PMID: 33025256]

Deidda, S., Tora, L., Firinu, D., Del Giacco, S., Campagna, M., Meloni, F., Orrù, G., Chessa, L., Carta, M.G., Melis, A., Spolverato, G., Littera, R., Perra, A., Onali, S., Zorcolo, L., Restivo, A. (2021). Gastrointestinal coronavirus disease 2019: epidemiology, clinical features, pathogenesis, prevention, and management. *Expert*

Rev. Gastroenterol. Hepatol., 15(1), 41-50.
[http://dx.doi.org/10.1080/17474124.2020.1821653] [PMID: 32955375]

Ducarme, G., Maire, F., Chatel, P., Luton, D., Hammel, P. (2014). Acute pancreatitis during pregnancy: a review. *J. Perinatol., 34*(2), 87-94.
[http://dx.doi.org/10.1038/jp.2013.161] [PMID: 24355941]

Fong, Z.V., Pitt, H.A., Strasberg, S.M., Molina, R.L., Perez, N.P., Kelleher, C.M., Loehrer, A.P., Sicklick, J.K., Talamini, M.A., Lillemoe, K.D., Chang, D.C. (2019). Cholecystectomy During the Third Trimester of Pregnancy: Proceed or Delay? *J. Am. Coll. Surg., 228*(4), 494-502.e1.
[http://dx.doi.org/10.1016/j.jamcollsurg.2018.12.024] [PMID: 30769111]

Gayam, V., Chobufo, M.D., Merghani, M.A., Lamichhane, S., Garlapati, P.R., Adler, M.K. (2021). Clinical characteristics and predictors of mortality in African-Americans with COVID-19 from an inner-city community teaching hospital in New York. *J. Med. Virol., 93*(2), 812-819.
[http://dx.doi.org/10.1002/jmv.26306] [PMID: 32672844]

Giannouchos, T.V., Biskupiak, J., Moss, M.J., Brixner, D., Andreyeva, E., Ukert, B. (2021). Trends in outpatient emergency department visits during the COVID-19 pandemic at a large, urban, academic hospital system. *Am. J. Emerg. Med., 40*, 20-26.
[http://dx.doi.org/10.1016/j.ajem.2020.12.009] [PMID: 33338676]

Guldner, G.T., Magee, E.M. (2020). Grey-Turner Sign. *StatPearls.* Treasure Island (FL): StatPearls Publishing.
[PMID: 30485001]

Gürleyik, G., Gürleyik, E. (2003). Age-related clinical features in older patients with acute appendicitis. *Eur. J. Emerg. Med., 10*(3), 200-203.
[http://dx.doi.org/10.1097/00063110-200309000-00008] [PMID: 12972895]

Hammer, H.F. (2021). Management of Chronic Diarrhea in Primary Care: The Gastroenterologists' Advice. *Dig. Dis., 39*(6), 615-621.
[http://dx.doi.org/10.1159/000515219] [PMID: 33588424]

Hughes, DL, Hughes, A, White, PB, Silva, MA (2021). Acute pancreatitis in pregnancy: meta-analysis of maternal and fetal outcomes. *Bri. J. Surg., 109*(1), 12-14.
[http://dx.doi.org/10.1093/bjs/znab221]

Husby, S., Bai, J.C. (2019). Follow-up of Celiac Disease. *Gastroenterol. Clin. North Am., 48*(1), 127-136.
[http://dx.doi.org/10.1016/j.gtc.2018.09.009] [PMID: 30711205]

Jones, S., Ranzenberger, L.R., Carter, K.R. (2021). Appendix Imaging. *Stat Pearls.* StatPearls Publishing.Treasure Island (FL):
[PMID: 31751093]

Kim, D.W., Suh, C.H., Yoon, H.M., Kim, J.R., Jung, A.Y., Lee, J.S., Cho, Y.A. (2018). Visibility of Normal Appendix on CT, MRI, and Sonography: A Systematic Review and Meta-Analysis. *AJR Am. J. Roentgenol., 211*(3), W140-W150.
[http://dx.doi.org/10.2214/AJR.17.19321] [PMID: 30040469]

Lei, H.Y., Ding, Y.H., Nie, K., Dong, Y.M., Xu, J.H., Yang, M.L., Liu, M.Q., Wei, L., Nasser, M.I., Xu, L.Y., Zhu, P., Zhao, M.Y. (2021). Potential effects of SARS-CoV-2 on the gastrointestinal tract and liver. *Biomed. Pharmacother., 133*, 111064.
[http://dx.doi.org/10.1016/j.biopha.2020.111064] [PMID: 33378966]

Li, J., Huang, D.Q., Zou, B., Yang, H., Hui, W.Z., Rui, F., Yee, N.T.S., Liu, C., Nerurkar, S.N., Kai, J.C.Y., Teng, M.L.P., Li, X., Zeng, H., Borghi, J.A., Henry, L., Cheung, R., Nguyen, M.H. (2021). Epidemiology of COVID-19: A systematic review and meta-analysis of clinical characteristics, risk factors, and outcomes. *J. Med. Virol., 93*(3), 1449-1458.
[http://dx.doi.org/10.1002/jmv.26424] [PMID: 32790106]

Machado, N.O. (2016). Laparoscopic Repair of Bochdalek Diaphragmatic Hernia in Adults. *N. Am. J. Med.*

Sci., 8(2), 65-74.
[http://dx.doi.org/10.4103/1947-2714.177292] [PMID: 27042603]

Millet, I., Sebbane, M., Molinari, N., Pages-Bouic, E., Curros-Doyon, F., Riou, B., Taourel, P. (2017). Systematic unenhanced CT for acute abdominal symptoms in the elderly patients improves both emergency department diagnosis and prompt clinical management. *Eur. Radiol., 27*(2), 868-877.
[http://dx.doi.org/10.1007/s00330-016-4425-0] [PMID: 27271919]

Park, S.K., Lee, C.W., Park, D.I., Woo, H.Y., Cheong, H.S., Shin, H.C., Ahn, K., Kwon, M.J., Joo, E.J. (2021). Detection of SARS-CoV-2 in Fecal Samples From Patients With Asymptomatic and Mild COVID-19 in Korea. *Clin. Gastroenterol. Hepatol., 19*(7), 1387-1394.e2.
[http://dx.doi.org/10.1016/j.cgh.2020.06.005] [PMID: 32534042]

Radia, T., Williams, N., Agrawal, P., Harman, K., Weale, J., Cook, J., Gupta, A. (2021). Multi-system inflammatory syndrome in children & adolescents (MIS-C): A systematic review of clinical features and presentation. *Paediatr. Respir. Rev., 38*, 51-57.
[http://dx.doi.org/10.1016/j.prrv.2020.08.001] [PMID: 32891582]

Reimer, RP, Heneweer, C, Juchems, M, Persigehl, T (2021). Bildgebung bei akutem Abdomen – Teil 1 : Fallbeispiele häufiger organbezogener Ursachen: Leber, Gallenblase, Pankreas, Milz und Gefäße [Imaging in the acute abdomen - part 1 : Case examples of frequent organ-specific causes: liver, gallbladder, pancreas, spleen and vessels]. *Radiologe, 61*(5), 497-510.
[http://dx.doi.org/10.1007/s00117-021-00843-1]

Sahin, Y. (2021). Celiac disease in children: A review of the literature. *World J. Clin. Pediatr., 10*(4), 53-71.
[http://dx.doi.org/10.5409/wjcp.v10.i4.53] [PMID: 34316439]

Tan, S.Y.T., Teh, S.P., Kaushik, M., Yong, T.T., Durai, S., Tien, C.J., Gardner, D.S. (2021). Hypertriglyceridemia-induced pancreatitis in pregnancy: case review on the role of therapeutic plasma exchange. *Endocrinol. Diabetes Metab. Case Rep., 2021*, 21-0017.
[http://dx.doi.org/10.1530/EDM-21-0017] [PMID: 34013888]

Vandertuin, L., Vunda, A., Gehri, M., Sanchez, O., Hanquinet, S., Gervaix, A. (2011). Invagination intestinale chez l'enfant: une triade vraiment classique? *Rev. Med. Suisse, 7*(283), 451-455. [Intestinal intussusception in children: truly a classic triad?]. [French.].
[PMID: 21452514]

Ward, D., Hashmi, D.L., Zhitnikov, S. (2021). Successful laparoscopic cholecystectomy at 32weeks of pregnancy - A case report. *Int. J. Surg. Case Rep., 84*, 106119.
[http://dx.doi.org/10.1016/j.ijscr.2021.106119] [PMID: 34167073]

Whang, B. (2018). Thoracic Surgery in the Pregnant Patient. *Thorac. Surg. Clin., 28*(1), 1-7.
[http://dx.doi.org/10.1016/j.thorsurg.2017.08.002] [PMID: 29150031]

Ye, L., Yang, Z., Liu, J., Liao, L., Wang, F. (2021). Digestive system manifestations and clinical significance of coronavirus disease 2019: A systematic literature review. *J. Gastroenterol. Hepatol., 36*(6), 1414-1422.
[http://dx.doi.org/10.1111/jgh.15323] [PMID: 33150978]

Zhang, R, Li, S, Wang, Y, Cai, W, Liu, Q, Zhang, J. (2021). Serum calponin 2 is a novel biomarker of tubal ectopic pregnancy. *Fertil Steril., Serum calponin 2 is a novel biomarker of tubal ectopic pregnancy., S0015-0282*(21), 00476-3.
[http://dx.doi.org/10.1016/j.fertnstert.2021.05.101]

CHAPTER 10

Extraabdominal Causes of Abdominal Pain

Abstract: Diabetes mellitus (DM), chronic renal failure (CRF), amyloidosis, sickle cell anemia (SCA) and acute intermittent porphyria are among diseases that can be associated with abdominal pain (AP) at some point in the course of the pathological process. Diabetic ketoacidosis (DKA) is a severe life-threatening syndrome characterized by fluid loss, electrolyte changes, hyperosmolarity and acidosis. These pathophysiologic factors can explain AP in patients with DKA. Vomiting and AP can also be initial manifestations of DKA even in euglycemic patients.

SCA is one of the most common autosomal recessive diseases classified in hemoglobinopathies. The disease is first recognized by history, then by peripheral smear and hemoglobin electrophoresis, and advanced studies. Splenic sequestration crisis is a severe complication of SCA that prompts emergent treatment, Opiate analgesia and hydration is the main treatment.

Patients with chronic renal failure (CRF) and end-stage renal disease are also prone to severe AP due to peritonitis which is triggered by continuous ambulatory peritoneal dialysis in vulnerable patients. Amyloidosis is mostly recognized with typical attacks *i.e.*, febrile episodes, exanthema, AP, myalgias and arthralgias.

Acute intermittent porphyria is an autosomal dominant disorder characterized by severe neurovisceral attacks of AP, nausea, vomiting, tachycardia, and hypertension in the absence of signs compatible with peritonitis. Management of mild attacks comprises symptomatic treatment, optimized calorie intake, and fluid replacement to beware dehydration.

Keywords: Abdominal pain, Acute intermittent porphyria, Amyloidosis, Chronic renal failure, Diabetes mellitus, Peritonitis, Porphyria, Sickle cell anemia, Splenic sequestration crisis.

DIABETIC KETOACIDOSIS (DKA)

DKA is a syndrome characterized by fluid loss, electrolyte changes, increased osmolarity due to high levels of plasma glucose, and a shift in blood pH to acidosis. All these reasons may trigger AP along with dehydration in the peritoneum. As a result, the acute AP emerges and can be seen as an entity that can masquerade all other etiologies of AP.

Ozgur KARCIOGLU, Selman YENİOCAK, Mandana HOSSEINZADEH & Seckin Bahar SEZGIN

DKA occurs with either a sudden increase in the need for insulin (such as pneumonia, other infections, stress, overwork) or a decrease in insulin production and secretion (such as pancreatitis, pancreatic insufficiency, sudden cessation/decrease in previously used insulin therapy).

Although DKA is mostly seen in childhood diabetes, which we call type I diabetes, it is also seen in seniors with type II. DKA may be the first sign of diabetes in one of 4 cases.

The severity of the clinical findings in DKA is not proportional to the level of hyperglycemia.

The main findings of DKA are dehydration, Kussmaul breathing, and unconsciousness. Ketones in the urine and high blood sugar associated with low pH also support this. Of note, children with Type-I Diabetes and severe DKA were found to be more likely to report vomiting, fatigue, and abdominal pain, but less likely to report polyuria, polydipsia, and polyphagia than those with mild/moderate DKA (Peng, 2021).

AP in the course of DKA is usually generalized and radiates throughout the abdomen, but sometimes it can be confined to a specific region.

Especially in children and those with communication problems, signs of dehydration should be sought by the physician (Table **1**). Interestingly, vomiting and AP can be initial manifestations of DKA even in euglycemic patients with long-term diabetes (Mumtaz, 2020)

Table 1. Evidence of significant dehydration (at least 5%).

• Extended capillary refill time (> 2 sec)
• Abnormal skin turgor
• Hyperpnea.
Adjunctive findings:
• Sunken eyes
• Dryness of mucous membranes
• Absence of tears
• Scammy extremities

Fluid replacement, correction of acidosis, and elimination of electrolyte imbalance which are the cornerstones of the treatment of DKA, will also treat pain. Likewise, altered mental status attributed to severe DKA also improves with treatment.

Alternative and additional diagnoses should also be excluded. ACS/AMI, CVA, acute heart failure, pyelonephritis, pneumonia, adrenal insufficiency, and thyroid problems that may trigger or accompany DKA should be investigated.

Wide-bore vascular access is opened bilaterally, preferably in the upper half of the body. There is no additional advantage of central vascular access. On the contrary, peripheral vascular access such as antecubital or external jugular veins should be preferred for rapid fluid infusion. 1 L of crystalloid fluid is given in the first hour, and 500 mL to 1 L of crystalloid fluid in the next several hours. Thus, 3.5-5 L is given in the first 5 hours. For the treatment of severe dehydration attributed to DKA, 6-12 L of fluid should be given in a total of 24 hours. Fluid therapy and insulin need to be administered simultaneously.

IV insulin infusion is given at a rate of 0.1 to 0.14 IU/kg/hour. When blood glucose readings fall below 250 mg/dL, insulin is stopped and 5% dextrose infusion is commenced. The HCO3 level should be kept above 18. The additional infusion of HCO3 is not helpful at pH values above 7.0 or 7.1, thus not indicated at all. On the contrary, it can deepen hypokalemia and cerebral complications.

- If serum K < 3.3 mEq/L, K replacement can take priority, insulin can be stopped and potassium solutions can be infused at 20-30 mEq/hour, with due caution.
- If serum K is between 3.3 and 5.3 mEq/L: 20 – 30 mEq K is put into each liter of IV crystalloids and administered to maintain blood K level between 4 and 5 mEq/L.
- If serum K > 5.3 mEq/L, K is not replaced, and the levels are frequently checked.

The Most Common Complications of DKA Treatment are Hypoglycemia and Hypokalemia

The serum phosphate level is also important. Levels below 1.5 mg/dl [0.48 mmol/L]), warrant oral replacement if the patient's consciousness is satisfactory to ingest the tablets.

If there is significant cerebral edema, 0.3 g/kg mannitol can be infused and titrated upwards. The patient must be admitted to the intensive care unit.

The reduction of ketone bodies in the urine is also one of the indicators that the treatment is successful, but it can also be misleading.

Non-diabetic ketoacidosis, on the other hand, is also a source of ketone bodies and can present with AP as well (Bashir, 2020). Starvation ketoacidosis and alcoholic ketoacidosis are subtypes of non-diabetic ketoacidosis.

Sickle Cell Anemia and Crisis

Sickle cell anemia (SCA) is one of the most common autosomal recessive inherited diseases in the world and is classified in hemoglobinopathies. HbS emerges as a result of the replacement of glutamic acid with valine at the 6th position of the β-globin chain.

SCA is between 0.3-0.6% in Turkey, but in some regions of southern Anatolia, this frequency reaches 3-44% (Arcasoy, 2003).

Symptoms of the disease usually appear after the sixth month of infancy. Fetal hemoglobin (HbF) is high in the blood until these months.

Diagnosis: SCA is first recognized by history, then by peripheral smear and hemoglobin electrophoresis, HPLC and certain DNA studies *via* PCR (Fig. **1**). Sickle cell disease is diagnosed by identification of significant quantities of HbS with or without an additional abnormal β-globin chain variant by hemoglobin assay or by identification of biallelic HBB pathogenic variants where at least one allele is the p.Glu6Val pathogenic variant (*e.g.*, homozygous p.Glu6Val; p.Glu6Val and a second HBB pathogenic variant) on molecular genetic testing (Bender, 2021).

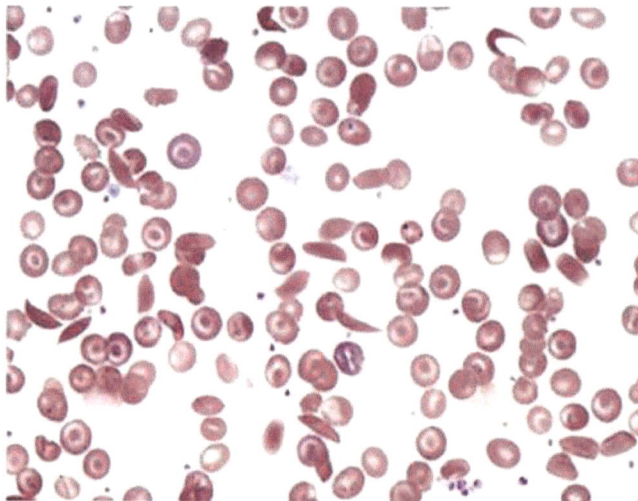

Fig. (1). Since sickled erythrocytes in patients with SCA do not have a normal shape, they both cause obstruction in small vessels and are retained by the spleen to be removed from the body. Thus, RBC life is reduced from 4 months to 20 days, which leads to anemia.

Blood viscosity increases due to sickling, resulting in microvascular occlusion, continuous hemolysis, and episodic vascular occlusions.

The most common reason for admission to the ED is painful crises (Vasoocclusive Pain Crisis). Silent cerebral infarcts have also been reported as high as 11% in those with SCA (Sayman, 2020). Stress, cold weather, working hard, being dehydrated, infection and pregnancy can trigger these crises in a patient with SCA who appears normal without these crises (Borhade, 2021).

Splenic sequestration crisis: It is a complication that mandates urgent treatment, characterized by sudden enlargement of the spleen, associated with shock due to volume loss, which is usually seen in young children. It is defined as an acute drop in hemoglobin level of 2 g/dL accompanied by splenomegaly (Kane, 2021). Fluid therapy, blood transfusion and splenectomy are recommended.

Management: The patient is usually in a severe clinical picture on presentation to the ED. Aggressive **analgesia** is usually achieved with opiates. Patient-controlled analgesia may be preferred. Sedoanalgesia with ketamine + midazolam can be an alternative to morphine or fentanyl. Meperidine is not used for this purpose. **Hydration** is the main treatment. In the first hour, a bolus of 10 ml/kg should be given, up to 3 L per day.

It is important to investigate and treat the cause that triggered the crisis. The percentage of HbS should be reduced below 30%.

Finally, complications should be investigated. **Exchange transfusion** may be necessary for severe patients who do not respond to the treatments mentioned.

Splenic Infarction (SI): It is one of the most important complications of SCA and crisis since it has long-term consequences. As a result of SI, the defense mechanisms against encapsulated bacteria (*e.g.*, pneumococci) are impaired, and the risk of serious infection/ sepsis arises (Overturf, 1999). Every patient with fever associated with SCA should receive broad-spectrum antibiotics (eg, 3rd generation cephalosporins) until the focus of infection and the causative agent are identified. Pneumococcal prophylaxis is important. Patients should be vaccinated against influenza.

How to Prevent Secondary Complications?

The following items will be useful in improving the outcomes of the disease and prevent complications (Bender, 2021).

- Aggressive education on the management of fevers
- Prophylactic antibiotics, including penicillin in children
- Immunizations
- Folic acid supplementation

• Iron chelation therapy for those with iron overload

Admission and discharge decisions

Patients who are adequately hydrated, do not require IV analgesia, and get meals themselves can be discharged. Patients with insufficient oral intake, requiring IV analgesia, those with complications, *e.g.* patients whose mesenteric ischemia cannot be ruled out should not be sent home.

Chronic renal failure (CRF) and end-stage renal disease are also severe metabolic diseases resulting in presentations with various clinical pictures. Severe AP due to peritonitis can be precipitated by **continuous ambulatory peritoneal dialysis (CAPD)** in vulnerable patients (Ounsinman, 2020).

Diagnosis and management: Demonstration of bacteria or yeasts *via* staining of CAPD samples, and isolation of causative agents in cultures will help establish the diagnosis and warrant emergent treatment. Immediate removal of the CAPD catheter and empirical treatment with broad-spectrum antimicrobials are necessary.

Autoinflammatory syndromes (AIS) such as **amyloidosis** are recognized with typical attacks *i.e.*, febrile episodes, exanthema, AP, myalgias and arthralgias. Boosted levels of the inflammatory serum markers such as CRP and systemic amyloid A (SAA) are expected during an attack (Blank, 2020). The geographical and ethnic origin of the patient and the patterns of the attacks are useful to establish the diagnosis. Colchicine represents an agent used in both diagnosis and treatment because it prevents attacks of FMF while other forms of AIS are unaffected. SAA deposition and involvement of the gastrointestinal canal explain the precipitation of AP in these patients.

Acute intermittent porphyria (AIP) is inherited as an autosomal dominant disorder characterized by severe neurovisceral attacks of AP, nausea, vomiting, tachycardia, and hypertension unaccompanied by signs compatible with peritonitis (Whatley, 2019). Acute attacks have a predilection for women. Altered mental status, seizures, peripheral neuropathy and hyponatremia can also be encountered in these patients. CRF, hypertension and hepatocellular carcinoma are among long-term complications of the disease. Some drugs including barbiturates, alcohol, endocrine diseases, stress, and infections precipitate acute attacks and limit themselves within weeks (Bonkovsky, 2014).

Management of mild attacks consists of symptomatic treatment, optimized calorie intake, and fluid replacement to beware dehydration.

Acute Neurovisceral Attacks are Intervened And Relieved with the Following

1. Stop chemicals that can precipitate acute attack;

2. Improve caloric intake by IV infusion when indicated

3. Avoid infusions of water in dextrose solutions.

4. Choose drugs to be used in the treatment of any infections vomiting, *etc.*

5. Use opiates liberally to manage acute and severe pain.

6. Management of dehydration and electrolyte disorders, especially hyponatremia.

7. Monitor neurologic status carefully and provide respiratory support as needed.

8. Human hemin (panhematin or heme arginate) administration is the specific treatment preferred to relieve acute neurovisceral attacks.

Familial Mediterranean fever (FMF) is known as an autoinflammatory syndrome inherited as an autosomal recessive entity. However, some studies pointed out that heterozygotes may also present with a whole array of the disease characteristics. The risk to sibs of inheriting two pathogenic variants and being affected is 1/4, should both parents be heterozygotes.

FMF comprises patients with either of two phenotypes: type 1 and type 2.

- Type 1 is defined as repetitive attacks of inflammation and serositis. This is manifested by fever, peritonitis, synovitis, pleuritis, pericarditis and meningitis. The presentations and severity differ in patients. The most serious complication recorded in these patients is amyloidosis, paving the way to renal failure in severe cases.
- Type 2 is diagnosed in the advanced stage of amyloidosis, which is the clinical presentation of FMF in a previously asymptomatic patient (Shohat, 2016).

Several mechanisms are launched to explain the cause(s) of organ involvements attributed to FMF. These include both subclinical inflammation and secondary (AA) amyloid deposition in the vessels and the myocardium which can evolve into acute myocardial infarction (AMI) with a poor prognosis. Polyarteritic lesions and Henoch-Schönlein vasculitis (HSV) are seen more significantly in FMF patients than in the general population with an increased frequency of mutations in the Mediterranean fever (MEFV) gene (Malik, 2021) (Table **2**).

The recognition of autoinflammatory syndromes including FMF warrants a high index of suspicion and evaluation of individual medical history. Age of onset and clinical features, in particular the self-limiting acute attacks, together with prodromal symptoms and trigger factors, are useful to suspect these disorders (Maconi, 2018) (Tables **3** and **4**).

Table 2. Most frequently observed mutations in the Mediterranean fever (MEFV) gene, by various ethnic groups (adapted fromAmbartsymian, 2012).

Mutations in different ethnic groups with FMF	
Arab	M680I, M694V, M694I
Armenian	M680I, M694V, V726A
Turk	M680I, M694V, V726A
Mizrahi Jews	E148Q, M694V
Ashkinazi Jews	E148Q, V726A
Sephardic Jews	E148Q, V726A, M680I, M694V

Table 3. FMF is to be included in patients with at least one of these signs and symptoms.

• Repetitive febrile attacks with, synovial, peritoneal and/or pleuritic inflammatory processes
• Erythema resembling erysipelas
• A history (and visible scars of) laparotomies for "surgical acute abdominal syndrome" without any evidence of pathology
• AA-type amyloidosis ensued after adolescence
• Positive response to colchicine
• Next of kin with FMF
• High risk ethnic group or geographical locations.

Table 4. Tel Hashomer clinical criteria devised to diagnose FMF in a suspected patient.

Fever AND:	• One major and one minor feature
OR	• Two minor features
Major features	• Fever
	• Abdominal or Chest pain
	• Joint pain
	• Skin eruption
Minor features	• Increased erythrocyte sedimentation rate (ESR) o >15 mm/h in men<50 years: o >20 mm/h in men between 50 and 85 years and in women <50 years: >20 mm/h o >30 mm/h in women between 50 and 85 years:
	• Leukocytosis (>11.0 x $10^3\mu$L)
	• Elevated serum fibrinogen concentration (>400 mg/dL])

A multicentric study in Turkey compared the findings in accord with new criteria in which FMF is diagnosed *via* the presence of two or more of five essential criteria (fever, abdominal pain, chest pain, arthritis, family history of FMF) (Ozçakar, 2011). The majority of the sample had heterozygous pM694V mutation (65%). The sensitivity of the new criteria set and that of the Tel Hashomer criteria in the multicentric sample were found to be 93% and 100%, respectively. Therefore, we can postulate that the sensitivity of the new criteria set is also high in patients who had a mutation at a single allele. Several criteria sets have been published, but the Tel-Hashomer criteria set of Israel is widely used for the diagnosis of FMF. Its sensitivity and specificity are more than 95% and 97%, respectively. A typical attack comprises fever (rectal - 38° C), pain due to inflammation, three or more recurrences of the attacks, and duration of 12 to 72 hours (Bhatt, 2021).

Tanatar *et al.* compared performances of three validated sets of diagnostic criteria for FMF (Tanatar 2020). New Eurofever/PRINTO classification criteria for FMF were similar and provide high utility in diagnosing/classifying patients with homozygous and compound heterozygous mutations. However, both Eurofever/PRINTO classification criteria and Tel-Hashomer criteria had significantly lower performance in heterozygous patients.

Case example. A 16-year-old girl from Turkey was diagnosed with soft tissue amyloidoma and systemic amyloidosis (Nalcacioglu, 2018). She was afebrile, and the rest of her vital signs were within normal limits (Fig. **2**). There were no positive signs including pretibial edema on examination. A histopathologic examination with Congo red and crystal violet dyes verified the presence of amyloidoma. Amyloid A protein was also positive on immunohistochemistry, with a renal biopsy compatible with AA amyloidosis. A detailed search for the etiology of systemic amyloidosis revealed heterozygous mutation in the FMF gene. Treatment with colchicine and anakinra was started after excluding the other causes of secondary amyloidosis.

Treatment of an acute attack consists of supportive measures, including infusion of IV saline and NSAIDs and/or paracetamol to relieve pain, treatment of febrile and inflammatory episodes with NSAIDs. Development of end-stage renal disease and relevant complications should be evaluated and managed accordingly, options including renal transplantation are to be individualized and assessed carefully.

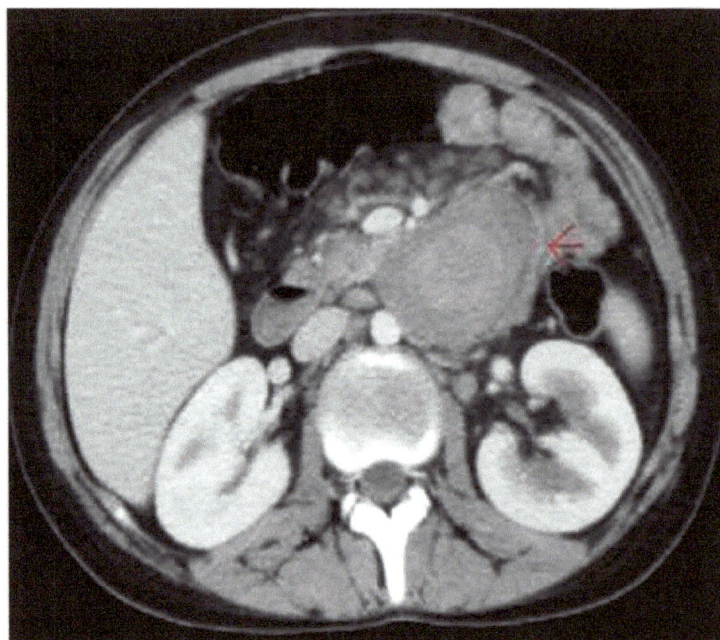

Fig. (2). A 44 x 62 mm irregular retroperitoneal mass with contrast enhancement and necrosis, compatible with amyloidoma (red arrow).

Colchicine is used to prevent primary manifestations of FMF. The mainstay of treatment for FMF is colchicine. It is an anti-inflammatory drug that inhibits tubulin polymerization and inhibits mitosis, leading to inhibition of neutrophil migration to inflammatory sites and stops the production of superoxide anion (Grattagliano, 2014).

Homozygous individuals for the pathogenic variant p.Met694Val or **compound heterozygous** for p.Met694Val should receive **lifelong colchicine treatment**. This approach prevents severe inflammatory attacks while alleviating amyloid deposition. Oral colchicine tablets are given 1-2 mg/day in adults and half the dose in children depending on age and weight.

Individuals who have infrequent inflammatory attacks and mild disease can be prescribed colchicine in an **outpatient** basis and be followed up in six months' intervals to detect proteinuria.

A Cochrane analysis revealed that colchicine appears to alleviate the rate and severity of attacks, especially when used three times daily (Wu, 2018). IL-1 antagonists such as anakinra can be associated with decreased levels of CRP in those unresponsive to colchicine.

Pregnancy and colchicine use: No differences were found between the treated group and the control group with respect to the rates of abortions, or malformations (Ben-Chetrit, 2010, Diav-Citrin, 2010). On the other hand, amniocentesis should be considered in pregnancies in mothers using colchicine.

Patients with renal transplant: Cisplatin may worsen symptoms of FMF, and cyclosporin A may precipitate untoward effects on renal transplant graft so that the relevant survival rates can decline (Shohat, 2016).

CONCLUSION

Extraabdominal causes of acute AP include important systemic disease processes with serious outcomes. Metabolic diseases DKA, CRF, SCA, amyloidosis and acute intermittent porphyria deserve attention to be ruled out from the DD of a given patient with AP. Most of these conditions can progress to more severe courses and even mortality if left untreated. Vital signs and findings on examination provide specific clues to diagnose these entities in most patients, while advanced studies including genetic counselling can be necessary for some patients such as those with porphyria.

Symptomatic treatment, pain management and fluid replacement are sufficient in selected patients with mild diseases, while aggressive resuscitation of severe metabolic acidosis and electrolyte imbalances will be mandatory in some situations such as DKA and acidotic end-stage renal disease with peritonitis following peritoneal dialysis.

REFERENCES

Ambartsymian, S.V. (2012). Myocardial infarction in patients with familial Mediterranean fever and cardiac lesions. *Georgian Med. News, 204*(204), 62-66.
[PMID: 22573751]

Arcasoy, A., Canatan, D. (2003). Dünyada ve Türkiye'de talasemi ve hemoglobinopatiler.

Bashir, B, Fahmy, AA, Raza, F, Banerjee, M (2020). Non-diabetic ketoacidosis: a case series and literature review. *Postgrad Med J., 138513.*
[http://dx.doi.org/10.1136/postgradmedj-2020-138513]

Ben-Chetrit, E., Ben-Chetrit, A., Berkun, Y., Ben-Chetrit, E. (2010). Pregnancy outcomes in women with familial Mediterranean fever receiving colchicine: is amniocentesis justified? *Arthritis Care Res. (Hoboken), 62*(2), 143-148.
[http://dx.doi.org/10.1002/acr.20061] [PMID: 20191511]

Bender, M.A. (2003). Sickle Cell Disease.*GeneReviews®.* (pp. 1993-2021). Seattle, WA: University of Washington, Seattle. [Internet]

Bhatt, H., Cascella, M. (2021). Familial Mediterranean Fever. *StatPearls.* StatPearls Publishing.Treasure Island (FL).:
[PMID: 32809589]

Blank, N, Schönland, SO (2020). Autoinflammatorische Syndrome und Amyloid-A-Amyloidose [Autoinflammatory syndromes and AA amyloidosis]. *Z Rheumatol., 79*(7), 649-659.

[http://dx.doi.org/10.1007/s00393-020-00778-3]

Bonkovsky, H.L., Maddukuri, V.C., Yazici, C., Anderson, K.E., Bissell, D.M., Bloomer, J.R., Phillips, J.D., Naik, H., Peter, I., Baillargeon, G., Bossi, K., Gandolfo, L., Light, C., Bishop, D., Desnick, R.J. (2014). Acute porphyrias in the USA: features of 108 subjects from porphyrias consortium. *Am. J. Med., 127*(12), 1233-1241.
[http://dx.doi.org/10.1016/j.amjmed.2014.06.036] [PMID: 25016127]

Borhade, M.B., Kondamudi, N.P. (2021). Sickle Cell Crisis. In: StatPearls [Internet]. Treasure Island (FL): StatPearls Publishing.

Diav-Citrin, O., Shechtman, S., Schwartz, V., Avgil-Tsadok, M., Finkel-Pekarsky, V., Wajnberg, R., Arnon, J., Berkovitch, M., Ornoy, A. (2010). Pregnancy outcome after in utero exposure to colchicine. *Am. J. Obstet. Gynecol., 203*(2), 144.e1-144.e6.
[http://dx.doi.org/10.1016/j.ajog.2010.02.063] [PMID: 20579964]

Grattagliano, I., Bonfrate, L., Ruggiero, V., Scaccianoce, G., Palasciano, G., Portincasa, P. (2014). Novel therapeutics for the treatment of familial Mediterranean fever: from colchicine to biologics. *Clin. Pharmacol. Ther., 95*(1), 89-97.
[http://dx.doi.org/10.1038/clpt.2013.148] [PMID: 23867542]

Kane, I., Nagalli, S. (2022). Splenic Sequestration Crisis. In: StatPearls [Internet]. Treasure Island (FL): StatPearls Publishing. PMID: 31985957.

Malik, J., Shabbir, A., Nazir, A. (2021). Cardiovascular Sequelae and Genetics of Familial Mediterranean Fever: A Literature Review. *Pulse (Basel), 8*(3-4), 78-85.
[http://dx.doi.org/10.1159/000516182] [PMID: 34307203]

Mumtaz, H., Shafiq, M.A., Batool, H., Naz, T., Ambreen, S. (2020). Diabetic Ketoacidosis in an Euglycemic Patient. *Cureus, 12*(8), e10065.
[http://dx.doi.org/10.7759/cureus.10065] [PMID: 33005499]

Nafile Sayman, E., Leblebİsatan, G., Leblebisatan, Ş., Bıçakcı, Y.K., Kılınç, Y., Barutçu, A. (2020). Silent cerebral infarct in sickle cell anemia patients of southern Turkey. *Turk. J. Med. Sci., 50*(8), 1887-1893.
[http://dx.doi.org/10.3906/sag-2003-192] [PMID: 32599969]

Nalcacioglu, H., Ozkaya, O., Genc, G., Ayyildiz, S., Kefeli, M., Elli, M., Aydin, O., Ceyhan Bilgici, M. (2018). Efficacy of anakinra in a patient with systemic amyloidosis presenting as amyloidoma. *Int. J. Rheum. Dis., 21*(2), 552-559.
[http://dx.doi.org/10.1111/1756-185X.13250] [PMID: 29239128]

Ounsinman, T., Chongtrakool, P., Angkasekwinai, N. (2020). Continuous ambulatory peritoneal dialysis-associated Histoplasma capsulatum peritonitis: a case report and literature review. *BMC Infect. Dis., 20*(1), 717.
[http://dx.doi.org/10.1186/s12879-020-05441-5] [PMID: 32993529]

Overturf, G.D. (1999). Infections and immunizations of children with sickle cell disease. *Adv. Pediatr. Infect. Dis., 14*, 191-218.
[PMID: 10079855]

Ozçakar, Z.B., Yalçınkaya, F., Cakar, N., Acar, B., Bilgiç, A.E., Uncu, N., Kara, N., Ekim, M., Kasapçopur, O. (2011). Application of the new pediatric criteria and Tel Hashomer criteria in heterozygous patients with clinical features of FMF. *Eur. J. Pediatr., 170*(8), 1055-1057.
[http://dx.doi.org/10.1007/s00431-011-1404-y] [PMID: 21287357]

Peng, W., Yuan, J., Chiavaroli, V., Dong, G., Huang, K., Wu, W., Ullah, R., Jin, B., Lin, H., Derraik, J.G.B., Fu, J. (2021). 10-Year Incidence of Diabetic Ketoacidosis at Type 1 Diabetes Diagnosis in Children Aged Less Than 16 Years From a Large Regional Center (Hangzhou, China). *Front. Endocrinol. (Lausanne), 12*, 653519.
[http://dx.doi.org/10.3389/fendo.2021.653519] [PMID: 33986725]

Shohat, M. (2000). Familial Mediterranean Fever. In: Adam, M.P., Ardinger, H.H., Pagon, R.A., (Eds.),

GeneReviews®.   (pp.   1993-2021).   Seattle,   WA: University   of   Washington, Seattle.https://www.ncbi.nlm.nih.gov/books/NBK1227/ [Internet] [Updated 2016 Dec 15]

Tanatar, A., Sönmez, H.E., Karadağ, Ş.G., Çakmak, F., Çakan, M., Demir, F., Sözeri, B., Ayaz, N.A. (2020). Performance of Tel-Hashomer, Livneh, pediatric and new Eurofever/PRINTO classification criteria for familial Mediterranean fever in a referral center. *Rheumatol. Int., 40*(1), 21-27. [http://dx.doi.org/10.1007/s00296-019-04463-w] [PMID: 31646357]

Whatley, S.D., Badminton, M.N. (2005). Acute Intermittent Porphyria. 2005 Sep 27 [Updated 2019 Dec 5]. In: Adam MP, Everman DB, Mirzaa GM, et al., editors. GeneReviews® [Internet]. Seattle (WA): University of Washington, Seattle; 1993-2022. Available from: https://www.ncbi.nlm.nih.gov/books/NBK1193/.

Wu, B., Xu, T., Li, Y., Yin, X. (2018). Interventions for reducing inflammation in familial Mediterranean fever. *Cochrane Database Syst. Rev., 10*(10), CD010893. [http://dx.doi.org/10.1002/14651858.CD010893.pub3] [PMID: 30338514]

CHAPTER 11

Abdominal Trauma and Pain

Abstract: Trauma is the most common cause of death in the young population, predominantly males. Abdominal trauma is a leading source of occult bleeding which is the second cause of early-phase deaths following major head injury. Uncontrollable bleeding constitutes the most common cause of preventable deaths especially if the management of shock is delayed. Penetrating trauma leads to significant morbidity and mortality, nonetheless, diagnosed more easily with its remarkable presentation.

The main goal in the evaluation of the abdomen in the acute setting is to uncover (*i.e.,* not to overlook) the injuries requiring surgery without delay, rather than to diagnose specific injuries in detail. Signs and symptoms of progressing shock states vary from patient to patient, and sometimes very subtle changes can herald impending doom.

The clinician should be proactive in detecting the injuries, using both evaluation findings and bedside ultrasound together with other advanced imaging techniques when necessary, keeping in mind that occult injuries can evolve in time insidiously. Ongoing intraabdominal bleeding is an ominous finding which precedes advanced hemorrhagic shock and needs to be sought for carefully in patients with trauma.

Keywords: Abdominal pain, Abdominal trauma, Bleeding, Computed tomography, Fluid management, Hemorrhagic shock, Injury, REBOA, Resuscitation, Rupture, Shock, Trauma, Ultrasound.

Abdominal trauma (AbT) is a type of injury that requires attention due to the difficulties in the evaluation as well as its course with a significant morbidity and mortality rate. Although the main title of AbT is a very general scope, there are countless different combinations of injury possibilities and presentations within this context. Likewise, inspection and examination have their own difficulties. Our goal in the evaluation of the abdomen is to identify (or not to miss) the injuries requiring surgery without delay, rather than to diagnose specific injuries. The most serious error in AbT is not missing a specific diagnosis, but the failure to pursue or delay the surgical intervention mandatory for stabilization. The most common preventable deaths occur as a result of uncontrollable bleeding due to delayed management. Many lesions are related to intra-abdominal injuries within the concept of the 'golden hour'.

Ozgur KARCIOGLU, Selman YENİOCAK, Mandana HOSSEINZADEH & Seckin Bahar SEZGIN

A focused history coupled with a complete physical examination and evaluation of the patient is essential. As a bedside test, point-of-care ultrasonography (USG/POCUS) is widely used by clinicians and is a regular part of physical examination. While diagnostic peritoneal lavage (DPL) was used in the past to evaluate abdominal trauma in the diagnosis of the unstable patient, it has now been almost abandoned with the development of both USG/POCUS and whole-body computed tomography (CT) scanning and MDCT. However, retroperitoneal injuries still represent a challenge in recognition in the emergency setting. CT imaging has replaced DPL in specific clinical situations and is invaluable in diagnosis. No test can replace the need for careful clinical evaluation and monitoring for the development of signs of serious injury. In recent years, diagnostic thoracoscopy and laparoscopy have been increasingly used in the evaluation and treatment of AbT (Table **1**).

Table 1. Indications for laparotomy in abdominal trauma.

Absolute (Prepare the OR immediately)
Ongoing severe hemodynamic instability, +/- positive FAST result
Generalized peritonitis (guarding, rigidity)
Evisceration
Relative indications (Consult trauma surgeon)
Free air image on X-ray or CT (can stem from thorax or other sources apart from abdominal trauma)
Signs of GI bleeding on NG or rectal exam
Penetrating abdominal trauma: firearm injuries (mostly operative) and stabbing wounds (can be operative)
Multisystem trauma + Ongoing hemodynamic instability, source of injury not defined yet

One of the most important points is to consider the victim as having multiple trauma, even in the case of presentation with significant AbT. The completeness of both the primary survey summarized with ABCDE mnemonic and the secondary survey formulated as "head-to-toe" is essential. Otherwise, non-abdominal vital injuries may be missed.

PATHOPHYSIOLOGY

Abdominal injuries mainly develop *via* two mechanisms: Blunt and penetrating trauma. It is also important to remember that these two types of injury can coexist. For example, a person with a stab wound on the chest may also have been bluntly beaten to lacerate his spleen. Similarly, there may be significant blunt trauma as well as penetration by sharp objects in a motor vehicle injury. Thus, the clinician should not set limit his/her vision with the easily seen.

Blunt Trauma

There are three mechanisms of injury by blunt trauma:

1. direct impact

2. crush injury

3. acceleration-deceleration injury. These types of injuries can also be found in a double or triple combination.

The abdomen consists of the peritoneal cavity and the extraperitoneal space. The extraperitoneal space includes the retroperitoneum and the extraperitoneal pelvis, which are hard to examine and evaluate, since their injuries usually cause minimal findings on physical examination. Peritoneal lavage is unreliable for injuries in this area and negative lavage may give a false sense of comfort. Ancillary secondary tests are more useful in the evaluation of the retroperitoneum and pelvis. Intravenous pyelography (IVP), upper GI contrast studies, cystography, angiography, and CT imaging will all be useful in selected cases. Oral and IV contrast-enhanced CT imaging is the single most useful test in the evaluation of retroperitoneal organs such as the kidney and pancreas (Fig. **1**). Although USG can also be used in the retroperitoneum, care should be taken in interpretation.

Rectal digital exam and stool occult blood test can be interpreted in selected cases to evaluate distal bowel injuries. Fresh blood coming directly to the finger on the digital exam may mean pelvic fracture and perforation of the rectum, which prompts further investigation.

Serum amylase level is a useful predictor of potential injury, but normal amylase level can be seen even in the presence of significant pancreatic injury.

In case of injury in the peritoneal space, there are usually obvious findings on physical examination of the abdomen, as the peritoneum responds to irritation very rapidly. Findings such as tenderness, guarding, or palpable mass raises suspicion of injury.

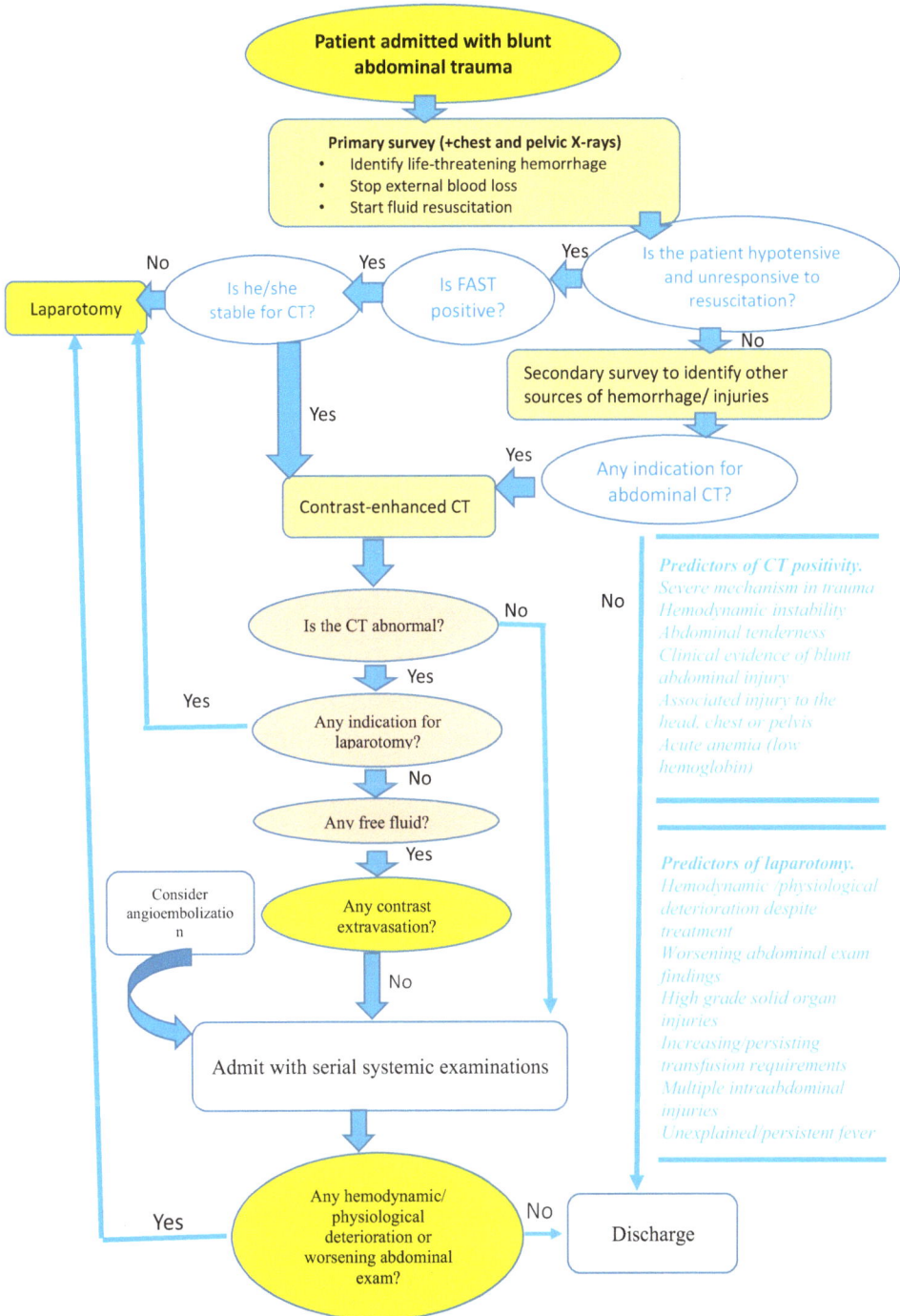

Fig. (1). The management algorithm proposed for blunt abdominal trauma.

Penetrating injuries can occur with gunshot or penetrating injuries. Among these, firearm injuries have a much more morbid and mortal course due to the difficulty in predicting the consequences, *i.e.*, the disproportion between the entry point and the extent of tissue damage, the extent of injury it causes inside the abdomen, and the extra-abdominal injuries. Although stabbing wounds may cause poor clinical outcome with certain critical injuries, it has a much more predictable course. One of the worst scenarios is pericardial tamponade and cardiac rupture in upper abdominal injury with long 'skewers' blades.

Three main mechanisms of damage have been proposed in gunshot wounds: 1. Direct penetration of the bullet into tissues 2. Fragmentation after direct impact 3. Impact on neighboring organs in the form of shock waves.

Gunshot wounds should be routinely explored. The extent of the damage can be observed much more clearly with the improvement of imaging technologies. Care should be taken for extra-abdominal injuries. Chest injuries with hemopneumothorax are possible when the bullet traverses the diaphragm. Of note, high velocity gunshot wounds can cause intra-abdominal injury without peritoneal penetration with the generation of shock waves.

In stabbing wounds, primary laceration of tissues occurs. Such penetrating injuries should be evaluated and explored by imaging, because of the high probability of false-negative laparotomy. For this reason, patients should be followed more selectively in trauma centers with experienced clinical follow-up and operation rooms.

Who should undergo laparotomy? The intervention is strictly indicated in patients with evisceration, signs of peritoneal irritation (guarding/rigidity), distension, and persistent hypotension. Imaging should be considered as an adjunct. In stabbing wounds, positive wound exploration is a sign of penetration through superficial fascia and an indication for laparotomy. Laparotomy will take priority in patients with suspicious findings and impaired consciousness or under the influence of drugs and/or substances.

Distracting injuries, and intoxication of the trauma victim constitute certain challenges in trauma management (Table **2**).

Table 2. Pitfalls in trauma management.

1. Concomitant drug and/or alcohol intoxication and head or spinal cord trauma represent a major limitation for the sensitivity of physical examination in identifying abdominal injuries. Therefore, the importance and priority of imaging increases in the presence of such co-morbidities.

(Table 2) cont.....

2. Distracting injuries are real challenges: Fractures of long bones such as tibia and femur, or injuries to spinal cord and thorax can precipitate severe pain and constitute a distracting injury for the patient as well as deceiving the physician. Even in the case of a very "red" injury, such as a bleeding open fracture tibial shaft, the physician should not waive the sequence of the primary survey with ABCDE followed by secondary survey and due investigations.
3. If 'duties' such as completion of laboratory work up and doing exactly what the consultant tells one to do are postponing the patient's stabilization, you are on the way to court. No instruction or work up can preclude evaluation of patient stabilization and vital injuries.
4. USG/POCUS is inappreciable, although it should be interpreted in the context of given injury. It should be kept in mind that it has user-dependent accuracy rates, and that there may be problems arising between the patient and the device. In cases in between, deficiencies should be complemented with additional examinations and consultations.
5. CT is used almost as standard, drastically reducing the missed injury rate. In women of childbearing age, CT should not be requested without a B-HCG result except in the presence of immediate life-threatening conditions. This is not the case in sudden life-threatening injuries, the risks, pluses and minuses should be evaluated individually.
6. Analgesia has no contraindications. Physical examination and stabilization of vital signs should be followed by analgesia and sedation in all painful situations, including trauma. The route to be chosen is the IV route, and the drug type is opiates in the acute phase. Short-acting agents should be prioritized to facilitate tracking the changes in the systemic examination findings. It is important to record the findings as is and not to discharge the patient by saying "the pain is gone" while still under the influence of analgesia.
7. Tetanus vaccination and, if necessary, antitetanic IgG serum administration should not be overlooked. The specific indications should be evaluated individually for the patient.
8. Due to the nature of diseases and injuries, there are more grays than black or whites in patient management and decision making. The physician should not hesitate to ask for consultation from the disciplines related to the injury. This is needed from the point of view of sharing both the responsibility and the workload items to be performed for the victim. *"The second couple of eyes is always better than a single".*
9. Decision making for a hospitalization is always a critical one. It will be safer to keep the patient in the hospital rather than sending home in cases where the stabilization is uncertain and "in between". For patients with social support, who are conscious and understanding, their return within a certain period of time and in case ofcertain occurrences (*e.g.* incessant severe pain, vomiting, unable to eat/drink, *etc.*) may represent a feasible and practical intermediate solution. The motto 'make mistakes for the benefit of the patient' or *'err on the patient's side'* will save you a lot of stomachache.

CLINICAL FINDINGS IN SPECIFIC ORGAN INJURIES

It should be kept in mind that different techniques will be used in various injuries in the evaluation of the patient with abdominal injury.

Hollow Viscera

Injury to these organs is serious and conveys significant morbidity and mortality. Blunt trauma resulting in sudden compression may cause hollow organ injury. When there are crushes or abrasions on the skin attached to the belt (seat belt sign), there is a high suspicion of severe internal organ injury (Fig. **2**).

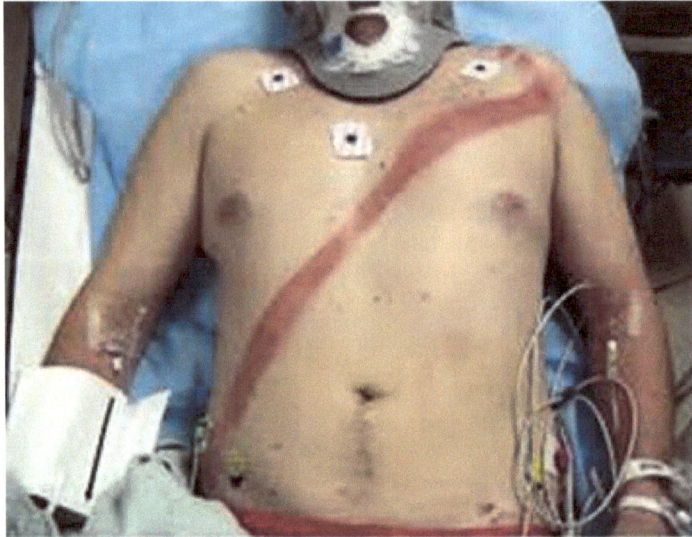

Fig. (2). The seat belt must be employed as it prevents many vital organ damage in multiple trauma, especially thoracoabdominal injuries. It is known that pancreatic injuries are statistically more common in patients with "seat-belt sign", but many vital injuries, including those that cause hemorrhagic shock, are prevented. The triangular-shaped belt is much more protective than the "lap belt" that covers only the abdomen.

A marked risk for sepsis emerges when visceral contents carrying bacterial flora are dispersed freely into the peritoneal cavity. Injuries to these organs often precipitate signs of peritonitis. Most of these injuries can be demonstrated with DPL and USG/POCUS, but it may be necessary to identify specific organ injuries with water-soluble contrast studies.

Stomach

Although the stomach is resistant to blunt traum, a distended stomach increases the risk of serious injury in acceleration-deceleration injuries, *e.g.*, motor vehicle accidents. Bloody drainage from the nasogastric tube is usually predictive of injury, although this drainage may be iatrogenic due to nasopharyngeal trauma *e.g.*, during tube insertion. CT is the mainstay tool for diagnosis (Fig. **3**). Contrast studies may sometimes be required to confirm the diagnosis.

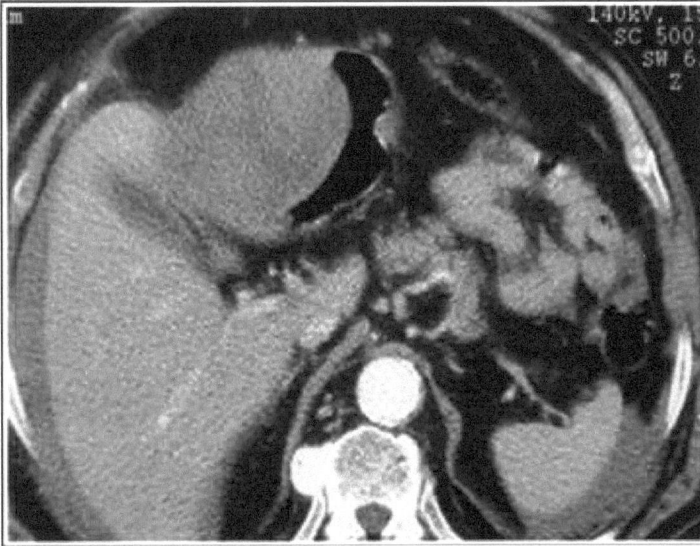

Fig. (3). Intramural gastric wall hematoma in an elderly patient who fell prone from his bed to the floor. It is remarkable that the GI passage is still possible from a narrow space. The patient can present with vomiting just after meals.

Small Intestine

Small bowel injuries resemble gastric injuries, they occur most frequently as a result of penetrating injury and generally show a favorable prognosis. In most cases, early peritoneal irritation occurs due to spillage of intestinal contents, which causes significant symptoms of small bowel injuries. Guarding and rigidity is identified in a typical patient. A deceleration injury can result in a bucket-handle tear of the mesentery or burst injury on the antimesenteric side. The intestine may lose its viability after a while, if the intervention is delayed. Expedient diagnosis is late in selected cases, especially in patients with head trauma and impaired level of consciousness. USG is valuable if done carefully and in experienced hands, although it can still be false-negative. CT is a good option and a "last stop" for diagnosis in suspected cases. A majority of small bowel injuries can be primarily repaired after local debridement. Resection and anastomosis may be mandated in larger injuries or cases that cause blood loss.

Duodenum

The retroperitoneal position of the duodenum complicates the diagnosis of injury. Injury is most common in the second part (36%). Signs and symptoms can sometimes ensue slowly and insidiously. Testicular pain and priapism are common because the sympathetic fibers of duodenum course adjacently to the gonadal vessels.

X-rays can be helpful when they are positive, while there is no point in a negative interpretation. Specific clues of duodenal injury are **retroperitoneal air on X-ray and elevated serum amylase**. Although the diagnosis cannot be made on amylase alone, persistently high amylase levels have been associated with poor prognosis and severe clinical course. An increase in lipase levels is associated with multiple organ failure after injury (Subramanian A, 2016).

The pathognomonic test for duodenal injury is the presence of extravasation on the contrast study. "Coil spring sign" on barium radiographs is diagnostic for intramural duodenal hematoma. CT with IV+oral contrast is the standard diagnostic method. Disadvantages are that it cannot be pursued in victims with unstable hemodynamics and the possibility of contrast nephropathy is possible.

Oral contrast may not adequately penetrate the duodenum on CT imaging and formal fluoroscopic evaluation may be required (Figs. **4** and **5**). **Visualization of intraperitoneal fluid is the most common radiological finding.** Duodenal injuries can range from intramural hematomas to crush injury or severe laceration. If the hematoma can be recognized without exploration, it can be managed nonoperatively. Intramural duodenal hematomas are very common after blunt trauma especially in alcoholics and in anticoagulant users.

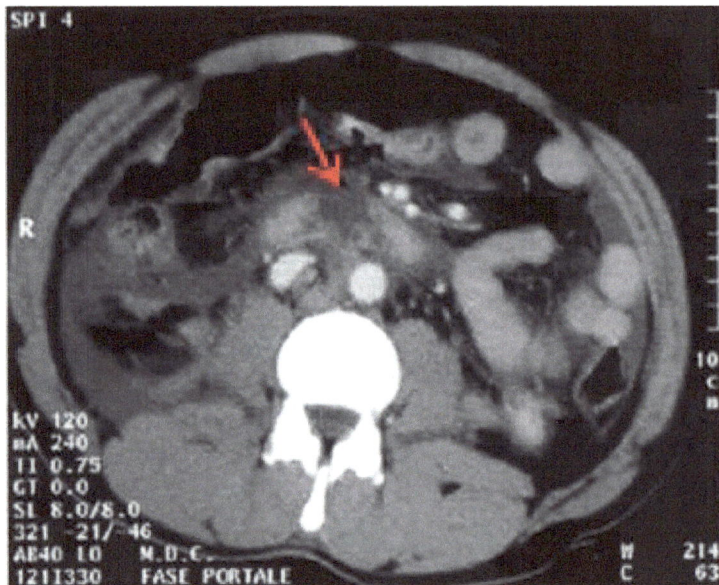

Fig. (4). Pre-op CT image showing rupture and separation of the 3rd part of the duodenum.

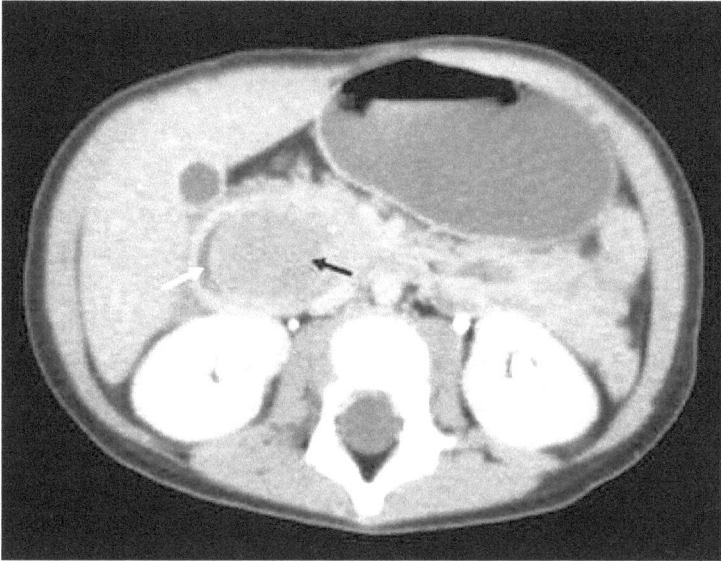

Fig. (5). Image of intramural duodenal hematoma in a child who fell down the stairs (black arrow). A small crescent-shaped passage can be provided in the duodenal lumen (white arrow).

Mortality and complications increase markedly with delayed surgery.

Large Bowels-Colon

The approach to large bowel injury is controversial. Excessive contamination may ensue due to delayed surgical treatment. In order to avoid this situation, it is necessary to suspect colon lesions in the early period and to investigate specifically. CT imaging with rectal contrast is the best modality to identify injuries expediently (Figs. **6** to **8**). If in doubt, gastrographin enema with fluoroscopy is the optimal test for evaluating colonic perforation. Barium irritates the peritoneal lineage and causes a brisk inflammatory response. If perforation is suspected, water-soluble contrast should be used. If there is still doubt, exploration should be done.

Some surgeons consider that most lesions can be sutured primarily. This approach is acceptable for early diagnosed left and right sided lesions with minimal contamination. Colostomy is often performed for severely injured left-sided lesions or heavily contaminated colonic injuries.

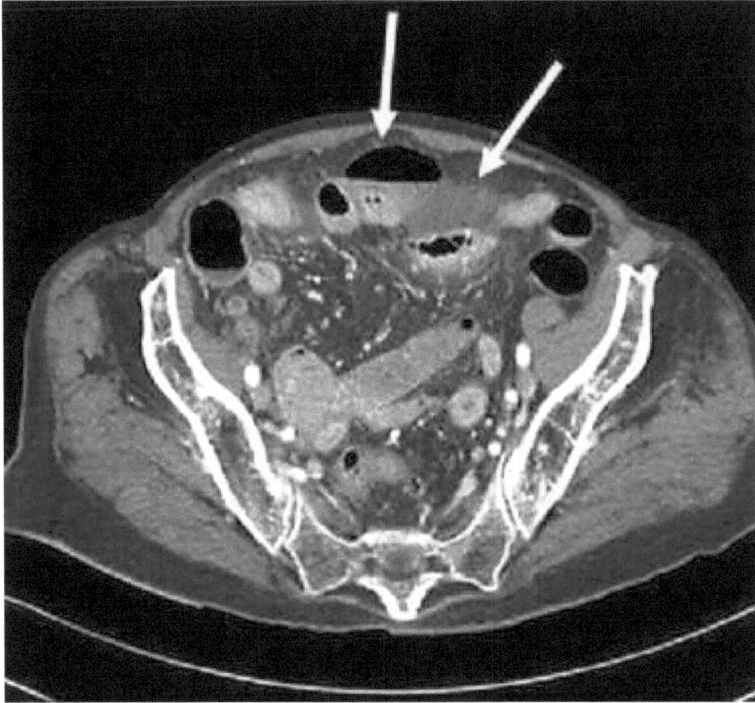

Fig. (6). Images of free air and fluid adjacent to the transverse colon in abdominopelvic CT. The patient was diagnosed with jejunal perforation.

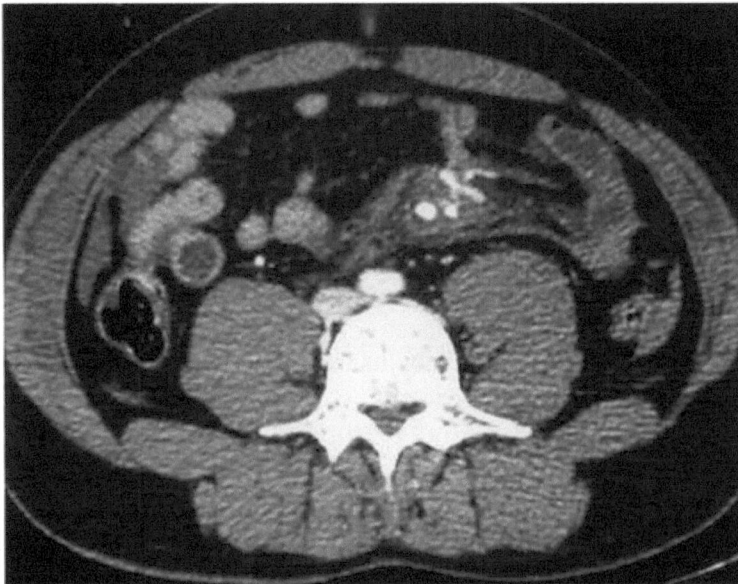

Fig. (7). Bowel and mesenteric injury. Mesenteric contrast extravasation and fatty streaks.

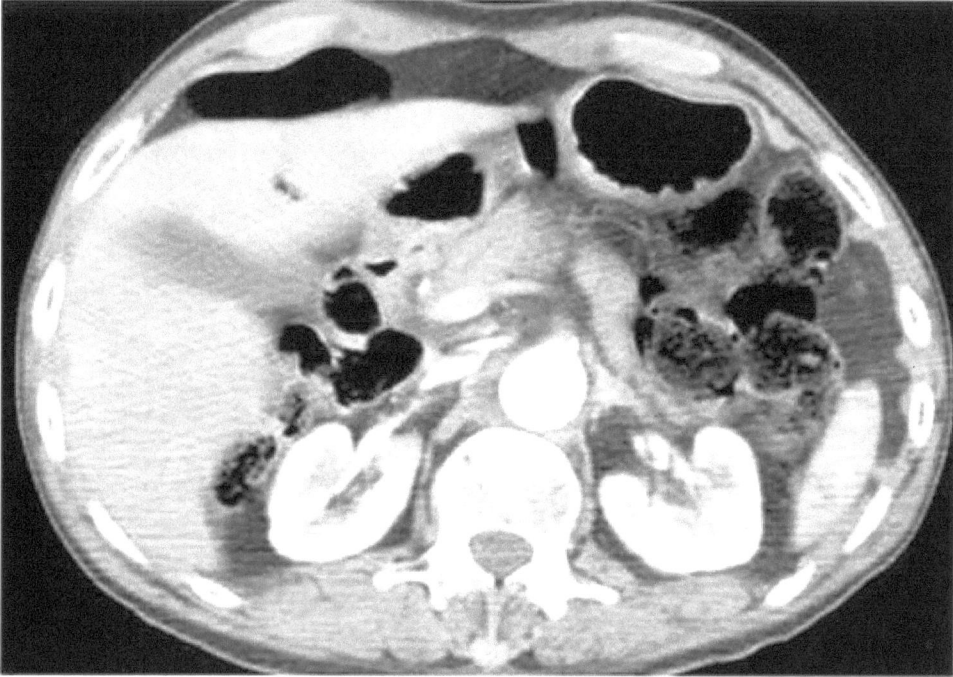

Fig. (8). Axial contrast CT yields the image of free air on the ventral aspect of the liver. Pneumoperitoneum is secondary to colonic injury.

Rectum

Preoperative diagnosis of rectal injuries is particularly important because it is difficult to diagnose peroperatively. The rectum is an extraperitoneal organ and its physical findings may not be obvious. With careful rectal examination, it should be evaluated whether there is bone penetration as a result of pelvic fracture.

An open pelvic fracture that goes unrecognized and leads to rectal injury will trigger rapidly developing sepsis and septic shock. In these patients, the surgical approach requires both the abdominal and perineal approach. If the diagnosis cannot be made before exploratory laparotomy, a repeat operation for the colostomy will be mandated. The approach includes preoperative broad-spectrum antibiotics, repair of associated injuries, drainage, and fecal diversion.

Gallbladder and Biliary Tract

Injuries of the gallbladder and its ducts are rare. Gallbladder injury is often caused by penetrating injury, but can also occur after blunt trauma in some cases. It often involves the incision near the papilla. Preoperative diagnosis of this injury is extremely difficult. It can also be recognized during exploration. Intraoperative cholangiogram provides definitive diagnosis in most cases.

Genitourinary System

Contrast studies are required for diagnosis if persistent microscopic or gross hematuria is present. Contrast-enhanced CT imaging is the best examination if time is available (Fig. **9**). Where this is not possible, rapid cystogram and intravenous pyelogram (IVP) in the resuscitation room (or in the radiology unit) are helpful. If there is time, oblique and lateral films such as postvoid films are valuable in injuries that are difficult to discern. IVP cannot be taken in an unstable/hypotensive patient, it should be employed after stabilization of the patient.

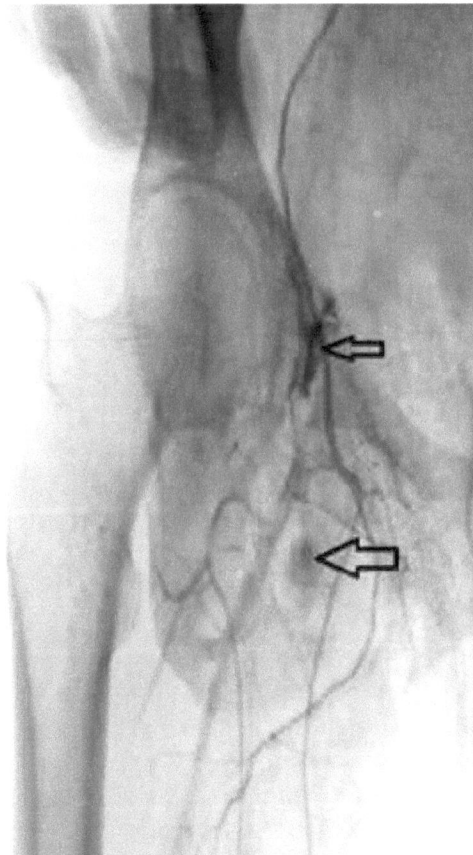

Fig. (9). Multifocal extravasation from internal iliac artery branch on CT-angiography section (arrows).

Dyes released in the urine, such as methylene blue and indigo carmine, may be helpful in determining the site of extravasation.

Solid Organs

Injury to solid organs primarily causes morbidity and mortality essentially with blood loss. Secretory products of these organs are a potential source of morbidity, although these are generally sterile and have a lower risk of infection. The blood loss can be severe and life-threatening. Surgical intervention is critical for the control of bleeding. On admission, there will be tachycardia and hypotension in addition to the abdominal findings. If the hemorrhage has accumulated in a limited area, a clinically palpable mass may develop that can be observed in radiological examinations. Of note, autogenous blood does not trigger a peritoneal irritation and the patient may not generate apparent findings on examination except for findings due to blood loss ensued in a long time. The net result may be a physician in the court advocating himself/herself as "but there was no guarding on examination on the deceased, and I did not think he/she will succumb to hemorrhagic shock at all".

Liver

The liver is frequently injured in both blunt and penetrating abdominal trauma. Mortality is high (50% to 100%) in this injury, and the key to survival is emergent control of bleeding. USG represents both a practical tool with repeatability and economical study applied at bedside, which helps recognize most hepatic injuries (Fig. **10**).

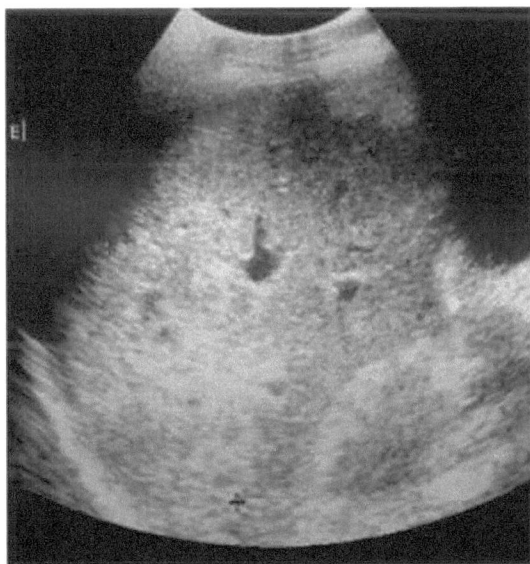

Fig. (10). Evaluation of hepatic contusion by USG. Hyperechoic post-traumatic areas are consistent with hematoma.

With CT imaging, some lesions can now be identified and managed nonoperatively (Figs. **11** and **12**). Total vascular isolation of the liver may be required in massive liver injury with caval or hepatic vein injury. Control is achieved with a shunt over the liver from the inferior vena cava. The vascular isolation of the liver is completed with the Pringle maneuver (occlusion of the vessels in the liver hilum). In some cases, vascular (aortic) control with thoracotomy before abdominal exploration prevents excessive blood loss due to evacuation of the tamponade.

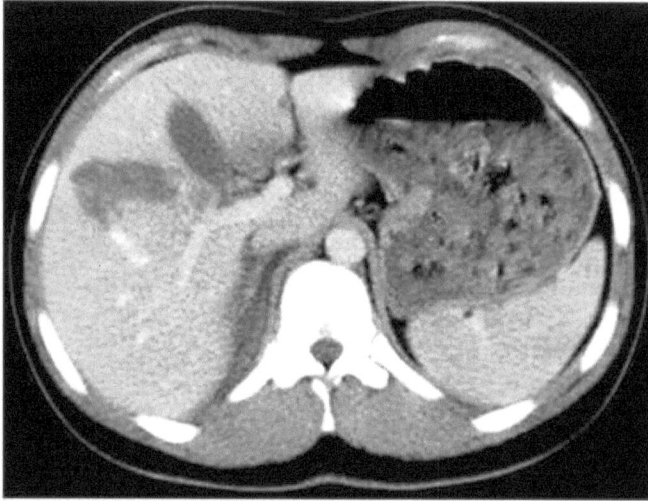

Fig. (11). In contrast-enhanced CT section, the hypodense area of the liver is consistent with hepatic contusion.

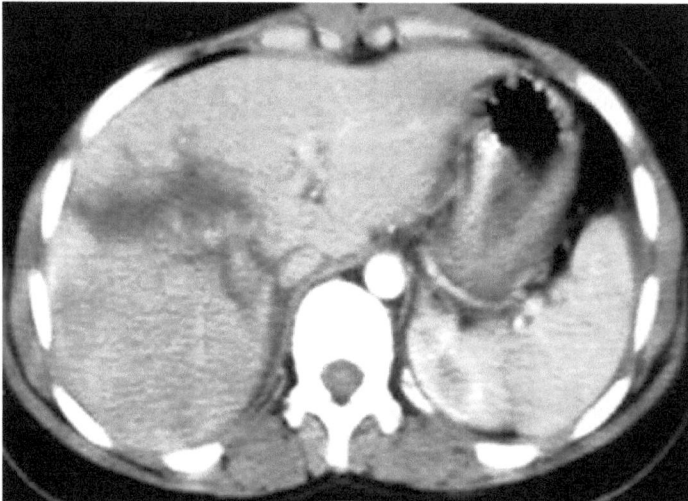

(Fig. 12) contd.....

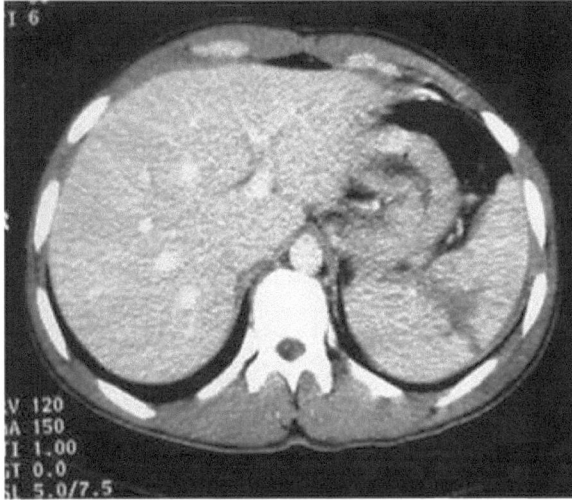

Fig. (12). Blunt liver injury. A. Complex hepatic lacerations with hypodense area in the liver on contrast-enhanced CT scan show hepatic fracture. B. Splenic fracture is diagnosed when laceration bands transsect the hypodens parenchyma and join the two sides of the hilum.

Hepatic packing becomes important when control cannot be achieved with other techniques or resection because the time required for major resection and the accompanying blood loss will not be appropriate. This is usually appropriate in presence of hypothermia and coagulopathy. Potential late complications of liver injury are biliary fistula, sepsis (intrahepatic or abdominal), hematobilia and vascular injury with pseudoaneurysm. Septic foci are usually recognized by CT imaging and treated with drainage. This can be done either surgically or with the guidance of CT or USG.

Hematobilia usually develops weeks or months after injury and trauma history should be specifically questioned. In this syndrome, signs include GI bleeding, jaundice, and colicky AP relieved by hematemesis. Besides the diagnostic application of selective angiography, it has uses to embolize fistula.

Spleen is the most frequently injured organ in blunt trauma and is usually associated with other intraabdominal injuries. Although splenectomy is the traditional treatment for splenic injuries, many publications mention the risk of postsplenectomy sepsis and there has been a trend towards a selective approach in recent years. Recent reports indicated that around 43% of the patients were managed non-operatively in developed centers (Jesani, 2020). In the same series, splenic artery embolisation was performed successfully in 4% of the cases and the overall hospital mortality was 10%. In some situations, splenectomy is still the treatment of choice, but spleen repair and non-operative monitoring are also indicated. American Association for Surgery of Trauma (AAST) has categorized these injuries to guide management approaches (Morell-Hofert, 2020) (Figs. **13** and **14**).

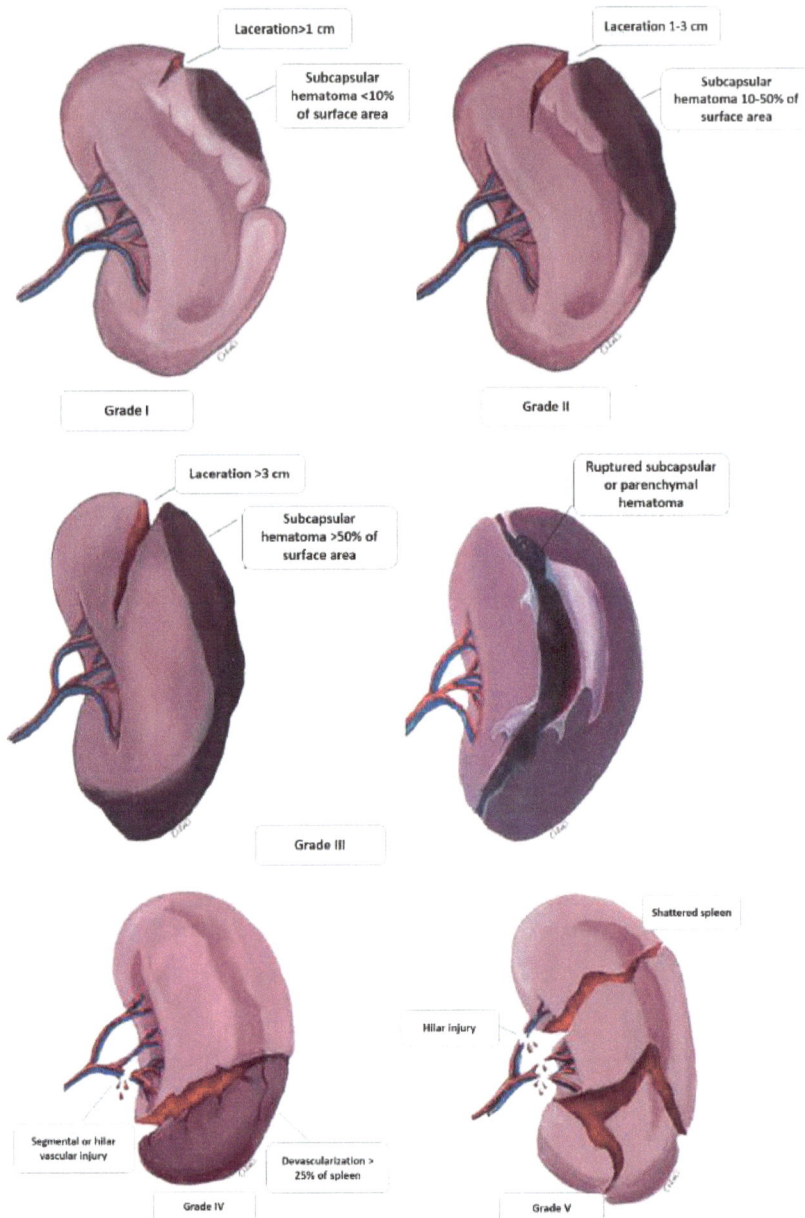

Fig. (13). Blunt splenic injuries can be classified by the system for predicting injury severity (Grade I to V) developed by the American Association for Surgery of Trauma (AAST).

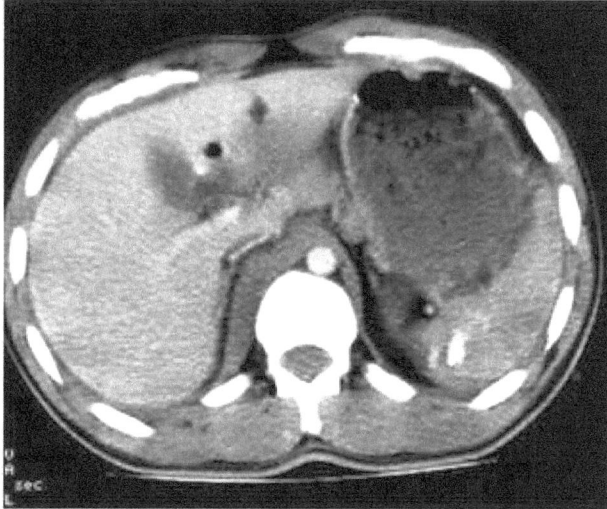

Fig. (14). Splenic injury on contrast-enhanced CT: Active contrast extravasation indicates active bleeding.

Delayed splenic rupture is a rare injury that develops in 1-2% of abdominal traumas. Rupture may develop following the original trauma. It resembles the symptoms of acute injury and is often diagnosed with imaging techniques. The late complications of spleen injuries are related to the treatment method. For example, secondary bleeding episodes or abscess formation may develop with spleen repair (splenorrhaphy) or non-surgical approach.

Late bacterial sepsis can be seen in children with splenectomy. The role of prophylactic antibiotics is uncertain in studies to date. Antibiotic prophylaxis is controversial in this situation. Vaccination should cover pneumococci, hemophilus influenzae and meningococci.

Pancreas

Pancreatic injury is most commonly triggered by penetrating trauma. However, crushing and damage can also ensue as a result of blunt injury. The classic scenario is the impact of objects such as a steering wheel or bicycle handlebars on the midepigastric region.

Pancreatic injuries include transections, contusions, and lacerations.

CT imaging is helpful in the diagnosis of these injuries, although it should be noted that some of them cannot be seen easily on CT. Indirect signs of injury are images such as fluid in the peripancreatic adipose tissue and thickening of the left anterior renal fascia (Soto, 2012).

Morbidity and mortality rates are extremely high when the diagnosis is overlooked or delayed. Exocrine secretions leaking from the pancreas have a strong irritative effect on the peritoneum. Autodigestion develops and creates a suitable environment for bacterial proliferation.

If the first CT is normal in patients with abnormal findings, a control CT should be taken 24-48 hours later.

If bile duct injury is suspected in stable patients, an endoscopic retrograde cholangiopancreatography (ERCP) study will assist in determining the anatomy. Surgical management of these lesions is difficult because the channels are small and difficult to distinguish. ERCP guidance can be helpful in this manner. Its greatest benefit is that it demonstrates the exclusion of major ductal injury because these lesions can be treated with drainage alone, without resection (Figs. **15** and **16**).

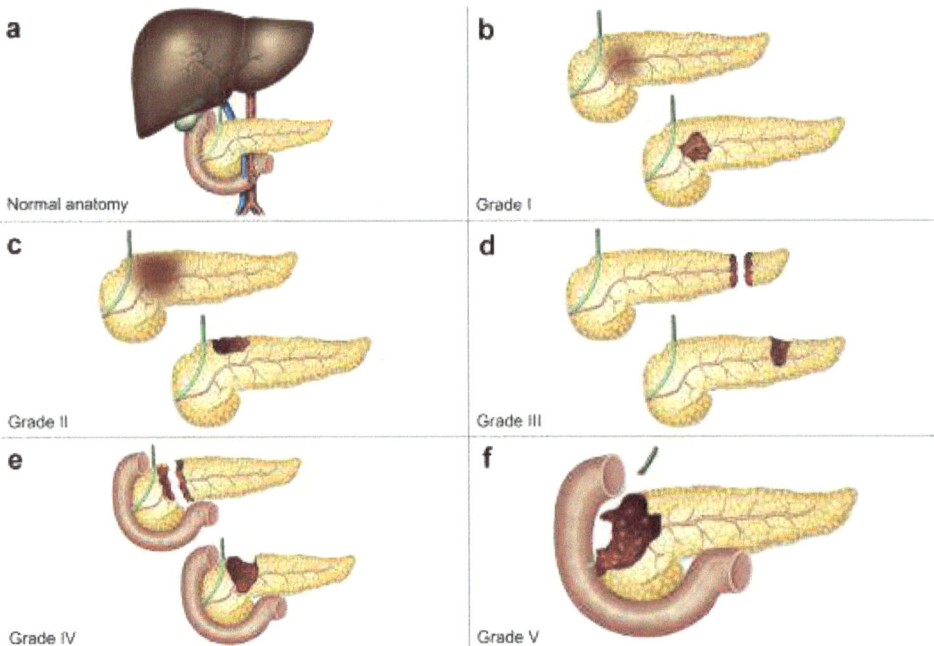

Fig. (15). The "organ injury scale" (OIS) was developed by the American Association for Surgery of Trauma (AAST) to reveal the severity of pancreatic injury.

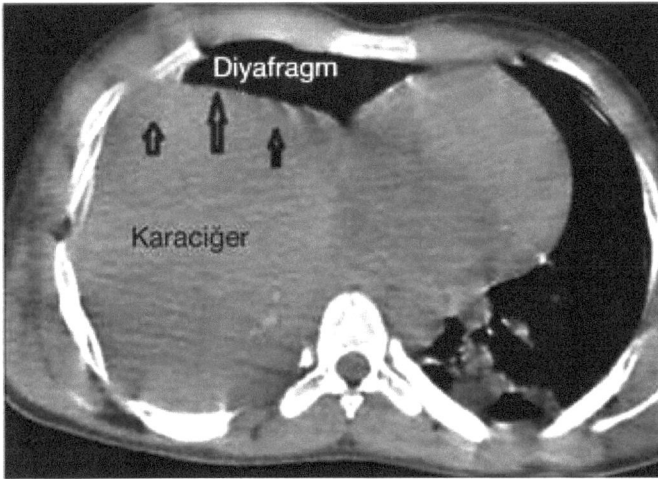

Fig. (16). In the trauma case, it is observed that the liver is in the right hemithorax after the rupture of the diaphragm.

Isolated pancreatic injury is rare in blunt trauma. There are many options for approach when it is associated with duodenal or biliary tract injury. Specific treatment depends on the combination of injuries.

Pseudocyst is a late complication in all types of pancreatic injuries.

Kidneys

Renal parenchymal injury usually presents with hematuria. Many kidney injuries can be managed without surgery, but diagnosis as soon as possible is essential. Before laparotomy or surgery, IVP or CT identifies major lesions. Most contusions and some lacerations can be managed without surgery. Renal vascular injuries can be diagnosed with selective angiography or contrast-enhanced CT. Indications for surgery are ongoing blood loss, laceration extending to Geroto's fascia, or loss of function.

Diaphragm

Diaphragm injuries are usually serious due to late recognition. In many cases there is no herniation, and the only finding may be elevation of the diaphragm or effusion hardly discernible on X-ray. Diaphragmatic injury is not expected to predominate in the clinical picture in a victim of trauma, which causes delay in diagnosis in most cases. The diagnosis is usually easy when there is herniation of the abdominal viscera into the thoracic cavity. Failure of the nasogastric tube to pass suggests this possibility. This injury is mostly seen on the left due to the protective effect of the liver on the right, but this is not the rule.

Diagnosis: Chest X-ray will be normal or nonspecific at a rate of 20-50%. USG/FAST may also aid diagnosis. In sonographic examination, the organ (spleen, intestines, liver) herniated to the thorax may be observed or the contours of the diaphragm may not be selected.

Diagnosis is often made by contrast studies and CT imaging (Figs. **16** and **17**). Helical CT is very helpful in diagnosis. CT is 78% sensitive and 100% specific for diaphragmatic ruptures on the left. It is 50% sensitive and 100% specific in right-sided ruptures. As it can be understood from this, CT is not 100% diagnostic, but it definitely ensures the exclusion of other diagnoses if there are relevant findings.

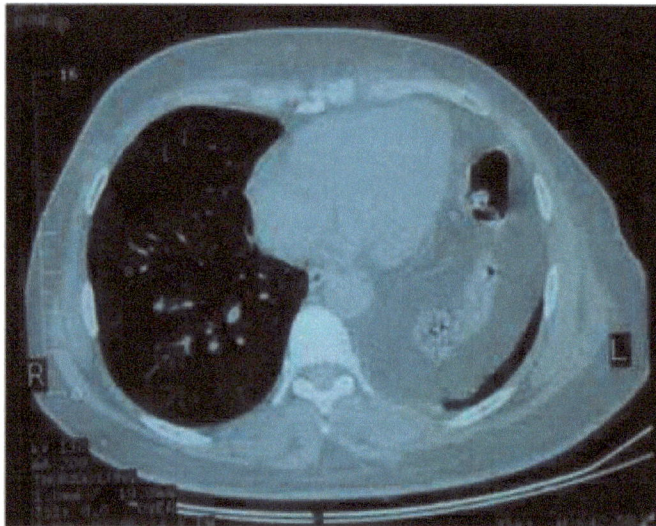

Fig. (17). In CT scans, displacement of the abdominal organs to the thorax on the left and the intraabdominal organs contacting the posterior thoracic wall are typical for diaphragm rupture.

Penetrating diaphragm injuries: These develop due to penetrating or gunshot wounds to the lower chest or upper abdomen, which can be anterior, lateral or posterior. AAST grading is provided in Table **3**.

Table 3. Diaphragm injuries can be classified according to the "American Association for the Surgery of Trauma-Organ Injury Scale".

Grade	Injury
I	Contusion
II	Laceration less than 2 cm
III	Laceration 2-10 cm
IV	Laceration greater than 10 cm + 25 cm2 tissue loss

(Table 3) cont.....

Grade	Injury
V	Laceration more than 25 cm2

Traumas resulting from stab wounds can initially be silent but lead to serious complications in the long term. The reason for the high number of left-sided injuries is that many attackers are right-handed.

Laparotomy is usually performed in its management because it often accompanies intraabdominal injuries. The frequency of follow-up of patients with diaphragm injury with non-surgical conservative treatment is around 12% to 60%. In chronic cases, presentation may be with symptoms of obstruction or bowel strangulation.

Eviscerations: Abdominal Wall Injuries

Penetrating abdominal wall injuries have always the potential for evisceration. Since these patients often harbor intraabdominal visceral injuries, full abdominal exploration is warranted. After the repair of the accompanying lesions, the abdominal wall defect is sutured. In cases where the only eviscerated organ is the omentum, more caution should be exercised as the appearance will be similar with subcutaneous fat. It is important to establish the correct diagnosis in terms of the necessity of laparotomy. Eviscerated organ must be covered with moist sterile dressing.

Vascular Structures

Arterial and/or venous injuries can be life-threatening by causing hemorrhage. In solid internal organ injury, the lesions present with signs of hypovolemia and rarely an abdominal mass. Since the person's own blood will not be irritant, there may be no guarding or rigidity in the abdomen. The strategy should focus on the early control of hemorrhage. "Military antishock trousers" (MAST) can be especially helpful in these lesions. This garment has a place in the field, in the ambulance environment, although not in the hospital. The use of a thoracotomy or intra-aortic Fogarty balloon to control the proximal aorta prior to abdominal exploration helps to minimize blood loss through termination of tamponade with MAST. The key to the surgical approach to all vascular injuries is proximal and distal control of the vessels.

Complications and Iatrogenic Injuries

Major problems as a result of abdominal injuries are either missed injuries or overtreatment of suspected injuries. Major risk is hemorrhage in missed solid organ and vascular injuries, and local infections or systemic sepsis as a result of leakage of contents into the peritoneum in hollow organ injuries. Negative laparotomy has low morbidity and is sometimes necessary to assure that there is no life-threatening injury. If indications are appropriate, the absence of a surgically correctable lesion does not implicate that surgery is unnecessary. Hyperthermia in extremely hot climates, hypothermia in other environments is a major risk for trauma patients. Trauma patients are sometimes brought to the ED from a cold environment, and cold blood transfusion, use of crystalloid solution for intravenous therapy at room temperature increase this risk. It is also affected by the fact that these patients have removed their clothing for a full physical examination. The patient's body temperature should be carefully monitored, preferably with a central thermometer. Fluid heaters, electric blankets, radiant heaters, warm lavage and warm-treatment rooms will help prevent this problem.

Abdominal Trauma: Management in the Emergency Department

History and Physical Examination

Evaluation with a focused history and detailed physical examination is essential. The history should include a brief medical history in addition to the injury. Paramedic personnel are especially important in providing information to patients with neurological and/or mental disorders with injuries. The condition of the vehicle and the position of other occupants in the motor vehicle are helpful in determining the severity of the injury mechanism. Previous illnesses, medications used, and allergies should be evaluated, as they can all affect diagnosis, management, and recovery.

Physical examination of the abdomen includes back, waist, lower chest and perineum, as well as rectal and vaginal examination. Such an examination is especially important in victims of serious trauma to disclose requirement of urgent exploratory laparotomy.

Shall we take a Radiograph in the Resuscitation Room?

Yes and no.

Pelvic injuries can cause a great deal of blood loss and are sometimes associated with severe intra-abdominal visceral or bony injury. In the presence of pelvic fracture, DPL should be performed with a supraumbilical incision without entering pelvic hematoma, which may cause false positive results. When urethral injury is suspected, a retrograde urethrogram should be performed before insertion of a Foley catheter. IVP and cystogram are useful in the presence of hematuria and if bladder rupture is identified, further investigation is unnecessary. Free air on X-ray indicates hollow organ injury and is an indication for laparotomy in presence of other suspicious findings for organ injury (Table **4**).

Table 4. Diagnostic imaging options in decision-making strategies in abdominal trauma.

Clinical status	Recommendation
1. mild: vital signs are normal, mechanism of trauma is low-energy, clinical evaluations do not reveal severe findings	CT can be canceled May not be transferred to trauma center CT imaging can show the severity and extent of injuries.
2. Stable: No major problems with primary examination or vital signs.	
3. Dynamic: SBP temporarily <105 mmHg or an ominous trend in vital signs	
4. Unstable: SBP permanently <105 mmHg, absent peripheral pulses, altered mental status	Resuscitate, get early surgical consultation Consider REBOA
5. Prearrest: SBP permanent <70 mmHg, loss of central pulse (carotid/femoral *etc.*)	Consider transport to operating room or trauma center CT is contraindicated

To REBOA or not to REBOA?

Resuscitative endovascular balloon occlusion of the aorta (REBOA) is a life-saving method that has been introduced in the agenda of medicine since the Korean wars 70 years ago, and which is escalated with the Iraq and Afghanistan wars in the 2000s. It has gained its deserved place in recent years with the advances in interventional radiology and other techniques. It is employed in non-compressible trunk (torso) injuries. REBOA can be used in many resuscitative conditions such as aortic aneurysm surgery, GI bleeding, postpartum hemorrhage, and trauma.

Indication of REBOA is to stop life-threatening hemorrhage and/or exsanguination without thoracotomy in isolated injuries under the diaphragm. Its main goal comprises prevention of cardiovascular collapse and severe shock in patients with or suspected hemorrhagic shock.

Mechanism: REBOA is initiated by advancing and inflating a balloon suitable for the patient's anatomy directly into the aorta after arterial puncture (Dubose, 2016). This technique allows time for the patient and surgical team/interventional radiology for the definitive operation. In this way, the distal circulation is cut off at once. The maneuver increases cardiac preload and proximal aortic pressure, resulting in augmented myocardial and cerebral perfusion, hence a reduced probability of collapse and arrest.

REBOA is particularly pursued for occlusion above the aortic bifurcation, distal to the renal arteries, known as zone III. Although its use is still being discussed, it should be known that it is a temporary method. Ideally, the definitive surgical approach is expected to be protocolized before the REBOA procedure is commenced.

Disadvantages and problems: With this maneuver there is a risk of ischemia of organs distal to the balloon, which can cause short- or long-term problems. It has been reported that the critical risk factor affecting lower extremity ischemia is the thickness of the sheath placed in arterial intervention (Ribeiro Jr. *et al.* WJES, 2018; Okada Y, 2016). For this reason, it is recommended to perform an intervention with a small sheath (4-5 Fr) in patients with a high risk of circulatory collapse. In order to prevent this problem, the "partial REBOA" (pREBOA) approach has also been developed.

Another issue is the effects of nitric oxide and other chemical toxic agents that pre-accumulate in the ischemic tissue after balloon deflation. Persistent hypotension and collapse can be seen at this stage. It is recommended to provide a suitable environment before deflating the balloon, and to prepare intensive care and operating conditions if necessary.

Ancillary Tests in Trauma: Imaging Studies

CT imaging is the best test to establish the diagnosis in most cases, although not a rule. The evaluation of the victim with trauma requires trained personnel. Oral or IV contrast material should be infused for optimal resolution, with their own drawbacks. Oral contrast should be given in two boluses. This is usually given through the nasogastric tube in the severe or critical patient. Before the first bolus examination, 900 ml of the 3.67% water-soluble contrast agent is given as soon as possible. A second bolus of 250 ml is given in the CT unit. IV contrast is given as a bolus during the examination: Iodinated IV contrast material is used in adults as 150 ml of 60% solution.

Studies are ongoing to outline the value of enema and contrast media to increase sensitivity in the assessment of suspected colon perforation.

The main advantage of CT imaging is a better evaluation of the retroperitoneum and the ability to show the localization of intra-abdominal injury more precisely before surgery.

Jejunal perforations are the most difficult entities to diagnose. This should be confirmed by CT imaging and evaluated in conjunction with the clinical situation (Fig. **18**).

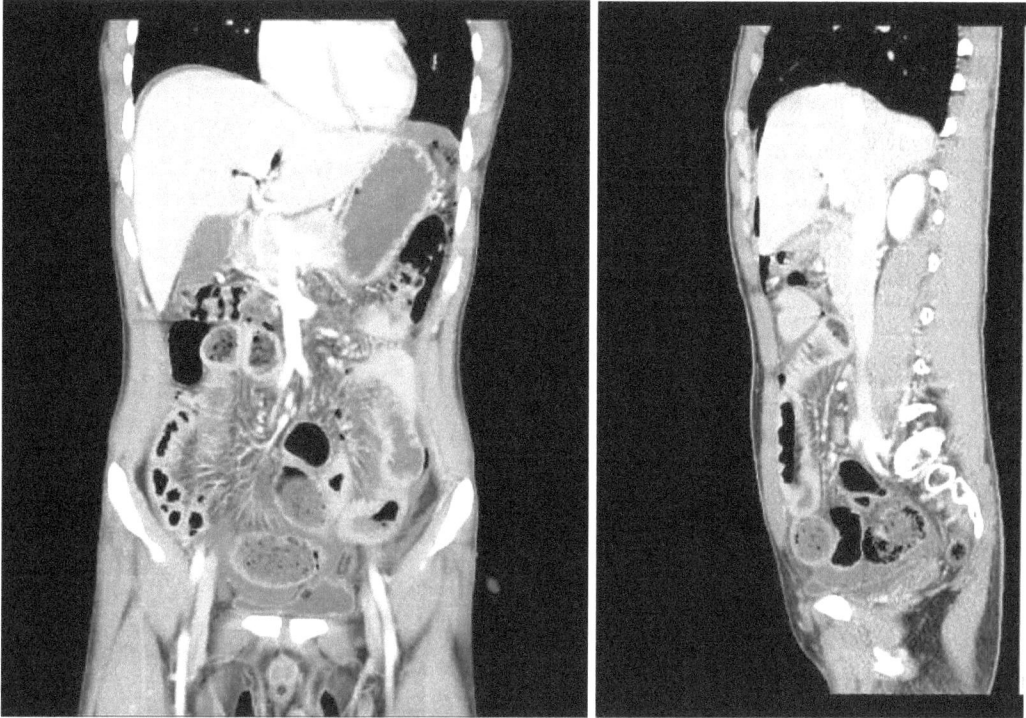

Fig. (18). Images of intraperitoneal free air and wall thickening in the jejunum in the coronal and sagittal sections of a 25-year-old patient with traumatic jejunal perforation who was injured by a heavy object falling on him.

USG

In trauma cases, focused USG examination is performed on predefined culprit areas, which is called **Focused Assessment with Sonography for Trauma (FAST).**

It has a sensitivity of 75% to 100% (weighted mean: 90%) and a specificity of 88% to 100% (weighted mean 95%) in distinguishing intraperitoneal free fluid. In other words, the presence of finding (free intraperitoneal fluid) is more valuable than its absence. The free fluid is easily detectable, especially when it is more than 500 mL. Its accuracy in detecting solid organ injury is lower.

Images from four basic windows are obtained as *sine qua non*. Since the examination of each region will take approximately 1 minute, USG can be completed in around 4 minutes in terms of revealing abdominal trauma, especially ruling out (and ruling in) hemoperitoneum. Therefore, this approach has been recognized as a **time-saving approach** in contemporary trauma management as other 'fancy' approaches like CT and MRI are more time consuming and mandate transfer of the patient to much less controlled areas like radiology suit. The right lateral subcostal position helps visualize the kidney-liver junction on the right (Morison's pouch) and is the most common and easy-to-use area for free fluid determination. Pericardial tamponade and cardiac injury are tried to be ruled out by examining the heart from the subxiphoid window. Up to 50 mL of fluid can be found in normal physiology, above which can be pathological in a patient without a history of disease of pericardium or adjacent structures (Fig. **19**) (Table **5**).

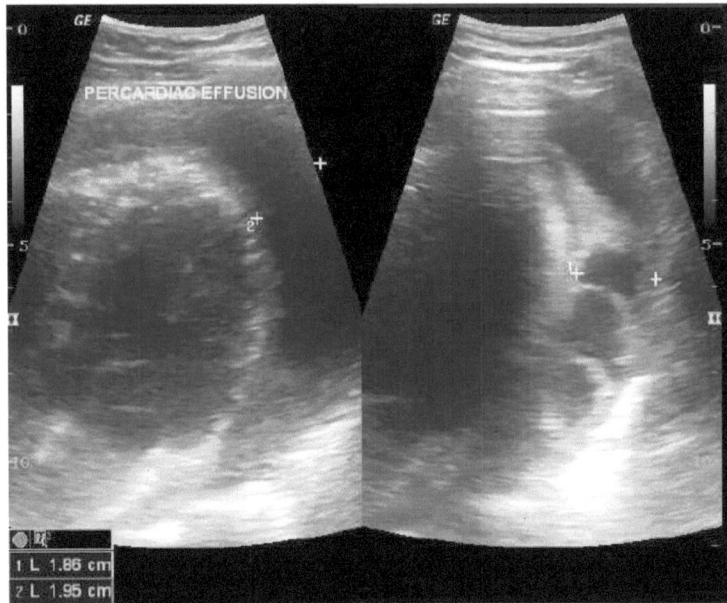

Fig. (19). Massive pericardial effusion image on USG.

Table 5. The thickness of the fluid collection in the pericardium will give an idea of the approximate amount of fluid.

• <5 mm: 50-100 mL
• 5-10 mm: 100-250 mL
• 10-20 mm: 250-500 mL
• >20 mm: >500 mL

Another approach is to report as little, moderate, or much fluid accumulation in roughly 3 groups:

- <10 mm: minor
- 10 to 20 mm: medium-moderate
- >20 mm: major or massive.

Surrounding the spleen is the third region to probe, and a perisplenic hematoma is sought. Finally, the perivesical (bladder) region and the Douglas space is examined. It is most commonly used in patients who need rapid evaluation and not stable enough to be transferred to the radiology room. However, it is also useful for serial follow-up of abdominal evaluation in stable patients. Serial evaluation with portable devices are easy and this approach minimizes the false-negative rates of this method. The accuracy of USG findings is user-dependent. It is accepted that a certain level of mastery has been reached after about 200 USG examinations.

Arteriography

Arteriography may be the best examination method for the evaluation of major vessel injuries. Contrast-enhanced CT replaces arteriogram in imaging renal arterial lesions. However, in pelvic fractures, for example, bleeding areas can be localized by arteriogram and hemorrhage control can be achieved with embolization. Although transesophageal echocardiography (TEE) and CT imaging are included in this evaluation, the aortogram remains the diagnostic test to exclude the probability of thoracic aortic injury.

Management

The approach to the patient with abdominal trauma cannot be simplified as a uni-dimensional method such that 'operation' or 'fluid resuscitation'. Although the approach is individualized according to the patient, the general principles are similar in all trauma cases. First of all, airway, respiration and circulation should be secured. For example, endotracheal intubation may be required to control the airway of a patient who is repeatedly vomiting and whose level of consciousness begins to deteriorate. By protecting the cervical spine (in-line stabilization) airway control should be provided. Respiratory support is given if necessary, intubation and positive pressure breathing are also included in this approach. This is followed by evaluation and support of the circulation. Fluid support is provided by multiple wide-bore (16 G) IV lines. Titration of the fluid in accord with the patient's general status and response to treatment is vital. The real infusion rate is proportional to the diameter of the catheter inserted. Blood samples are taken for laboratory tests. The so-called 'routine' trauma laboratory tests can include blood group and cross-match, complete blood count, electrolytes, glucose, amylase, urine analysis if renal trauma is also suspected, and, if deemed necessary, toxicological tests. Pregnancy test is requested in all women of child-bearing age. In addition to the basic work up, renal, hepatic and coagulation tests may be requested in those with severe trauma.

A nasogastric tube can be useful for both diagnostic and therapeutic purposes. A bloody aspirate is suggestive of nasopharyngeal or GI injury. Victims of trauma often have (or develop) gastric distension and nasogastric tube placement are necessary to prevent tracheal aspiration of gastric ingredients. Nasal insertion of the tube is contraindicated in patients with suspected facial injury with a fractured cribriform plate. In the presence of signs suggesting a urethral injury, a Foley catheter can be placed after excluding injury on the urethrogram. Blood in the urethral meatus or large perineal hematoma, scrotal ecchymoses suggest urethral tear and mandate advanced investigations.

In case of suspected pelvic fracture, a digital rectal exam can be performed before foley catheter insertion to determine the prostate position, although mewer guidelines recommend that the potential injuries should be ruled out by imaging modalities. A urethrogram is the imaging method of choice if any urethral injury could not be ruled out. IVP and cystogram should be ordered in case of macroscopic hematuria in adults, while microscopic hematuria can mandate the investigation in children. In the evaluation of more stable patients, CT imaging with contrast gives better results for renal parenchymal injuries. Renal function tests (blood urea and creatinine) should be noted to be normal before ordering contrast media injection in frail elderly, hypovolemic, dehydrated, and diabetic individuals.

Antibiotics effective against both aerobic and anaerobic microorganisms should be administered while the patient is in the ED, especially in penetrating injuries with suspected bowel injury. Often a single broad-spectrum antibiotic is administered intravenously, although in some cases empirical combined therapy may also be used.

Pain management and sedation: Pain management of each trauma victim should be planned individually and independently. There are no contraindications to the administration of painkillers. In cases with severe trauma, painful lesions such as fractures, chest or head trauma, potent analgesics -preferably opiates- should be administered, provided that the previous neurological examination is noted. Agents such as short-acting fentanyl take precedence. No side effects are expected when administered at a dose of 2-4 mcg/kg. The effect is evaluated every few minutes and titrated upwards if necessary. One should be cautious against chest wall rigidity and respiratory depression, and the patient should be monitored closely.

In cases with significant agitation and anxiety whose symptoms do not regress despite proper analgesic treatment, anxiolytics and sedatives should be added and titrated in accordance with the patient's clinical condition. Here, too, midazolam or etomidate are preferred to other agents.

Tetanus immunization is one of the essential tasks that should not be delayed during trauma management in the acute setting. In adult trauma patients, it is not easy to get the history of how many years ago the patient was vaccinated in the quagmire of the ED. In clean-looking wounds, 0.5 mL of tetanus toxin is injected into the deltoid muscle, whilst in dirty wounds, 500 IU of antitetanic globulin is injected into another muscle, preferably into the gluteal muscle. However, if the vaccination history in the last 5 years can be taken clearly in very clean wounds, general wound cleaning measures can be taken and vaccination can be delayed.

CONCLUSION

Abdominal trauma is to be evaluated both systemically and specifically, while temporal changes should also be searched for. Recurrent evaluations can disclose ongoing bleeding and prevent advanced hemorrhagic shock and resultant mortality. Laboratory values can be valuable in selected patients, while imaging studies can be used at the bedside and repeated as necessary, help establish operative indications. Dynamic evaluation and follow-up with necessary imaging studies provide vital clues in a patient with an initial phase of shock and expedite life-saving procedures like blood transfusions, REBOA, and operative interventions.

Pain treatment and sedation, tetanus immunization are also pursued in the proper management schemes.

REFERENCES

Abe, T., Uchida, M., Nagata, I., Saitoh, D., Tamiya, N. (2016). Resuscitative endovascular balloon occlusion of the aorta *versus* aortic cross clamping among patients with critical trauma: a nationwide cohort study in Japan. *Crit. Care, 20*(1), 400.
[http://dx.doi.org/10.1186/s13054-016-1577-x] [PMID: 27978846]

Brown, J.V., Yuan, S. (2020). Traumatic Injuries of the Pelvis. *Emerg. Med. Clin. North Am., 38*(1), 125-142.
[http://dx.doi.org/10.1016/j.emc.2019.09.011] [PMID: 31757246]

DuBose, J.J., Scalea, T.M., Brenner, M., Skiada, D., Inaba, K., Cannon, J., Moore, L., Holcomb, J., Turay, D., Arbabi, C.N., Kirkpatrick, A., Xiao, J., Skarupa, D., Poulin, N. AAST AORTA Study Group. (2016). The AAST prospective Aortic Occlusion for Resuscitation in Trauma and Acute Care Surgery (AORTA) registry: Data on contemporary utilization and outcomes of aortic occlusion and resuscitative balloon occlusion of the aorta (REBOA). *J. Trauma Acute Care Surg., 81*(3), 409-419.
[http://dx.doi.org/10.1097/TA.0000000000001079] [PMID: 27050883]

García Santos, E., Soto Sánchez, A., Verde, J.M., Marini, C.P., Asensio, J.A., Petrone, P. (2015). Duodenal injuries due to trauma: Review of the literature. *Cir. Esp., 93*(2), 68-74.
[http://dx.doi.org/10.1016/j.ciresp.2014.08.004] [PMID: 25443151]

Inoue, J., Shiraishi, A., Yoshiyuki, A., Haruta, K., Matsui, H., Otomo, Y. (2016). Resuscitative endovascular

balloon occlusion of the aorta might be dangerous in patients with severe torso trauma: A propensity score analysis. *J. Trauma Acute Care Surg., 80*(4), 559-566.
[http://dx.doi.org/10.1097/TA.0000000000000968] [PMID: 26808039]

Jesani, H., Jesani, L., Rangaraj, A., Rasheed, A. (2020). Splenic trauma, the way forward in reducing splenectomy: our 15-year experience. *Ann. R. Coll. Surg. Engl., 102*(4), 263-270.
[http://dx.doi.org/10.1308/rcsann.2019.0164] [PMID: 31909638]

Mama, N., Jemni, H., Arifa, N., Chavey, O., Kadri, K., Gaha, M., Hasni, I., Tlili, K. (2012). Abdominal Trauma Imaging. In (Ed.), Abdominal Surgery. IntechOpen.
[http://dx.doi.org/10.5772/50426]

Moore, L.J., Brenner, M., Kozar, R.A., Pasley, J., Wade, C.E., Baraniuk, M.S., Scalea, T., Holcomb, J.B. (2015). Implementation of resuscitative endovascular balloon occlusion of the aorta as an alternative to resuscitative thoracotomy for noncompressible truncal hemorrhage. *J. Trauma Acute Care Surg., 79*(4), 523-530.
[http://dx.doi.org/10.1097/TA.0000000000000809] [PMID: 26402524]

Morell-Hofert, D., Primavesi, F., Fodor, M., Gassner, E., Kranebitter, V., Braunwarth, E., Haselbacher, M., Nitsche, U.P., Schmid, S., Blauth, M., Öfner, D., Stättner, S. (2020). Validation of the revised 2018 AAST-OIS classification and the CT severity index for prediction of operative management and survival in patients with blunt spleen and liver injuries. *Eur. Radiol., 30*(12), 6570-6581.
[http://dx.doi.org/10.1007/s00330-020-07061-8] [PMID: 32696255]

Norii, T., Crandall, C., Terasaka, Y. (2015). Survival of severe blunt trauma patients treated with resuscitative endovascular balloon occlusion of the aorta compared with propensity score-adjusted untreated patients. *J. Trauma Acute Care Surg., 78*(4), 721-728.
[http://dx.doi.org/10.1097/TA.0000000000000578] [PMID: 25742248]

Okada, Y., Narumiya, H., Ishi, W., Ryoji, I. (2016). Lower limb ischemia caused by resuscitative balloon occlusion of aorta. *Surg. Case Rep., 2*(1), 130.
[http://dx.doi.org/10.1186/s40792-016-0260-4] [PMID: 27834057]

Ribeiro Junior, M.A.F., Feng, C.Y.D., Nguyen, A.T.M., Rodrigues, V.C., Bechara, G.E.K., de-Moura, R.R., Brenner, M. (2018). The complications associated with Resuscitative Endovascular Balloon Occlusion of the Aorta (REBOA). *World J. Emerg. Surg., 13*(1), 20.
[http://dx.doi.org/10.1186/s13017-018-0181-6] [PMID: 29774048]

Ribeiro Júnior, M.A.F., Brenner, M., Nguyen, A.T.M., Feng, C.Y.D., DE-Moura, R.R., Rodrigues, V.C., Prado, R.L. (2018). Resuscitative endovascular balloon occlusion of the aorta (REBOA): an updated review. *Rev. Col. Bras. Cir., 45*(1), e1709.
[http://dx.doi.org/10.1590/0100-6991e-20181709] [PMID: 29590238]

Søreide, K., Weiser, T.G., Parks, R.W. (2018). Clinical update on management of pancreatic trauma. *HPB (Oxford), 20*(12), 1099-1108.
[http://dx.doi.org/10.1016/j.hpb.2018.05.009] [PMID: 30005994]

Soto, J.A., Anderson, S.W. (2012). Multidetector CT of blunt abdominal trauma. *Radiology, 265*(3), 678-693.
[http://dx.doi.org/10.1148/radiol.12120354] [PMID: 23175542]

Subramanian, A., Albert, V., Mishra, B., Sanoria, S., Pandey, R.M. (2016). Association Between the Pancreatic Enzyme Level and Organ Failure in Trauma Patients. *Trauma Mon., 21*(2), e20773.
[http://dx.doi.org/10.5812/traumamon.20773] [PMID: 27625999]

CHAPTER 12

Treatment and Resuscitation of the Patient with Acute Abdominal Pain

Abstract: Provision of airway patency, effective breathing and gas exchange and circulatory functions producing adequate perfusion (ABC) are vital elements in all emergent and critical patients. Initial resuscitation should begin with control in a primary survey both in the field and in the hospital in the management of the patients with abdominal pain. In a patient whose respiratory patency is under threat, evaluation and management of the inflammatory process in the abdomen should not be considered before this is resolved. Differential diagnosis and proper management of abdominal pain follow the primary survey, resuscitation and resolution of vital threats. IV fluid therapy and pain management are commenced as prompted by the general condition. Prehospital providers should operate in communication with the command control center in this context. "Tubes or fingers for all orifices" can be accepted as a general approach for the moribund patient to monitor the clinical course. In the hospital, the emergency physician should relieve the pain expediently after evaluating and recording the initial vital signs and findings on systemic examination. Antiemetic therapy and other symptomatic measures should be individualized for the given patient.

Keywords: Abdominal pain, Airway, Breathing, Circulation, Management, Resuscitation.

As in all emergency and critical patients, initial resuscitation should begin with airway, breathing and circulation (ABC) control in a primary survey both in the field and in the hospital (Table **1**). In a patient whose respiratory patency is under threat, evaluation and management of the inflammatory process in the abdomen should not be considered before this is resolved.

MANAGEMENT IN THE HOSPITAL

When performing the first-line resuscitative interventions for diseases that will require operative treatment, a quick contact should be made with the general surgery consultant (+cardiovascular surgery for vascular pathologies, +OB/GYN

Ozgur KARCIOGLU, Selman YENİOCAK, Mandana HOSSEINZADEH & Seckin Bahar SEZGIN

for gynecological or obstetric problems). About 1/3 of patients with AP presenting to the ED are consulted, and eventually around 1/10 are hospitalized. For this reason, the education of front-line physicians about AP is critical.

Table 1. Treatment steps and mainstays in the prehospital area. EMS command control center (CCC) instructions are followed throughout all procedures.

IV fluid therapy is started as prompted by the general condition. Two wide-bore (16-14G) vascular accesses should be opened from the antecubital or equivalent area in the upper half of the body. Femoral or calf veins are not preferred.
Cardiac rhythm and pulse oximetry are monitored continuously.
Give supplemental O2. Additional O2 is given by 100% face mask or nasal cannula based on findings if SpO2 is below 94%, or in those with symptoms such as fever, tachycardia, agitation, ischemic chest pain, or unconsciousness.
IV analgesic agents, preferably opiates (morphine/fentanyl) are titrated to effect.
Since abdominal pain may be a sign of ACS, especially over the age of 40, an ECG should be obtained and interpreted.
Anti-emetics (preferably ondansetron and/or H1 antagonists or metoclopramide 10 mg *via* slow infusion) may be given.
Antibiotherapy should be started as early as possible according to local protocols in patients who are prepared to undergo operation and in those with suspected sepsis. Empirical combination therapy takes priority in emergency situations.
Insert NG tube.
Monitor urine output with a Foley catheter.
Admit the patient to intensive care / general surgery beds.

Hypovolemic or septic shock should be rapidly recognized and resuscitated. In addition, perhaps more important is the recognition of the case that will succumb to shock (eg ruptured spleen or ruptured aneurysm) even though clinical findings of shock are not obvious.

How much of which Liquid Should we Give in Which Way?

Since there may be external (bleeding, vomiting, diarrhea) or internal (sequestration to the third cavities in the abdomen) fluid loss, the volume status should be evaluated urgently and fluid replacement should be initiated as soon as possible. Crystalloid fluids (normal saline and lactated Ringer's solution) take priority for initial resuscitation. Colloid fluids have not been found to have any advantage over crystalloids, on the contrary, they can cause coagulation problems (*e.g.*, Dextran solutions).

For this, at least two antecubital wide-bore (16 or 14 G) vascular accesses must be opened. Peripheral wide vascular access is superior to central catheters in almost every aspect except for indications of CVP monitoring.

20 mL/kg formula is a concrete strategy that can be employed initially in every case including weight extremes in hypovolemic patients with the poor general conditions. In an elderly patient with suspected heart failure, the behavior of not giving fluid paves the way to hypovolemia and hypotension. In these cases, starting with 100 to 150 ml/hour, the response to fluid resuscitation can be titrated within a few hours by monitoring the inferior vena cava with bedside USG. In other hypovolemic/hypotensive cases, a bolus of 20 mL/kg of fluid can be infused. For patients with acute blood loss, the 10 mL/kg formula for the initial dose of blood transfusion is more suitable.

A nasogastric (NG) tube is indicated for evacuation and decompression of gastric contents since aspiration may be common in acute abdominal syndromes with persistent vomiting such as mechanical bowel obstruction and pancreatitis. Caution should be exercised in the insertion of NG catheter in EVB, for it may rarely trigger bleeding. Nonetheless, it is not contraindicated. It should be inserted after endotracheal intubation in patients with impaired consciousness. In patients with injuries to the head and/or maxillofacial area involving the midface, it should not be inserted without ruling out a basilar fracture of the skull.

In critically ill patients, who may be prone to hypovolemia, monitoring urinary output *via* catheterization will be useful. The same is true in cases such as postrenal obstruction, and/or prostatism. In cases where there is difficulty in defecation due to anal/rectal mass, and/or fecaloma(s), a rectal tube can be placed to ease excretion.

ACUTE PAIN MANAGEMENT

In cases presenting with acute AP, the emergency physician should relieve the pain expediently after evaluating and recording the initial vital signs and findings on systemic examination. There are no contraindications for cessation of pain in a patient with pain. A point to be noted is that acute AP of inflammatory origin can be disguised or 'masked' by anti-inflammatory agents and cause misdiagnosis. Therefore, some authors emphasized that NSAID group drugs such as ketorolac and tenoxicam should not be used in undiagnosed patients with AP. A meta-analytic study disclosed that postoperative IV ketorolac infusion may provide substantial pain relief for most patients, but further research may impact this estimate (McNicol, 2021). Adverse events are recorded at a slightly higher rate when compared to placebo and other NSAIDs.

Opiates, on the other hand, can be used safely after initial evaluation as they have no such drawbacks. Fentanyl is the most widely used safe agent because it is a short-acting and potent agent with predictable analgesic effects. Almost no side effects have been reported at a dose of 2-3 mcg/kg. It is also an advantage that there is no histamine discharge compared to other opiates and morphine. However, it should be titrated in accordance with the patient's findings. Caution should be exercised concerning spasm of Oddi in those with risk groups (previous gallbladder disease, gallstones or sludge, indigestion, *etc*).

The value of the parasympatholytics, *i.e.*, scopolamine-like group, which is introduced as 'spasmolytic', in those with AP is not clear except those pointed out in small post-operative studies and endoscopy. In brief, these are not a remedy in general, for an undiagnosed patient with AP in the acute setting. Care should be taken for anticholinergic side effects in the use of this group of agents.

H_2 receptor blockers such as ranitidine have no relief in cases with AP, including gastritis and thus should not be considered in the first-line treatment. Proton pump inhibitors (PPI, -prazole group) can be given *via* IV route in cases where hyperacidity is considered to be the main cause of AP and in those deemed high-risk for GIB.

For pain thought to be due to functional bowel diseases including IBS, quaternary ammonium derivatives such as otilonium bromide or L-type calcium channel blockers (pinaverium bromide) can be considered and started for long-term treatment not only for pain but also for the correction of general symptomatology.

Can we Use Medical Cannabis for Chronic Noncancer AP?

Those with chronic noncancer pain require a comprehensive pain management procedure which cover many aspects of the disease and individual properties into account. **Medical cannabis** is advocated by many authors and is also experienced in many countries for selected patients. North America champions in the use of the agents with this indication. The agent, namely, **Delta---tetrahydrocannabinol (THC)** is the psychoactive compound derived from *Cannabis sativa*. It is known to modulate pain perception *via* interaction with cannabinoid receptors (Chang, 2021).

Cannabis-based medicines are promoted in **neuropathic pain** especially when the other established treatments fail to relieve pain after careful analyses and multidisciplinary assessment (Hauser 2018). Likewise, CAG recommended cannabinoids to control GI symptoms including AP if conventional therapies are unsuccessful (Andrews, 2019). Moderate-quality evidence supported the use of cannabinoids for the treatment of chronic AP. Medical cannabis is also advocated in the treatment of chronic pain in general and for the specific conditions of neuropathic pain, chronic pain in people with HIV, and chronic AP (Chang, 2021).

However, many studies recommended against the use of cannabis as the first- or second-line therapy in chronic AP.

MANAGEMENT OF VOMITING

Metoclopramide

Using its prokinetic properties, it can be given in cases such as postoperative adynamic ileus or subileus, and in cases where bowel movements decrease, *e.g.*, in those vomiting accompanied by migraine. It should not be used in other cases such as those with AGE. It should not be given *via* a rapid IV infusion in a shorter time than 15 minutes, otherwise, akathisia will occur in most cases.

5-HT3 Antagonists

These agents, also known as the ondansetron group, are effective in almost all types of vomiting (excluding motion sickness), including post-operative vomiting and those attributed to chemotherapy. In a study we conducted in 1999, its adjuvant effectiveness in renal colic cases was also shown (Ergene, 1999). Ondansetron can be started at 4 mg IV in children and 8 mg in adults. It can be administered if there is robust indication during pregnancy.

In pediatric gastroenteritis, Hartman *et al.* emphasized that ondansetron may also be prescribed if needed to prevent vomiting and improve tolerance of oral rehydration solutions, after being used in intravenous treatment (Hartman 2019).

Parenteral infusion of another 5-HT3 antagonist, granisetron has been demonstrated to be highly efficacious in the control of emesis consequent to intestinal obstruction caused by metastatic cancer (Tuca, 2009). It can also be used effectively in patients refractory to other antiemetics.

Oral granisetron (1 mg) has been shown to be more effective and well tolerated with minimum adverse effects compared with ondansetrons in children with acute lymphoblastic leukemia (Siddique, 2011). Granisetron transdermal system (GTS) appears to be a beneficial delivery system for patients with gastroparesis. It was moderately effective in reducing nausea and/or vomiting in 76% of gastroparesis patients in a case series (Midani, 2016).

On the other hand, some specific patient groups with vomiting may require other agents. For example, haloperidol was found more useful than ondansetron in the acute treatment of cannabis-associated hyperemesis as studied in randomized trials (Ruberto, 2021).

Patients receiving emetogenic chemotherapy constitute a distinct group with special needs in terms of antiemetic treatment. An oral suspension containing 2 mg granisetron and 16 mg dexamethasone was administered to chemotherapy-naive patients before emetogenic chemotherapy (Jordan, 2005). Complete control of acute vomiting was achieved in 60% to 72.7%. Researchers reported that granisetron/dexamethasone is an active prophylaxis of nausea and vomiting and compares favourably with data reported on IV administration.

Shall I Admit the Patient to the Hospital?

First, do not hesitate to seek support and advice from your senior, specialist, or other specialty (often general surgery) in case of a "mysterious patient" or when you feel "in-between". In these suspicious cases, decide to admit the patient, rather than discharge, whenever possible. Some patients can be discharged and arranged for repeat examination in well-controlled environments, provided that the patient's general condition is acceptable and social support can help the patient should any deterioration occurs. This strategy can facilitate more efficient use of hospital beds and EDs in case of limited resources.

Pitfalls and Pearls in the Management of AP

- Some conditions such as the use of certain drugs (steroids, NSAIDs), debility and/or obesity may make peritoneal findings to appear more indistinctly.
- Use of beta-blockers and some other drugs may mask the signs of hypovolemic/ hemorrhagic shock (i.e., hinder tachycardia).
- Absence of fever does not exclude infection in most cases, especially in those with unstable clinical findings.
- If severe abdominal pain inconsistent with physical findings is identified, consider diagnoses such as mesenteric infarction, aortic rupture/dissection, acute pancreatitis, ovarian cyst torsion (with ischemia).
- In some patient groups (such as ITP, malaria, infectious mononucleosis), splenic rupture may occur with seemingly trivial injuries.
- Give the tetanus vaccine to the patient with a laceration and the antibiotic to the patient who will go to the operation as early as possible.
- Women are pregnant until proven otherwise. Always ask for a pregnancy test.
- Men over the age of 40 are having a heart attack until proven otherwise. Always ask for an ECG and assume coronary syndrome.
- Do not make a discharge decision solely based on the leukocyte count. Even septic patients can have a normal leukocyte count.
- The elderly must not be discharged, as a rule, they can be discharged

exceptionally after everything is ruled out.
- Asking for consultation is sharing responsibility. Ask for it.
- Beware of a distracting injury. It is present in many patients and leads to misdiagnosis. The injury you see easily is not the only injury.
- The imaging method you choose may not be the best choice for the given patient. *e.g.*, Noncalcified gallstones can only be seen on MRI, diaphragmatic hernia can be missed in many examinations. X-ray can diagnose very few diseases like bullet injury or bowel obstruction. CT is expensive albeit not very sensitive for gallstones.
- If 'duties' such as completing laboratory examinations and doing exactly what the consultant says, cause delay or overlooking the patient's stabilization, you are on the way to the court.
- No instruction or work up can preclude patient stabilization and management of vital injuries.
- There are no known contraindications to giving painkillers to individuals in pain. Including those people known to be "addicts".
- If you need to administer an antiemetic, give a 5HT3 antagonist (-setron), if available. May combine with metoclopramide in those with paralytic ileus or migraine vomiting.
- Do not send the patient home with her/his pain, saying that there is nothing wrong. If you have to discharge, give her/him your phone to be awakened in the dawn.
- Be concerned for the patient who comes back more than once in a few days and as a rule, do not discharge them easily again.
- Do not discharge the patient with AP that you took over at the visit, without really getting to know her/him.
- Check the blood sugar of the patient whose general condition is poor but you could not diagnose, do everything including NG, Foley, consultation and broad work up for broad DD.
- Make sure the patient is really "well" before discharge. Ask directly him/her if everything goes alright.
- Do not discharge the patient writhing in AP. Do not discharge "the pain" home.
- Central catheter, gastric lavage, arterial blood gases and direct abdominal radiographs are ordered more than necessary. Be careful.
- "Should I consult?" If so, discuss the patient with either your senior or your consultant.
- "Shall I admit?" If you ask yourself, put the patient to bed, not at home.
- Painkillers are administered IV in the emergency setting. Do not use IM pain relievers.
- Never administer IM diclofenac. It is neurotoxic.
- Scopolamine is not used as a pain reliever against AP in the acute setting.

- Each patient comes with a lawyer and a judge.
- Do not discharge the patient for whom you administered opiate analgesia before the effect of the agent expires, because the pain will occur again and the patient may deteriorate without an established diagnosis.
- The ill patient needs you as the monitor and caretaker. So don't send her/him to radiology. Go together with her/him.
- The most important diagnostic method is your repeat examinations, not the radiology suit.
- Ranitidine, scopolamine, thiocolchicoside and diclofenac are drugs that should rarely be used in the acute setting. Such as silk suture, diagnostic peritoneal lavage and venous cut-down.

CONCLUSION

Many different entities can present with acute abdominal pain. A wide spectrum of conditions from benign and self-limited illness to surgical emergencies can be distinguished *via* a carefully focused history and thorough evaluation. Laboratory and radiological techniques serve as an important adjunct to establish a diagnosis in most situations. Subgroups based on age, gender, sociodemographic features can help clinicians narrow the list of possible diagnoses. Most specific diagnoses may require consultation with a specialist to plan management and disposition decisions.

REFERENCES

McNicol, E.D., Ferguson, M.C., Schumann, R. (2021). Single-dose intravenous ketorolac for acute postoperative pain in adults. *Cochrane Database Syst. Rev., 5*(5), CD013263.
[http://dx.doi.org/10.1002/14651858.CD013263.pub2] [PMID: 33998669]

Chang, Y., Zhu, M., Vannabouathong, C., Mundi, R., Chou, R.S., Bhandari, M. (2021). Medical Cannabis for Chronic Noncancer Pain: A Systematic Review of Health Care Recommendations. *Pain Res. Manag., 2021*, 8857948.
[http://dx.doi.org/10.1155/2021/8857948] [PMID: 33613794]

Häuser, W., Finn, D.P., Kalso, E., Krcevski-Skvarc, N., Kress, H.G., Morlion, B., Perrot, S., Schäfer, M., Wells, C., Brill, S. (2018). European Pain Federation (EFIC) position paper on appropriate use of cannabis-based medicines and medical cannabis for chronic pain management. *Eur. J. Pain, 22*(9), 1547-1564.
[http://dx.doi.org/10.1002/ejp.1297] [PMID: 30074291]

Andrews, C.N., Devlin, S.M., Le Foll, B., Fischer, B., Tse, F., Storr, M., Congly, S.E. (2019). Canadian association of gastroenterology position statement: Use of cannabis in gastroenterological and hepatic disorders. *J. Can. Assoc. Gastroenterol., 2*(1), 37-43.
[http://dx.doi.org/10.1093/jcag/gwy064] [PMID: 31294362]

van Randen, A., Laméris, W., Luitse, J.S., Gorzeman, M., Hesselink, E.J., Dolmans, D.E., Peringa, J., van Geloven, A.A., Bossuyt, P.M., Stoker, J., Boermeester, M.A. OPTIMA study group. (2011). The role of plain radiographs in patients with acute abdominal pain at the ED. *Am. J. Emerg. Med., 29*(6), 582-589.e2.
[http://dx.doi.org/10.1016/j.ajem.2009.12.020] [PMID: 20825832]

Eng, K.A., Abadeh, A., Ligocki, C., Lee, Y.K., Moineddin, R., Adams-Webber, T., Schuh, S., Doria, A.S. (2018). Acute Appendicitis: A Meta-Analysis of the Diagnostic Accuracy of US, CT, and MRI as Second-

Line Imaging Tests after an Initial US. *Radiology, 288*(3), 717-727.
[http://dx.doi.org/10.1148/radiol.2018180318] [PMID: 29916776]

Ergene, Ü., Fowler, J.R. (1999). O. Karcioglu, Z. Kirkali. Ondansetron for primary pain relief in ureteral colic. Süleyman Demirel Üniv. Tıp Fak. *Dergisi, 6*(1), 27-30.

Hartman, S., Brown, E., Loomis, E., Russell, H.A. (2019). Gastroenteritis in Children. *Am. Fam. Physician, 99*(3), 159-165.
[PMID: 30702253]

Tuca, A., Roca, R., Sala, C., Porta, J., Serrano, G., González-Barboteo, J., Gómez-Batiste, X. (2009). Efficacy of granisetron in the antiemetic control of nonsurgical intestinal obstruction in advanced cancer: a phase II clinical trial. *J. Pain Symptom Manage., 37*(2), 259-270.
[http://dx.doi.org/10.1016/j.jpainsymman.2008.01.014] [PMID: 18789638]

Siddique, R., Hafiz, M.G., Rokeya, B., Jamal, C.Y., Islam, A. (2011). Ondansetron versus granisetron in the prevention of chemotherapy induced nausea and vomiting in children with acute lymphoblastic leukemia. *Mymensingh Med. J., 20*(4), 680-688.
[PMID: 22081189]

Midani, D., Parkman, H.P. (2016). Granisetron Transdermal System for Treatment of Symptoms of Gastroparesis: A Prescription Registry Study. *J. Neurogastroenterol. Motil., 22*(4), 650-655.
[http://dx.doi.org/10.5056/jnm15203] [PMID: 27400689]

Ruberto, A.J., Sivilotti, M.L.A., Forrester, S., Hall, A.K., Crawford, F.M., Day, A.G. (2021). Intravenous Haloperidol Versus Ondansetron for Cannabis Hyperemesis Syndrome (HaVOC): A Randomized, Controlled Trial. *Ann. Emerg. Med., 77*(6), 613-619.
[http://dx.doi.org/10.1016/j.annemergmed.2020.08.021] [PMID: 33160719]

Jordan, K., Grothey, A., Kegel, T., Fibich, C., Schöbert, C. (2005). Antiemetic efficacy of an oral suspension of granisetron plus dexamethasone and influence of quality of life on risk for nausea and vomiting. *Onkologie, 28*(2), 88-92.
[http://dx.doi.org/10.1159/000082523] [PMID: 15662112]

SUBJECT INDEX

www.ingramcontent.com/pod-product-compliance
Lightning Source LLC
Chambersburg PA
CBHW050806220326
41598CB00006B/132